Perimenopausal and Geriatric Gynecology

Perimenopausal and Geriatric Gynecology

Hugh R.K. Barber, M.D.

Director
Department of Obstetrics and Gynecology
Lenox Hill Hospital
New York

Macmillan Publishing Company
New York
Collier Macmillan Canada, Inc.
Toronto
Collier Macmillan Publishers
London

Macmillan Publishing Company
866 Third Avenue, New York, NY 10022

Collier Macmillan Canada, Inc.
Collier Macmillan Publishers • London

Printing: 1 2 3 4 5 6 7 8

Year: 8 9 0 1 2 3

Library of Congress Cataloging-in-Publication Data

Barber, Hugh R. K., 1918–
    Perimenopausal and geriatric gynecology.

    Includes bibliographies and index.
    1. Menopause. 2. Geriatric gynecology.
I. Title. [DNLM: 1. Genital Diseases, Female–
in old age. 2. Menopause. WP 140 B234p]
RG186.B37   1988   618.97′81   87-32512
ISBN 0–02–305880–3

I dedicate this book to my late parents Elizabeth Frances and Thomas Francis Barber, who brought me into the world after their fortieth birthday. They encouraged me in my studies and athletic career. Unfortunately, I was unable to repay them for their help during their lifetime. This dedication is my way of thanking them and expressing my appreciation for their sacrifices on my behalf. May God bless them.

Contents

Preface

The logical question is, what is geriatric medicine and geriatric gynecology? Geriatric medicine is the prevention, diagnosis, care, and treatment of illnesses and disabilities in an older person. Geriatric gynecology is a subdivision of the overall emerging specialty of geriatric medicine. This approach to promoting the health of older patients takes into account the interaction of diseases, medications, the environment, personal and social problems, and age. Perimenopausal gynecology and geriatrics acknowledge the favorable and unfavorable elements of aging, but they stress that physical and mental deterioration are not inevitable consequences of the aging process and that there are positive aspects to growing older.

Some changes occur naturally as people grow older. There is a decrease in mean body mass (primarily muscles and bones) as opposed to fat and total body weight, muscles lose elasticity, blood pressure tends to increase, and the ability to metabolize sugar tends to decrease.

Currently, no official subdivision of gynecology has been designated as geriatric gynecology, but it is obvious that this field is assuming increasing importance, requiring special knowledge, techniques, and skills within the discipline of obstetrics and gynecology. The greatest number of cases must still be diagnosed and treated by nongynecologic gerontologists. It is the purpose of this book to establish guidelines to help the practitioner. Every clinician has an obligation, despite a heavy workload, to exercise self-discipline and to maintain high standards of professional knowledge. Based on training and personal integrity, the medical profession has developed continuing medical education programs that enable the clinician to deliver the best health care that is available. This book is designed to serve the needs of both continuing education and the optimal delivery of health care. The gynecologist is the principal physician and often sees elderly patients who have a variety of problems. It is important for gynecologists to take care of the problems that they feel comfortable treating and to refer patients to the appropriate specialist when they believe that greater expertise is needed.

Treating the elderly is often complex. These patients tend to have several diseases or disabilities at the same time. Some diseases behave differently in the elderly than in younger patients; for example, an older person may have a heart attack without pain or appendicitis without abdominal tenderness. Other diseases that are common in the elderly, such as cancer and osteoporosis, rarely affect younger people. In addition, older patients respond differently to medications than do younger patients and may require carefully coordinated prescriptions. The elderly may take longer to recuperate after an illness and must be monitored carefully to prevent further problems or relapses during recovery. Finally, fears of death, loss of a spouse and friends, and retirement from income-producing work may have to be taken into account in planning the care of older patients.

At the beginning of the twentieth century, 4 percent of all Americans (3 million) were 65 years old or more. That figure has now grown to more than 10 percent (23 million), with those over the age of 75 increasing from 900,000 to 11 million. Census projections indicate that by the year 2000 there will be 31 million people over the age of 65 and 13 million over the age of 75 in the United States. Those who are now 75 and over constitute the fastest-growing segment of the U.S. population. By 2030, nearly one in five Americans may be over the age of 65. By the time the present medical students and residents are in their midcareer years, they will have spent over half of their time with patients 65 years of age and over.

A 1977 survey by the American Medical Association reported that only 629 physicians cited care of the elderly as one of their major specialties. Although interest in geriatric medicine is growing, many medical schools do not offer structured courses in the overall care of the geriatric patient. Even fewer offer clinical experience with generally healthy and chronically ill older patients in the community, the hospital, or the nursing home. Given hospital trends, it seems essential that all health professionals prepare students and residents to handle the special needs and problems of the aged.

To know how to grow old is one of the most difficult chapters in the great art of living. Programs in gerontology will provide the guidance physicians need to assist their patients—and eventually themselves—in growing old successfully. They will not be dedicated to survival alone, but rather to achieving a full life in their later years.

On May 13, 1974, the Research on Aging Act was signed into law. This legislation authorized the establishment of the National Institute on Aging (NIA) for the conduct and support of biomedical, social, and behavioral research and training related to the aging process, as well as the diseases and other special problems and needs of the aged. This broad mandate presented an exciting opportunity to support studies on the physiologic, psychologic, social, educational, and economic aspects of aging in order to study the aging process effectively as a whole. The NIA is concerned not only with the extension of life but with the improvement and quality of life. It is firmly committed to basic research that includes research in molecular or cellular aging and immune biology, as well as fundamental investigations of the interpersonal and social aspects of human experience. The NIA has directed its energies to broad areas. It is interested in preventative medicine, individual and family lifestyles, personal, and social and physical fitness—including exercise, dietary habits, and the adverse effects of so-called recreational drugs such as tobacco, alcohol, and caffeine.

To date, the NIA has concentrated on basic biology (80 percent) and, to a lesser degree, on social and behavioral science (16 percent). Although very little research (4 percent) has been done in clinical investigation, it is obvious that some of the most central insights concerning geriatric medicine will be developed in this field.

The NIA has encouraged many scientists to pursue aging research and supports researchers throughout the field of aging. Currently, the NIA funds over 600 grants on topics ranging from cell aging to senile dementia. It also conducts its own research, primarily at the Gerontology Research Center in Baltimore, Maryland. One of its major activities is the Baltimore Longitudinal Study of Aging, in which nearly 1000 male and female volunteers return every 12 to 24 months for extensive physiologic, behavioral, and intellectual testing and measurement. The NIA has also established a Geriatric Medicine Academic Award designed to encourage faculty and curriculum development, as well as research in geriatric medicine. In October 1979, the NIA announced a Geriatric Dentistry Academic Award to stimulate the development of a curriculum in geriatric dentistry in those schools that do not have one and to strengthen and improve the curriculum in those school that do. They have also established other awards that bear upon geriatric medicine. These include (1) the Clinical Investigator Award, which offers funds enabling the recipient to make the transition from clinical training to a career in independent biomedical research; (2) the Special Initiative Grant, which stimulates high-quality research in gerontology by supporting pilot studies leading to the creation, expansion, or modification of problems in aging research and training; and (3) the NIA Academic Award, which bridges the gap between the initial period of postdoctoral study and a formal academic appointment for individuals with high potential for research and teaching careers in clinical areas.

A physician who treats older patients must be well informed and skilled, compassionate and sensitive, and capable of coordinating a variety of medical and social services. The physician must be able to recognize unusual symptoms in the elderly; be prepared for adverse interactions among diseases and disabilities; and be able to employ, with precautions, a variety of medicines. The physician must be willing to assist the patient in utilizing community resources to cope with poverty, handicaps, or loneliness. The physician must also be an understanding and perceptive listener. Above all, the physician caring for aged patients must not view them as disease-ridden or as hopeless and depressing cases, but as people who, with proper care, may be able to lead happier, healthier, and more independent lives.

The gynecologist is the principal physician for the postmenopausal and geriatric patient. It is evident that there is a need for a new subspecialty in the field of obstetrics and gynecology. It should be designated *geriatric* or *gerontologic gynecology.* The postmenopausal woman has many pelvic problems, several of which require surgery. The aging patient often has prolapse of the uterus, enterocele, cystocele, and/or rectocele. These conditions are usually the result of previous childbearing, and as the patient grows older, with the attenuation of tissue, the problems become evident. Repair of these herniations is necessary in order to improve the quality of life. Sometimes, with marked prolapses that are affecting the urinary system, it is important to prevent further damage of the urinary tract. The geriatric patient who requires surgery must have a very careful evaluation of the cardiac, pulmonary, and renal systems.

Postmenopausal bleeding must always be investigated and should always be diagnosed by careful pelvic examination and a fractional curettage. This should be done even if the patient is receiving estrogen replacement therapy. The screening and monitoring can usually be carried out as an office procedure.

The ovary grows too old to function but never grows too old to form a cancer, and the peak incidence is at age 77. Patients with continued gastrointestinal upset who have had a negative gastrointestinal investigation should be suspected of having ovarian cancer. The geriatric patient with ascitic fluid must always be investigated for ovarian neoplasm. Ascites may be secondary to heart failure, liver failure, or tuberculosis. Cardiac diseases and osteoporosis are the two most debilitating problems that can afflict the geriatric patient. Prophylaxis for osteoporosis should be practiced in all women, starting at approximately age 40. The use of estrogen in the immediate postmenopausal period, unless contraindicated, will prevent or at least delay the onset of osteoporosis and will decrease its severity. Estrogen replacement therapy also reduces the flushes, flashes, insomnia, night sweats, and dry vagina accompanying the menopause. Eliminating the night sweats and insomnia will relieve the patient's fatigue and depression.

Proper diet and weight control, as well as a structured exercise program, can protect the cardiovascular system. These patients should be encouraged not to smoke and to limit their intake of alcohol.

Since the breast is part of the upper genital tract, the gynecologist taking care of the elderly must learn to examine the breast very carefully and to teach the patient breast self-examination. The physician must be familiar with the guidelines that have been established for screening of the breast and must be prepared to order the appropriate test on a yearly basis.

The problem of ageism must receive increasing support. It must be done in this decade. To increase the awareness of the medical profession (all specialties), crash courses should be established under the direction of the NIA. To qualify for a license or renewal of a license to practice medicine, physicians must be required to participate in one of these courses. The physician would not be qualified as a specialist, but the instruction would provide an awareness of the problems. The first responsibility of the medical profession is to educate its physicians to the problems of ageism and how to cope with them. The medical profession must strike a balance between its great opportunities and great responsibilities. Structuring sensitive as well as practical programs to help the elderly may be the medical profession's finest achievement.

Acknowledgments

To the resident staff in obstetrics and gynecology at Lenox Hill Hospital I am grateful for the help, suggestions, and stimulation they have provided.

To Dr. Irving Buterman and Dr. Alfred Fields I want to express my thanks for the coverage they provided for my private patients, allowing me to spend more time in the preparation of this book.

To Marcia Miller and Ruzena Danek I am most grateful for their help and encouragement. Their typing and editorial skills have been invaluable. It is difficult to express my gratitude adequately, and therefore, I can only say, thank you so much for your help.

To Shirley Dansker, Ruth Hoffenberg, and their library staff, I am deeply indebted for their cooperation and help. They were most helpful in searching the literature, as well as providing copies of articles that I felt might be helpful in my writing.

I am grateful to Patricia Kuharic of the Department of Medical Photography; Lenox Hill Hospital; for the preparation of illustrations.

To my wife, Mary Louise, I am grateful for the patience she showed during this time and for her help. Her support has sustained me in this project.

To my co-workers, Bridie McGuire and Ann McGuire, who do such a magnificent job in organizing my private practice and, therefore, provide time for me to devote to the writing of this book, I am most grateful. Thank you so much, Bridie and Ann, and may God bless you.

To Alys von Lehmden-Maslin I express my thanks for helping me begin the writing of this book.

To Isadore Rossman I am very grateful for the help and encouragement he gave me in writing this book and for the stimulation he provided me for the writing of a chapter for his own book, *Clinical Geriatrics.*

To PW Communications, the publisher of "The Female Patient," thank you for allowing me to publish editorials relating to the aging population. My particular thanks go to Lucy Kavaler and Dympna Burkhart for the encouragement they have given me.

To the Macmillan Publishing Company and Ms. Alice Macnow, I express my thanks for their help and encouragement in preparing this book.

FIGURE	*ACKNOWLEDGMENT*
2-3, 3-1, 3-2, 5-1, 8-3 to 8-7	Courtesy of Patricia Kuharic, Lenox Hill Hospital, Department of Medical Photography.
8-1, 8-2	© Copyright 1954. CIBA-CEIGY Corporation. Reproduced with permission from THE CIBA COLLECTION OF MEDICAL ILLUSTRATIONS by Frank H. Netter, M.D. All rights reserved.
11-1, 11-2, 13-2	© Masson Publishing USA, Inc. Used by permission.
11-3 to 11-10	Courtesy of the American Cancer Society and Henry P. Leis, Jr., M.D.
12-1 to 12-3	From Friedrich, Eduard G., Jr., *Vulvar Disease,* 2nd edition, Philadelphia, W.B. Saunders Co. Reproduced with the permission of W.B. Saunders Co. and Eduard G. Friedrich, Jr., M.D.
14-1	Courtesy of Ayerst Laboratories.
14-2 to 14-4	Reprinted with the permission of Barbara Lowenstein, Associates.
17-1	Masters, W.H., and Johnson, V.E. *Human Sexual Response.* Boston: Little, Brown, 1966. Used by permission.
18-1 to 18-3	From Eliopolous, Charlotte, *Gerontological Nursing,* Philadelphia, Lippincott. Reproduced with the permission of Lippincott and Charlotte Eliopolous.

Perimenopausal and Geriatric Gynecology

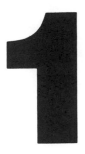# Introduction

Only stay quiet while the mind remembers
The beauty of fire from the beauty of embers.

On Growing Old
John Masefield

According to *Dorland's Illustrated Medical Dictionary, geriatrics* is defined as pertaining to the treatment of the aged. At present, it has taken on an expanded meaning in the United States. There is a great deal of work in progress on the anatomy of aging and changes related to aging.

On May 31, 1974, the Research on Aging Act was signed into law. This legislation authorized establishment of the National Institute of Aging (NIA) for the conduct and support of biomedical, social, and behavioral research and training related to the aging process and to the diseases and other special problems and needs of the aged. A great deal of research has been stimulated by this act.

Gerontology is emerging as a specialty in the United States, as well as in other countries. It is a specialty whose time has come. At the beginning of the twentieth century, 4 percent of all Americans (3 million) were 65 years old or more. That figure has now grown to more than 10 percent (23 million), with the segment of the population over 75 increasing from 900,000 to 11 million. This trend indicates that by the year 2000 there will be 31 million people over 65 and 13 million over 75 in the United States (Table 1-1). Many other developed and developing countries are experiencing similar growth in their elderly population. This phenomenon has significantly changed medical practice. Physicians now see clinical prob-

Table 1-1. Increase in the "Old Old" Population (in Millions)

AGE	1960	1970	1980	1983
Total				
65+	16.7	20.1	25.7	27.4
65-69	6.3	7.0	8.8	9.0
70-74	4.8	5.5	6.8	7.4
75-79	3.1	3.9	4.8	5.3
80-84	1.6	2.3	3.0	3.3
85+	0.9	1.4	2.3	2.5

(Data from the US Bureau of the Census, Current Population Reports, series P-25, Nos. 519 and 949, 1985)

lems increasingly related to the aging process. It has also become essential to understand the effects of aging on normal, healthy individuals aged 70 or more. At this point, it is important to structure a plan to deal with the serious social, economic, and personal consequences of this aging population. The medical profession must face the challenge and the professional responsibility of guaranteeing that this population does more than survive. The fruitful middle and later years of life must be extended so that the aging will live creatively and remain productive contributors to society. Much has been achieved, but the specialty of gerontology is still in its infancy. There are programs and organizations, however, that are concerned with the problems of an aging population.

Years ago, families stayed together; children grew up and lived out their adult lives in the same neighborhood. The elderly continued to be protected within the family environment. They often became the sages of their community—love, respected, and never abandoned. This situation has changed, and in our very complex society there is no haven for the aged.

As physicians, we must recognize that the young, up to puberty, and the elderly beyond 65 have certain physiologic characteristics in common. Since the endocrine system has not started to function at its maximum, the child or adolescent has a decreased immunologic response and an increased susceptibility to illness. The same holds true for the elderly. As their hormone levels fall, their receptiveness to disease rises.

Just a few years ago came the recognition that pediatric patients were being neglected, and many efforts were made to solve their problems. Now we are beginning to realize that senior citizens also face many crises and that far less has been done for them. In this context, it is of interest to review the historical development of pediatrics and family medicine.

DEVELOPMENT OF SPECIALTIES

Specialties do not develop according to an immutable law of progression or out of any one functional arrangement. They develop at different times and for different reasons. Some, like radiology, may focus on a piece of machinery; others, like urology and neurology, on a part or system of the body; still others, like ophthalmology, on particular techniques.

Pediatrics and family medicine are both organized around societal interests. In their early days, both were stimulated by government activity

—pediatrics as part of the child welfare movement early in this century, family medicine through recent federal grants for training.

Organizational progression of a medical specialty usually starts with a few individuals who meet informally to share common interests. This is followed by the establishment of a formal association. Later, chairs are established in medical schools, and practitioners who limit their practice or consultation to the one field and conform to the standards of the field are scrutinized by regulatory bodies. This is followed by a movement to include the specialty in the medical curriculum and by testing programs, residencies, and certification.

Geriatric medicine is on the first rung of this organizational ladder. Unfortunately, it has been at this stage in the United States for at least 70 years; an effort must now be made to push it beyond this level. Numerous individuals are interested in various aspects of the field, but relatively few regard themselves as full-time geriatricians. The progression from mutual interest to formal recognition as a medical specialty is slow. It is a social and political process and is sometimes fraught with conflict. Pediatrics is a good example.

The situation may be clarified by tracing the historical development of pediatrics as the basis for comparision. Pediatrics began to develop in the 1850s, growing out of various movements that focused on increasing public awareness of the status of children in American society. Then, in the latter part of the nineteenth century, efforts to combat infant diarrhea, an extremely serious problem, led to the clean milk movement and other measures to promote infant hygiene. The first full-time chairmanship of a pediatric department was established at Johns Hopkins University in 1912. The earliest pediatricians were not full-time specialists but general practitioners who were interested in children. Pediatric specialization at first was concentrated on research, and later on preventive medicine and the child health movement. The federally supported maternal and infant programs established in the 1920s attracted pediatricians. Pediatricians took an active role in the political battles between supporters and opponents of such programs. In the 1930s, the specialty of pediatrics began to coalesce. There were 1500 full-time pediatricians in the United States and several hundred part-time practitioners at the beginning of that decade. At that time, the American Academy of Pediatricians was formed as an action group to establish qualifications for pediatric practitioners.

The founding of the American Board of Pediatrics in 1933 provided an opportunity to set up standardized residency programs. Progress was slow, and pediatrics did not come into its own until the decline of the general practitioner following World War II.

Although there was considerable interest in geriatric medicine, the lack of a formal organization distinguished geriatrics from other medical fields, including pediatrics. The first American textbook on geriatric medicine appeared in 1914. It was written by a pathologist, Dr. I. L. Nascher, who was credited with coining the term *geriatrics* in 1909. Dr. Nascher concentrated on unusual physiological and pathological problems of aging and described geriatric patients in a somewhat unappealing light. Little appeared from that time on in the field of geriatrics until 1929. That year, a new textbook appeared and received a fair amount of attention. This was *Old Age: The Major Involution,* written by another pathologist, Dr. Alfred Scott Warthim, who also saw aging in rather grim terms. Early American writers on geriatrics have been pessimistic. The pattern was hardly broken until the 1940s, when there was an upsurge of public interest, both in the diseases of old age and in the status and conditions of the elderly. The founding of the American Geriatric Society in 1942 and of the Gerontology Society in 1945 reflected this interest. Both organizations took a much broader and brighter view of the conditions of the aged and the problems of aging than the early textbook writers had done. A new era for geriatrics opened in 1943 with the appearance of a major textbook for general practitioners, *Geriatric Medicine: Diagnosis and Management of Disease in the Aging and in the Aged,* edited by Edward J. Stieglitz. The book was modern in that it combined work on the biology of aging with the clinical and socioeconomic problems of aging individuals. By considering health as well as disease, it presented a much more optimistic view of aging than the previous American textbooks had done. From 1943 to the late 1950s, little was accomplished in geriatric medicine. Today geriatrics is viewed in terms of the intractable problems of aging and the necessary attempt to deal with the consequences of living longer. It is now more acceptable to think of life not as a simple curve of growth, maturity, and decay but as a continuing cycle.

In the later years of life, multiple disorders are present as the body's protective mechanisms, such as immunity, are compromised. Symptoms present differently in the old, and the untrained clinician may miss the diagnoses. For example, (1) an older person with hyperthyroidism may appear apathetic, not hyperactive; (2) tuberculosis may proceed in silence; (3) appendicitis may occur without the characteristic abdominal tenderness at McBurney's point, without fever, and without an elevated white blood cell count; and (4) an older person may even have a heart attack without chest pains and may instead appear to be confused, disoriented, and the victim of a stroke.

There is also the problem of cost. The United States spent some $118.7 billion on health care in 1975. Of this staggering figure, some 50 percent, or $60 billion, went for chronic disease, and one-third of all acute-care hospital beds were used by old people. There were 1.2 million patients in 23,000 nursing homes in 1975—more than in our more than 7500 voluntary hospitals. This has more than doubled in the 1980s, and Congress is working feverishly to contain the cost of medicine and Social Security reimbursements. Nearly one-fourth of all drugs consumed in this country were used by older Americans. Most of the office visits in the United States are made by the elderly.

Geriatric medicine includes the prevention, diagnosis, care, and treatment of illness and disability in older persons. This approach to promoting the health of the older patient takes into account the interaction of diseases, medication, environment, personal and social factors, and age. Geriatrics acknowledges the favorable and unfavorable elements of aging, but it

4

stresses that physical and mental deterioration are not an inevitable consequence of the aging process and that there are positive aspects of growing older.

PERIMENOPAUSAL AND GERIATRIC GYNECOLOGY

In this book, the phase in the life of a woman that marks the transition from the reproductive period to the period in which reproductive function is lost will be referred to as the *climacteric*. This stage is characterized by progressive endocrine changes that lead to the *menopause,* the final menstrual period that signals the end of cyclic ovarian function. The *perimenopause* is defined arbitrarily to include the last few years of the climacteric and the first year after the menopause. Geriatric gynecological problems will be designated as beginning at the age of 65. However, even in gynecology, it is becoming more and more difficult to refer to the senium as beginning in the 65th or even the 60th year of life and to designate all female patients an aged women from this time on. The first phase of geriatric gynecology might thus correspond approximately to the late menopause, with the senium beginning only after the 70th year or even later.

THEORIES OF AGING

Throughout time, people have proposed methods and theories to prevent aging, and throughout time the facts have proved them wrong. What constitutes the aging process? How is it defined? Terminology is often lacking, making it difficult to discuss aging.

In a biologic sense, growth and development represent the opposite of aging: a growing and developing organism is moving toward greater efficiency and size. As a biologic term, *aging* is used to identify changes taking place over time and finally ending in death. The changes reveal a decline in body efficiency, a change in body structure, arrest of the growth process, and reversal of size. Primary aging involves the biologic changes occurring in humans and animals; they are initially determined by heredity but are modified by the environment. These inborn processes are called *aging. Secondary aging* is defined as disabilities caused by accidental damage and illnesses.

The modern concepts of aging include body components with the crucial factors in the aging process. Exhaustion has been proposed as an explanation of aging. It is based on the assumption that a living organism contains a fixed supply of energy not unlike that contained in a coiled watch spring. There are biologic theories including autoimmunity, the air–earth theory, and the free radical theory. Assuming that there is validity to the free radical theory of aging, scientists have proposed that human or animal life spans might be increased by the intake of antioxidants that tie up the free radicals and inactivate them. Vitamin C is the most widely known and used antioxidant.

Psychologic and behavioral theories of aging are almost as numerous and diversified as biologic ones. Although the psychologic and behavioral theories are not well accepted, it has been reported that the state of late adulthood is important. The basic conflict arises between two beliefs: the belief that one's life can be useful and successful versus a sense of despair and a fear of death. More work is needed in this field.

Sociologic theories of aging are considered with the changes that affect social status, social roles, and economic conditions during the adult years. Consequently, social theories of human aging are directly related to the society's structure, its habitual patterns of functioning, and the repetitiveness of social values, changes, and technological advances. There is little doubt that successful aging includes accepting the inevitable reduction in social and personal interactions and recognizing the need to maintain one's activities.

Caloric restrictions have proved to be the most effective method of delaying senescence in the rodent; convincing data on caloric restriction in human beings has not yet been obtained. The mechanism for the augmented life span induced by caloric restriction is unknown.

The existence in primates of a cerebral clock with diurnal and lunar cycles is well known. A similar central determinant of menopause in aging may be present, presumably also at the level of the hypothalamus. It is possible that the prolongation of life in rats by caloric restriction may in fact be mediated by a control center in the hypothalamus. It has been shown that the administration of L-dopa may reinstate cyclic ovarian steroid production in old rats and prolong the life span in mice. The life cycle, including puberty and senescence, may in fact be centrally controlled and mediated by changes in catecholamine synthesis and metabolism. This may offer an explanation for the function of the cerebral clock.

GENETICS

Aging may result from altered gene structure or gene action. Injury to deoxyribonucleic acid (DNA) and somatic cells may be either spontaneous or introduced by outside agents such as chemicals and ionizing radiation. One theory of aging suggests that there are intrinsic differences among species in their susceptibility to mutational injuries because of genetically determined differences in the enzymatic machinery that replicates and repairs DNA. Thus, long-lived mammals seem to have more efficient enzymes for at least one system for repairing DNA. The importance of errors inherent in DNA replication and other types of somatic mutation needs to be evaluated. Does mutation in somatic cells depend on numbers (of generations) or on time (age)? When somatic mutations occur, are they randomized or do they grow as clones? Can prevention or repair of nuclear damage be facilitated by chemicals or other agents? Since aging may bring about errors in any of these processes, the importance of errors needs to be evaluated and steps taken to correct them.

A great deal of work has been done on human cells. Experiments have demonstrated the mortality of human diploid cell lines. Using cultured fetal lung cells, it has been demonstrated that after approximately 50 doublings, they fail to replicate further. Further investigations found that the cells from progressively older subjects exhibited fewer doublings and that adult cells showed only 20 doublings before death. It was estimated that approximately 54 population doublings would be required to produce from a single cell the entire number of erythrocytes and leukocytes needed for 60 years of life. These estimates correspond remarkably to findings of cell longevity in vitro.

Few people in the United States live to be 100. However, there are some centenarians in three other parts of the world. One group lives in a small village in Equador called Vilcabamba. The second group, the Hunzukuts, occupies the Karakoram range in Kashmir, and the third group, the Abkhazians, lives in the autonomous republic of Georgia in the southern Soviet Union. Time and genetics probably play a key role in prolonging their life, but no hard data are available on these subjects.

Undoubtedly, genetics plays a great role in longevity. The old people are born to parents who often live past 80. Since these people are living in isolated areas, gerontologists feel that isolation safeguards their gene pool, since there is very little intermarriage with persons in neighboring communities. These people consume about 1900 calories per day, compared to 3300 for the average American. Most Americans consume more protein and fats than the persons in Vilcamba and Hunza. These people are never obese, nor do they suffer from malnutrition. On a workup, the plasma cholesterol levels of those who live to be more than 100 years of age averages less than half the accepted normal amount for Americans aged 50 to 60.

However, many elderly Abkhazians are heavy smokers and drink red wine and vodka regularly. They eat a mixed diet that consists of milk, vegetables, fruit, and meats. Their daily caloric intake is approximately 1800 per day. Many Abkhazians live to 100 years of age, in spite of their smoking and drinking habits, and, unlike the Hunzukuts and elderly citizens of Vilcabanba, are obese. Although the Abkhazians, Hunzukuts, and Vilcabanbas are being intensely studied, no definitive conclusions can be drawn at this time.

CLIMACTERIC, MENOPAUSE, GERIATRICS

The most dramatic event in the life of a woman at the end of her reproductive span is the cessation of menstrual periods, which is referred to as the *menopause*. The ovary is the principal actor in the menopause. It contains primordial follicles that represent the primary reproductive unit. These follicles are also important in the production and maintenance of steroids. When they are exhausted or become resistant to the hormone gonadotropin, the amount of circulating estradiol drops, and with this comes the changes associated with the menopausal and postmenopausal years. Since there is a negative feedback of estrogen to the pituitary, follicle-stimulating hormone (FSH) and luteinizing hormone (LH) increase in amount and the hypothalamus loses its tonic and pulsatile stimulation of the pituitary gland.

After the menopause, the ovaries are smaller and more fibrotic and usually exhibit pits on their surfaces. Besides the diminution of primary and differentiating follicles, ultrastructural studies indicate a great increase in fibroblasts and connective tissue throughout, especially in the cortex, where germinal structures are largely absent. The advanced follicles identified in postmenopausal ovaries are usually undergoing atretic changes. An abundance of stromal cells is seen in postmenopausal ovaries, and in vitro experiments indicate that these cells are the source of androgens. The ovary shows varying degrees of avascularity. Eventually, the ovary becomes an inert residue that consists of connective tissue, and it clings to the posterior leaf of the broad ligament. Its color changes from pink to pure white. It shrinks to $2 \times 1.5 \times 0.5$ cm, and in some cases it may be as small as $1.5 \times 0.75 \times 0.5$ cm. Its wrinkled surface resembles that of the gyri and sulci of the cerebrum.

SYSTEMIC CHANGES

Although the cessation of menstrual periods and the diminished secretion of estrogen are the most dramatic aspects of the menopause, there are also changes of varying degrees in other organ systems.

Central Nervous System

With advancing age, there is a decrease in the number of neurons in the brain, which results in a slowing of the reflexes and a diminution in the senses of smell, taste, and hearing. The neuromuscular reflexes are dimmed, and this change, together with a decrease in vision, leads to a greater number of falls among the elderly. The other problem is that elderly people do not adjust to environmental changes and are particularly sensitive to the cold. Another problem of the elderly—and these may be influenced by the change in lifestyle and the sociology of society—are a great deal of depression and a sense of loneliness.

Cardiorespiratory System

Cardiorespiratory problems are common during the gerontolic period. There is a decrease in cardiac output and an increase in arteriosclerosis and atherosclerosis, as well as peripheral vascular resistance and hypertension. The lungs lose a great deal of their elasticity, and there is a decrease in vital capacity. Elderly patients are more susceptible to pollutants and to respiratory infections. A change in the cardiopulmonary system is important when preparing the elderly patient for surgery.

Gastrointestinal System

The gastrointestinal system undergoes changes. The elderly patient often complains of dyspepsia, increased gas, stomach distention, and constipation. There is usually decreased motility of the bowel, as well as decreased absorption through the mucosa. These changes are all important in the postoperative management of the geriatric patient. Gallstones, gastrointestinal cancer, and diverticulitis occur with increasing frequency among the elderly. It is important to understand the nutrition of the elderly.

Some of these patients suffer from overnutrition, consuming foods that lack essential nutrients but contain large amounts of sugar, saturated fats, salt, cholesterol, phosphates, and calories. Such a diet is accompanied by obesity, high blood pressure, strokes, osteoporosis, and gastrointestinal upsets. The elderly often suffer from undernutrition. The essential nutrient deficiencies predispose the patient to anemia, weakness, brittle bones, infection, gum disease, loss of teeth, and depression.

Urinary Tract

The urinary tract causes many problems for the aged. Bladder capacity is decreased, the bladder is usually more irritable, and this increased irritability, together with the atrophic changes in the urethra, leads to increased urinary tract infections. After age 60, the glomerular filtration rate drops, as does renal blood flow. The distal renal tubules become more sensitive to the antidiuretic hormone, and these patients suffer from systemic symptoms secondary to this increased absorption of water. The changes in glomerular filtration rate and plasma flow have a direct bearing on the use of medications. Drugs that are excreted by the kidney may reach toxic levels if the average dose for the premenopausal patient is used. Personality changes and evidence of dementia may be related to drug toxicity.

Skin and Its Appendages

The integumentary system consists mainly of the skin and its appendages. The skin consists of three distinct compartments—the epidermis, the dermis, and subcutaneous fat. The major aging changes in the gross morphology of the skin include dryness, which presents as roughness, wrinkling, atrophy, uneven pigmentation, and a variety of proliferative lesions. The most striking and consistent histological change is flattening of the dermoepidermal junction, with reduction in the number of interdigitating papillae and rete pegs per unit skin surface. This results in a considerably smaller contiguous surface between the two compartments, and presumably less communication and nutrient transfer and less resistance to external forces. The number of sweat glands and the growth of fingernails are also reduced. The subcutaneous fat is decreased, which leads to visible changes. The skin is prone to develop common dermatosis, and treatment is often more difficult than in the premenopausal patient.

Musculoskeletal System

The musculoskeletal system in the aged is markedly altered. The muscles degenerate and are replaced by fat and collagen. The musculoskeletal system of the aged patient is more prone to rheumatic disorders, orthopedic problems, particularly of the lower extremity, geriatric aspects of the foot and ankle, and a variety of degenerative changes.

HORMONAL CHANGES

The most dramatic change of the menopause is the withdrawal of estrogen. In the premenopausal period, the principal circulating estrogen is

17β-estradiol. Estradiol is produced both by direct ovarian secretion and by peripheral conversion of testosterone and estrone. Androgens, estrogen, progesterone, and gonadotropin secretion all change with the menopause, mostly because of cessation of ovarian follicular activity.

Androgens

During the reproductive and premenopausal years, the principal ovarian androgen is androstenedione, which is the major secretory product of the developing follicles. With the menopause, the androstenedione secretion drops by about one-half of the level in the premenopausal patient. However, the postmenopausal ovary continues to secrete testosterone, and the drop is only slightly below that seen in the premenopausal patient. The hilar cells and luteinized stromal cells responding to LH stimulation produce the testosterone. The drop in estrogen with the continued secretion of testosterone by the ovary may account for the defeminization and hirsutism seen in the geriatric patient. It is therefore accepted that the endogenous hormonal milieu of the postmenopausal woman is primarily androgenic.

Dehydroepiandrosterone (DHEA) and dehydroepiandrosterone sulfate (DHEA-S) levels begin to decline after the menopause and finally reach a level that may be 80 percent lower than that in the premenopausal patient. The principal source of these androgens is the adrenal glands, with the ovary contributing very little. Since adrenal androgen secretion dips to such a low level, this period has been called the *adrenopause.*

Estrogen

Following the menopause, estrogen secretion drops. The principal circulating estrogen of the premenopausal woman is 17β-estradiol. In the premenopausal woman, approximately 95% of circulating estradiol is derived from the ovary. In the postmenopausal woman, estrone is the most common estrogen. Most estrone results from the peripheral conversion of androstenedione, which occurs in fat, muscle, liver, bone marrow, brain, fibroblasts, and hair roots. The peripheral conversion of estrone, and to a lesser extent testosterone, account for most of the estradiol in the postmenopausal woman. It has been shown that no matter how atrophic the endometrial cells are, estrone is converted by an enzyme into estradiol in the cell, and the cell is then subjected to the same estrogenic stimulation as the premenopausal cell.

Progesterone

Postmenopausal progesterone levels drop dramatically and are only about one-third of those found during the follicular phase. The source of the progesterone is presumably the adrenal gland. The value of progesterone in the postmenopausal period has recently been demonstrated by the finding that women who are cycled with progesterone have a lower rate of endometrial cancer than those who are not. A progestogen challenge test proposed by Gambrell has been devised to identify postmenopausal women at greatest risk for endometrial adenocarcinoma. The use of this test in untreated postmenopausal women has identified many women who are at increased risk. It has been concluded that the use of this test and the continued use of progestogens in climacteric women who respond with withdrawal bleeding will reduce the risk of endometrial carcinoma in both estrogen-treated postmenopausal women and those with increased endogenous estrogens.

Gonadotropins

In the postmenopausal woman and the geriatric patient, the FSH titer is elevated because of lack of a negative feedback mechanism from the ovary. FSH values of 40 mIU/mL or more are generally associated with failure of ovarian function, and values greater than 100 mIU/mL indicate menopause with relative certainty. The hypothalamus loses both its tonic and pulsatile burst of stimulation of the pituitary.

Exogenous Estogens and Endometrial Cancer

It has been estimated that approximately 25 percent of women of menopausal age have symptoms severe enough to warrant estrogen therapy. Although the evidence is not conclusive, it is suggested that replacement estrogen therapy produces long-term metabolic benefits by reducing the incidence of stroke, heart attacks, osteoporosis, and fractures. It has been shown that estrogen reduces the level of low-density lipoproteins (LDL) and very-low-density lipoproteins (VLDL) and elevates that of high-density lipoproteins (HDL). HDL is more important in protecting the patient against a heart attack than LDL and VLDL.

A number of case control studies have indicated, however, that this treatment is associated with an increased incidence of endometrial cancer, with a risk ratio between 5 and 15. These figures, although alarming, should not discourage the physician from using estrogen replacement therapy when indicated. The common symptoms that are closely related to decreased estrogen function include flushes, flashes, sweats, insomnia, and dry vagina. The flushes and insomnia often lead to fatigue and depression. As the patient grows older, the flushes, sweats, and insomnia disappear but the dry, atrophic vagina worsens. The use of progesterone, particularly medroxyprogesterone acetate, augments the effect of estrogen in controlling menopausal symptoms and osteoporosis and does not interfere with the level of HDL.

The quality of life for the postmenopausal and geriatric patient can be significantly improved by active investigation and treatment of gynecologic disorders such as postmenopausal osteoporosis, the various pelvic relaxations, and urinary tract problems. Control of vasomotor symptoms is easily accomplished by using estrogen; each patient requires an individual dose schedule. Sexuality in later life is a healthy sign, and free discussion should be held between the patient and the physician.

URINARY INCONTINENCE

Urinary incontinence is an especially significant problem, both socially and medically, in the aged. It is important to make a correct diagnosis and institute proper treatment for these patients. Since women spend one-third of their life in the estrogen-deprived state, a considerable number of women will require major surgery for the handicaps inherent in aging. Disorders of the female genital tract are certainly not among the major causes of death. Yet they give rise to important illnesses, producing discomfort and disability, and therefore warrant treatment. Most of the gynecologic complaints of elderly women are related to genital prolapse. Surgery can be carried out in these patients, particularly if the vaginal route is employed, without increased morbidity and mortality.

OSTEOPOROSIS

Osteoporosis has become a national health hazard. There are approximately 20,000 deaths each year among patients with hip fractures caused by this condition. The patient predisposed to osteoporosis is a postmenopausal woman who is slender, with very fair skin and small bone structure. There are other contributing factors that may predispose to osteoporosis, namely, a family history of the disease, nulligravida, lack of physical activity, poor diet, calcium deficiency, vitamin D deficiency, smoking, use of alcohol, change in estrogen balance, and change in calcium metabolism. Prophylaxis should start at age 35 in the high-risk group and at menopause in others. The patient should be instructed in the use of a well-balanced diet, adequate exercise, and control of smoking and the use of alcohol. Calcium and hormones should be administered according to the physician's judgment.

Therapy for established disease includes calcium supplements, vitamin D, estrogens, androgens, fluoride, and calcitonin. Treatment should be carried out under controlled supervision. Osteporosis cannot be cured, but the patient can be made more comfortable by treatment. Progression of osteoporosis may be slowed, if not prevented. Dual photon absorptiometry is a method for identifying patients with bone loss and for monitoring those under treatment.

Osteoporosis is a disfiguring, discouraging, and painful condition that is seen in the postmenopausal years. It has often been called the *silent disease.* Technically, this is because it produces absolutely no symptoms until the fracture occurs. Therapy is now available to control, if not reverse, osteoporosis.

SEXUALITY

The Victorian concept of sexuality stops with the menopause. It is a myth, with no basis of reality. Most older people want and are able to lead an active, satisfying sex life. With age, women do not ordinarily lose their physical capacity for orgasm or men their capacity for erection and ejaculation. However, there is a gradual slowing of responses, especially in men. This process is currently considered a part of normal aging but perhaps may eventually be treatable and even reversible.

A pattern of regular sexual activity, which may include masturbation, helps to preserve sexual ability. When problems occur, they should not be viewed as inevitable, but rather as a result of disease, disability, drug reactions, or emotional upset, and as requiring medical care. Women generally experience little serious loss of sexual capacity due to age alone. Those changes that occur, involving flexibility and lubrication of the vagina, can usually be traced directly to lowered levels of the hormone estrogen during and after menopause. In the past, women who had severe problems were usually advised to use a lubricant. However, there are now hormone creams available that, when applied externally and at the introitus, reverse atrophy of the vagina and restore these women to a normal sex life. Lubrin an unscented, colorless, convenient vaginal lubricating insert has proved helpful as a lubricating agent.

GERIATRIC MEDICINE

Although the geriatric period is generally considered as starting at age 65, geriatric medicine is concerned principally with people at least 75 or 80 years of age who have reached the point at which aging itself is likely to present clinical problems. Before that time, disability and frailty are generally the result of specific illnesses. After 75, however, various parts of the body deteriorate and thus generate problems.

Gerontology, the study of normal aging, helps us to know what to expect as patients grow older. Much of physiological aging consists of a series of losses. Hearts lose vigor in reserve power, lungs grow more rigid and less efficient, bones grow brittle, muscles become thinner and weaker, and strength fades. The senses, especially hearing and vision, diminish measurably. The age of geriatric medicine has arrived.

Geriatrics or gerontology is fast emerging as one of the most important specialties of the future. It has been stated that the proper study of geriatrics begins with pediatrics. Translated, this means that the whole is the sum of the parts. A geriatric patient represents a total life's experience.

The NIA is attempting to strike a balance between the extension of life and the quality of life. The NIA appreciates the fact that basic research includes not only biologic research in molecular or cellular aging and immune biology but also fundamental investigations of the interpersonal and social aspects of human experience. It has directed attention to preventive medicine, as well as individual and family life styles and personal, social, and physical fitness. A wide range of activities are being investigated, including exercise, dietary habits, and the adverse effects of the so-called recreational drugs like tobacco, alcohol, and caffeine. The geriatric patient is touched by every aspect of life, including cultural factors, religion and ethics, health, nutrition, physical environment, transportation, social services, communication, legal services, education, recreation and culture, civic participation, commerce, employment, and economic support.

The demographic and social characteristics of the old are changing. Reductions in mortality and fertility have markedly changed the age distribution of the United States. Compared to a total population increase of 2.5 times from 1900 to 1970, the number of persons aged 65 and above has increased 7 times. This group now constitutes about 10 percent of the

Table 1-2. Sex Ration in Population 65 Years and Older

YEAR	NUMBER OF MALES PER 100 FEMALES
1910	101.1
1920	101.3
1930	100.5
1940	95.5
1950	89.6
1960	82.8
1970	72.1
1980	67.6
1983	67.1

(Data from the US Bureau of the Census, based on US Census of Population: 1950, 1960, and 1970, part B; and Current Population Reports, series P-25, No. 949)

total population, but over the next 50 years it is expected to make up between 12 and 16 percent. There are now about four persons under age 20 for every one person over age 65. If zero population growth is reached in the United States within the next 50 years and then maintained, that ratio will become 1.5:1. About one-third of the older population is very old, 75 years or more. This proportion will stay about the same for the foreseeable future if mortality rates remain constant. If they do, there will be about 12 million of the very old by the year 2000. If mortality rates decline, however, the number of very old persons may grow as high as 16 or 18 million. A 65-year-old man can now expect, on the average, to live to 78; a woman of 65, to 82 (Table 1-2). By the year 2000, life expectancies for 65-year-olds may increase by another 2 to 5 years. The average age expectancy has been steadily increasing since the turn of the century. However, the maximum age that humans can achieve is approximately 120, years and this has remained fairly stationary for centuries.

GERIATRIC GYNECOLOGY

Geriatric gynecology is emerging as a new specialty in the field of gynecology. The most frequent symptom that results in hospital admission is genital bleeding. The management of genital displacement in elderly women is very common. Urinary incontinence is frequently associated with genital displacement, and constitutes not only a medical problem but also a social and nursing problem, especially in the very old patient. Patients with large cystoceles have retention of urine rather than incontinence of urine (unless it is overflow incontinence) and are subject to more bladder infections. It is important to make a correct diagnosis. In studying the geriatric patient, it is difficult to separate the various genital prolapses and urinary problems. They should rightfully be placed together as genitourinary problems. Pruritis vulvae is also one of the most frequent symptoms in geriatric gynecologic pathology.

The geriatric patient is often reluctant to have a gynecologic examination and must be educated to the need for periodic examination. The patient must be told that carcinoma of the genitalia or breast can occur at any age; for example, cancer of the ovary peaks in incidence at age 77. Many older women recognize that they have atrophic vaginal and vulvar tissue and that an examination may be painful. Therefore, they are inclined to avoid routine examinations. It is important that the patient receive as little discomfort and pain as possible during the examination. The geriatric woman requires an empathetic physician that can listen well, evaluate well, and make an educated judgment about therapeutics.

In the lower genital tract, which includes the vulva, vagina, and cervix, there is usually an atrophic condition. If there is any type of bleeding with evident benign pathology present, however, it must not be assumed that the benign process accounts for the bleeding. It is imperative that a careful examination be carried out to identify any potential malignancy that may be present. The upper genital tract consists of the endometrium, ovary, and breast. it is commonly appreciated that geriatric patients are at high risk for developing a malignancy. It is important to make an accurate diagnosis and carry out treatment as promptly as possible.

Genital prolapse, consisting of cystourethroceles, uterine descensus, rectocele, enterocele, and/or retention of urine or stress incontinence, is frequently seen in the elderly patient. Symptoms related to one area must be carefully identified with other structures, and the patient must have an evaluation of her genitourinary problem. The genital and urinary systems should not be separated.

MAJOR GYNECOLOGIC SURGICAL PROCEDURES IN THE AGED

Medical advances in diagnosis and treatment and a better understanding of physiology and pathophysiology in the elderly now justify the performance of major operations in this group. Reports from numerous authors have shown that age alone does not contraindicate surgical intervention if due regard is paid to the patient's general condition. Better anesthesia and antibiotics have resulted in greater security in the postoperative period. The operation should be kept as brief as possible because the prolonged lithotomy position invites even more complications than does prolonged anesthesia. Miniheparinization should be carried out in these patients, starting the evening before surgery and continuing through surgery and for the first few postoperative days. As the geriatric population increases, women will no longer accept age as a barrier to active life, and more elective surgery will be demanded by patients and performed by gynecologic surgeons. Contradications to surgical intervention should not include age.

Disorders of the female genital organs are certainly not among the major causes of death. Yet they give rise to important illness-producing discomfort and disability, and therefore warrant treatment. Most of the gynecologic complaints of elderly women are related to genitourinary problems. These patients tolerate vaginal surgery quite well.

The gynecologist taking care of geriatric patients must truly be the primary care physician for these patients. A great number of medical disorders may occur beyond the realm of expertise of the physician and the physician should then direct them to the proper specialist.

The geriatric patient admitted to a hospital often becomes disoriented. Well-meaning but unprepared professionals may not know how to react. If geriatric beds were placed in a specific area of the hospital, it might be easier for medical personnel with special training to set up a coordinated management plan. This section could be arranged so that a family member or friend could stay with the patient at night to ease fears, anxieties, and apprehensions. Short of this, the family should bring in familiar articles from the geriatric patient's home so that the patient does not feel isolated.

Every elderly person, healthy or ill, must deal with changes in human relationships. Old friends die or enter nursing homes, and children move away. Often the elderly must move, too, leaving lifelong friends behind. Some must give up their houses or apartments where they have lived for a long time and go into nursing homes. If one asks the elderly what problem bothers them most, the answer usually is loneliness. There is no one to share the present or remember the life that was pleasant and happy but is now gone. They sit and stare, gaze off into space, and sometimes weep. No modern medicines can alleviate this problem. Physicians must find ways of helping the old form new relationships or adjust better to being alone.

A whole new health team, including people from all disciplines, must be created to care for the elderly. Patience and compassion are even more necessary than in other areas of health care. The elderly may need six meals a day and sleep at 4-hour intervals. Professionals must not assume that age is invariably associated with senility and that patients do not know what they are talking about. Diagnosis can be missed when that attitude is taken. Of course, an old patient may be confused and disoriented, and may not display the same symptoms and responses as younger patients. A woman of 86 may have a heart attack without the classic accompanying symptoms. Her state might be incorrectly considered normal for her age. Another example is the patient who complains of malaise and confusion and is treated with tranquilizers. What she really has may be appendicitis without the classic symptoms of abdominal tenderness, fever, and a high white blood cell count. It is apparent that physicians do not know what signs and symptoms to look for in their elderly patients. The reason is simple: these symptoms are not taught in medical schools. The medical profession looks to the NIA to help train physicians in the care of the elderly.

The gynecologist must be alert to many changes that occur when treating the elderly. The question is often raised: who among us would think of advising the elderly not to eat cheddar cheese and drink Chianti at the same meal? Yet, the pressor effect produced by this combination could blow out a weakened artery and cause a stroke. Frequently a physician will encourage an old patient to take a drink without finding out whether another physician has prescribed a mood-stabilizing tranquilizer. The addition of a drink at dinner may cause the patient to faint, perhaps become unsteady, and fall and break a hip. Drug overdose in a geriatric patient is particularly likely to occur if the drug remains active in the body until it is excreted by the kidney. Dehydration, congestive heart failure, or urinary retention may create a real problem if digitalis or oral hypoglycemic agents are prescribed. Barbiturates may increase nocturnal restlessness and produce a hangover that makes the elderly inattentive, mentally confused, and unsteady on their feet the next day. Phenothiazines often decrease anxiety, hallucinations, and delusions but may induce a Parkinson-like syndrome. Given the current level of knowledge of gerontology, it is difficult to even advise the elderly on such basic matters as what clothing to wear or how much exercise to undertake. Hopefully, as studies progress and more physicians contribute their ideas to the literature, a systematized and rational approach to the care of the geriatric patient will evolve.

It is obvious that aging is a developmental process. As patients grow older (aging process):

time seems to race
cognitive thinking increases
sleeping decreases (insomnia)
the sleep/wake rhythm becomes diverse
eating patterns become more varied
a sharper sense of taste develops

REFERENCES

Andrew, W. 1956. Structural alterations with aging in the nervous system. *J. Chronic Dis.* 3:575.

Barber, H. R. K. and E. A. Graber. 1971. The PMPO syndrome (postmenopausal palpable ovary syndrome). *Obstet. Gynecol.* 38:921.

Becker, P., and H. Cohen. 1984. Functional approach to the care of the elderly. *J. Am. Geriatric Soc.* 32(12):923.

Blatt, M. H. G., H. Wiesbader, and H. S. Kupperman. 1953. Vitamin E climacteric syndrome. *AMA Arch. Intern. Med.* 91:792.

Calkins, E. 1981. Aging of cells and people. *Clin. Obstet. Gynecol.* 24:165.

Chestnut, C. H. 1984. An appraisal of the role of estrogens in the treatment of postmenopausal osteoporosis. *J. Am. Geriatric Soc.* 32:604.

Comfort, A. 1979. *The Biology of Senescence,* ed 3., Elsevier, New York, p. 265.

Erlik, Y., I. V. Tataryn, D. R. Meldrum, P. Lomax, J. G. Bajorek, and H. L. Judd. 1981. Association of waking episodes with menopausal hot flushes. *JAMA* 245: 1741.

Fink, P. J. 1980. Psychiatric myths of menopause, in: *The Menopause: Comprehensive Management* (B. A. Eskin, ed.), Masson Publishing USA, New York, p. 111.

Hart, R. W., and R. B. Setlow. 1974. Correlation between deoxyribonucleic acid excision-repair and life-span in a number of mammalian species. *Proc. Natl. Acad. Sci. USA* 71: 2169.

Hayflick, L. 1965. The limited in vitro lifetime of human diploid cell strains. *Exp. Cell Res.* 37:614.

Hayflick, L., and P. Moorhead. 1961. The serial cultivation of human diploid cell strains. *Exp. Cell Res.* 25:985.

Jazzmann, L. J. B. 1976. Epidemiology of the climacteric syndrome, in: (S. Campbell, ed.), *Management of the Menopause and Post-Menopausal Years,*

Lancaster, MTP Press, p. 285.

Judd, H. L. 1976. Hormonal dynamics associated with the menopause. *Clin. Obstet. Gynecol.* 19:775.

Kannel, W. B., M. C., Hjortland, P. M. McNamara, and T. Gordon. 1976. Menopause and risk of cardiovascular disease: The Framingham Study. *Ann. Intern. Med.* 85:447.

Mohr, D. M. 1983. Evaluation of surgical risk in the elderly: A correlative review. *J. Am. Geriatric Soc.* 31:99.

Nascher, I. L. 1914. *The Diseases of Old Age and Their Treatment.* Blakeston & Son, Philadelphia.

Osbourne, J. L. 1976. Postmenopausal changes in micturition habits and in urine flow and urethral pressure studies, in: *The Management of the Menopause and Post-Menopausal Years* (S. Campbell, ed.), MTP Press, Lancaster, p. 285.

Peluso, J., G. Breitenecker, and E. S. E. Hafez. 1979. Atresia of ovarian follicles and ova, in: *Human Ovulation* (E.S. E. Hafez, ed.), Elsevier-North Holland Biomedical Press, Amsterdam, p. .

Piscitelli, J. T., and R. T. Parker. 1986. Primary care in the postmenopausal woman. *Clin. Obstet. Gynecol.* 29(2): 343.

Renshaw, D. 1985. Sex, age and values. *J. Am. Geriatric Soc.* 33(9): 635.

Resnick, N., and V. Y. Subbarao. 1985. Management of urinary incontinence in the elderly. *N. Engl. J. Med.* 313:800.

Rossman, I. 1986. The anatomy of aging, in: *Clinical Geriatrics,* ed. 3 (I. Rossman, ed.), J. B. Lippincott, Philadelphia, p. 364.

Somers, A. 1985. Toward a female gerontocracy? in: *Current Social Trends in the Physical and Mental Health of Aged Women* (M. Haug, A. Ford, and M. Schaefer, eds.), Springer Publishing Co., New York, p. 16.

Wallach, J. 1978. Osteoporosis in the female, in: *Advances in Obstetrics and Gynecology,* (R. M. Caplan and W. J. Sweeney III, eds.), Williams & Wilkins Co., Baltimore, p. 567.

Young, E. A. 1983. Nutrition, aging and the aged. *Med. Clin. North Am.* 67:295.

Young, J. Z. 1971. *An Introduction to the Study of Man.* Clarendon Press, Oxford.

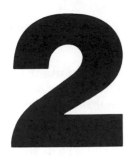 # History and Physical Examination

INTRODUCTION

Geriatric patients are often afflicted with poor eyesight and poor hearing. Many chatter on and are very talkative, and it is difficult to get them to answer a question directly. Other patients seem to be withdrawn and introspective, and particularly on the first interview have difficulty concentrating on the questions they are asked. It is important not to underestimate the sensitivity of these patients. Many of them, because of their frailty and often because of arthritic changes in their hands, do not appear neat. No matter what their physical appearance is, it is most important to maintain a professional manner tempered with kindness and warmth. After greeting the patient, if the nurse or secretary has not introduced her, it is very important to introduce yourself and address the patient as either "Mrs." or "Miss." Once the patient–physician relationship is established, many of these patients respond much better when they are called by their first name. However, at the first introduction, some elderly patients look upon this practice as disrespect.

The confidence of the patient must be gained, a relaxed and friendly atmosphere must be created, and the physician must be prepared to take time when taking a history from an elderly patient. A consultation room that has an environment that resembles a home puts these patients more quickly at ease.

Since many of these patients are hard of hearing, it is important to speak directly to them and ask them if you are talking loudly enough. Most patients appreciate this consideration. A significant number of elderly women may be unable to give a history of their obstetric and gynecologic experience or the age at which menopause occurred. These patients are often not certain whether they have ever had hormone therapy. Their past medical and surgical histories are often difficult to obtain. It is useful if a relative or a close and trusted friend of the patient is available. However, this is not always possible. Some elderly patients may complain of, or be referred for, so-called vaginal bleeding, but on close questioning are uncertain whether the bleeding is coming from the urethra, the vagina, or the anal area.

Fortunately, many elderly patients are fully alert and possess excellent recall. Thus, an accurate obstetric, menstrual, postmenopausal and gynecologic history can usually be taken. The patient should be asked about drug ingestion, particularly hormones, tranquilizers, blood pressure pills, and mood stabilizers. It is also important to explore the patient's eating habits and nutrition. Many patients in this age group do not realize that they have a very poor diet, which often leads to fatigue, depression, and an anemia that may be difficult to explain.

Epidemiologic data suggest that anxiety disorders are exceedingly common, occurring more frequently in women than in men in all age groups. It is estimated that approximately 5 percent of all women, at some time in their lives, will have an anxiety disorder of sufficient severity to interfere with their usual functioning. An estimated 10 to 15 percent of women over the age of 65 experience anxiety that is sufficiently severe to warrant medical intervention. Anxiety in the elderly may present as neurologic, gastrointestinal, cardiovascular, or respiratory symptoms. The most common genitourinary symptoms are pruritis vagina, and/or ani, or dyspareunia.

The Victorian concept that all sexual activity ends at the time of menopause is totally inaccurate. Many studies have shown that men, and particularly women, are able to function sexually late in their lives. Therefore, it is very important to ask the patient about sexual function. If the inquiry is approached in an open but concerning manner, it reinforces the patient's regard for the physician. Very often this allows the patient to talk freely about herself and about things that may be bothering her. It establishes confidentiality and improves the patient–physician relationship.

Sexuality and sexual function in the menopausal and postmenopausal years are now receiving a great deal of attention in the literature. It seems that women who are sexually active in this period of their lives are approximately 22 pounds heavier than those who are not. Thus, in terms of estrogen storage and conversion as well as sexual activity, some adiposity is probably important. This conclusion focuses attention on the importance of diet and nutrition in some age-related processes. Kinsey reported that sexual activity in unmarried women remains relatively constant until age 55, whereas that of unmarried men declines progressively from adolescence. Among married couples as well, the frequency of sexual intercourse appears to decline in similar fashion with aging. Kinsey observed that in women, age has no effect on sexual activity until very late in life, and that the subsequent reduction in sexual activity may be due primarily to diminution in the sexuality of the male partner. This can be elicited by discrete questioning of the patient. It will allow her to talk about her interest in sexual matters and provide the opportunity for the physician to offer counselling.

AN OUTLINE OF THE HISTORY

There are some differences in the format of the patient's history. However, the chief complaint and present illness, the general evaluation and past history, a review of systems, and a personal and social history are essential.

Chief Complaint

It is important to identify the reason for the patient's visit. In the geriatric patient there are usually a series of complaints. After the patient has given all of these complaints, it is important to ask her tactfully to identify the most important one. Once this has been done, the others, which may or may not be related to one another, will be explored. It is also important to determine whether this is a chronic condition that has suddenly gotten worse or whether it is a totally new symptom. Therefore, it is very important to spend extra time exploring the chief complaint with the patient. It immediately gives the patient a sense that the physician is truly interested in her problem and permits a better interview.

Systemic Review of General Health

It is always good to start with generalities by asking about the patient's sense of well-being and whether there has been any change in the ability to carry out normal activities. This offers an opportunity to find out what drugs are being taken. At this point, it can tactfully be suggested that the patient bring in every bottle or container of drugs that she has at home for evaluation at the next visit.

Since cardiovascular problems occur to some degree in most postmenopausal and geriatric women, it is important to start by inquiring about problems in this area. The cardiovascular changes that occur with aging include decreased cardiac output, progressive arteriosclerosis, increased peripheral vascular resistance, and hypertension. Shortness of breath is sometimes difficult to identify as solely a problem of the cardiovascular system. It may be confused with fatigue; conversely, angina may be identified as arthritis in the shoulder. It is important to inquire whether these symptoms continue while the patient is at rest or only during exercise. Patients who complain about shortness of breath may have poor cardiac function or chronic obstructive pulmonary disease. It is important to inquire about cigarette smoking and environmental pollutants, as well as the patient's occupation and working conditions, past and present.

The gastrointestinal tract also gives rise to a variety of symptoms in the elderly. Poor bowel function secondary to decreased motility of the bowel, poor abdominal musculature, and the lack of well-regulated bowel habits all contribute to this problem. It is important to ask if there has been any change in eating or bowel habits and to pursue any change that has occurred. There may be decreased absorption from the bowel, which may lead to a variety of conditions including anemia. The elderly patient is more inclined to have gallstones, gastrointestinal cancer, diverticulosis, or hiatal hernias, but rarely an ulcer. It is important to ask about the color of the stool and about whether any blood is present. Black stools may be secondary to the iron that the patient is taking. The caliber of the stool should be explored. Although the history is valuable, laboratory testing is necessary as well.

Respiratory symptoms in the elderly may be due to cardiac insufficiency or to a problem in the lung itself. It is known that pulmonary compliance, vital capacity, alveolar surface area, and resistance to infection diminish with age. It is very important to inquire about cigarette smoking, environmental pollution, and whether the patient has been exposed by occupation to any contaminant that may have an effect on the respiratory system. The patient must be asked whether the present symptoms have been of long standing and unchanged, if there has been a recent change, or if the symptoms are new.

Postmenopausal and geriatric women often complain of frequency, burning on urination, nocturia, and a variety of distressful urinary symptoms. Special attention must be paid to bleeding at the time of urination. The history is valuable in evaluating the urinary tract. A differential diagnosis must include stress incontinence, urgency incontinence, and total incontinence. This is usually determined by an evaluation of the history. The patient with urinary symptoms often complains of local discomfort around the vulva of dryness, itching, and occasional burning, which may be secondary to estrogen deprivation. This condition can be better evaluated at the physical examination and by a study of the laboratory tests. The Pap smear is useful in determining the estrogen titer by evaluating the vaginal cytology.

It is important to ask about past illnesses and their method of treatment. Most of the illnesses will be uncovered by reviewing each organ system, as outlined previously. However, the patient will often state that she has diabetes, high blood pressure, a metabolic disorder, or a skin disease.

Operations

It is important to ask about the number and types of operations the patient has had. It is well to start off by asking if the patient has ever had a tonsil operation or an appendectomy. It allows the patient time to recall the operations she has had and the reasons for them, whether there were any postoperative complications, and the length of hospitalization. At this time, it is important to ask about radiation therapy. Although not common today, radiation therapy was once used for acne, thymic enlargement, and certain dermatologic conditions overlying the chest. All of these treatments predispose the patient to malignancy, and it is important to know the age at which it was given, the area in the body to which the radiation was given, and the result. In the geriatric patient, it is important to ask whether radiation to the pelvis was ever employed. At one time, a low dose of radiation was given to the ovaries to help correct infertility and to control heavy vaginal bleeding. The question about whether the patient had ever received transfusions is important. Up to 10 or 15 years ago, blood was freely given for a variety of conditions, and the so-called one transfusion has been known to lead to a variety of problems. Patients have developed chronic hepatitis, and those with non-A, non-B hepatitis may progress slowly to an advanced cirrhosis, while those who have had hepatitis B may develop a malignancy of the liver.

The history of the hormone therapy that might have been given is important. It is vital to ask about thyroid, estrogen, progesterone, cortisone, and the pill. It was fashionable about 15 to 20 years ago to give thyroid for a variety of conditions, this was usually done without an adequate workup. Therefore, it is important to explore this area with the patient.

The obstetric history is important. The patient should be asked about the number of pregnancies, the number of children, and whether there were miscarriages, induced abortions, or ectopic pregnancies. If the patient gives a history of any abnormal bleeding in the first trimester with evacuation of the uterus, it is important to find out whether there was any molar pregnancy at the time, and if so, whether it was treated.

A menstrual history is important in the menopausal and geriatric patient. The patient should be asked about her last menstrual period; if it occurred before age 35, the patient probably had ovarian failure. Those who have menstruated regularly, particularly if their menstruation was heavy late into the fifties, are at risk for endometrial cancer. The presence of menopausal symptoms should be brought out in the questioning. The most important, of course, are flushes, flashes, insomnia, night sweats, dry vagina, fatigue, and depression during the menopausal years. The history also provides an opportunity to return to the question of whether the patient had hormone therapy. The age of onset of menstruation and the age of menopause are important to document. Having rejected the Victorian concept that all sexual activity ends at the end of menopause, it is important to find out whether there is any postcoital bleeding and/or discomfort. If the inquiry is approached in an open, discerning manner, it reinforces the patient's regard for the physician. This is an important part of the interview.

The nervous system, as well as the musculoskeletal system, should be reviewed. The patient should be asked about the slowing of her reflexes and the diminution in the senses of smell, taste, touch, hearing, and vision. Neuromuscular coordination faults account, at least in part, for the greater number of accidents incurred in the elderly.

Personal and Social History

A short personal and social history may bring out some interesting things about the patient. Patients are usually very eager to talk, and although it is time-consuming, it is most important to hear them out. It is worthwhile to ask them to describe a typical day or days; this gives the physician an insight into the physical and psychiatric limitations of the patient. It also provides an opportunity to find out about the diet, the number of meals eaten each day, the emotional stability, and the patient's living conditions. It is important to be discreet and inquire about the patient's financial history so that a judgment can be made regarding the limits of therapy at home and how the patient can best take advantage of the different programs that have been established by the federal government for the elderly.

PHYSICAL EXAMINATION

Gynecologic Examination

The geriatric patient is often reluctant to have a gynecologic examination and must be educated to the need for periodic examinations. Many older patients recognize that they have atrophic vaginal and vulvar tissue and know that the examination may be painful. Therefore, they are inclined to avoid routine examinations. It is important that the patient be subjected to as little discomfort and pain as possible during the examination.

Although not a direct part of the gynecologic examination, the weight, blood pressure, and a brief outline of the general overall appearance of the patient should be recorded. It is important to examine the eyes and ears, as well as the throat and teeth. The supraclavicular area should be carefully palpated because it may be the site of a metastasis from a cancer located in the lung or anywhere in the abdomen. The thyroid should be carefully palpated to make sure that there are no hard nodules present (Fig. 2-1).

The heart should be examined and the rhythm identified. It should be determined whether there are any murmurs, and the types of sounds that are present must be recorded. The lungs should be carefully examined by percussion and auscultation.

The breasts must be carefully examined with the patient lying down, and special attention must be given to each quadrant of the breast, the subareolar area, and the axilla. The patient should also be examined while sitting or standing.

The spine should be gently pounded, as well as the costovertebral angles. Tenderness in this area may indicate that the patient has a pyelonephritis that will require careful follow-up. While this is being done, the extremities can be observed for any changes, and the elderly patient with a foot problem can be referred for help. Those with a foot problem often stumble, and in this age group there is an increased risk of fracture of the wrist as well as of the hip.

THE PELVIC EXAMINATION: SUMMARY OF GUIDELINES

The pelvic examination is part of a continuum that includes a careful history and complete physical examination. If a complete systemic evaluation is not possible, the following essential points are covered:

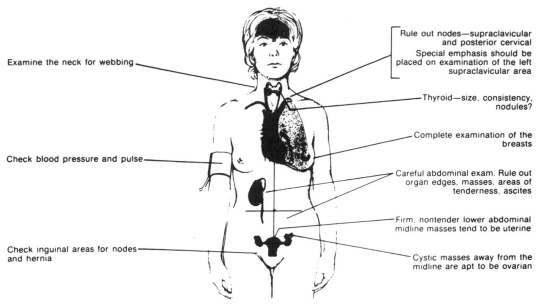

Examine the neck for webbing

Check blood pressure and pulse

Check inguinal areas for nodes and hernia

Rule out nodes—supraclavicular and posterior cervical
Special emphasis should be placed on examination of the left supraclavicular area

Thyroid—size, consistency, nodules?

Complete examination of the breasts

Careful abdominal exam. Rule out organ edges, masses, areas of tenderness, ascites

Firm, nontender lower abdominal midline masses tend to be uterine

Cystic masses away from the midline are apt to be ovarian

Figure 2-1. The pelvic examination.

The abdomen should be carefully inspected and then examined. It should be noted whether there is any enlargement of the liver, spleen, or kidney or any other abdominal masses. Frequently the elderly patient has a distended bowel, and poor musculature almost gives the impression of soft masses, particularly in the area of the large bowel. Inguinal areas should be carefully evaluated to make sure that there are no nodes or hernias in this area. Although inguinal hernias are not common in the female, femoral hernias do occur more commonly in the female than in the male.

Pelvic Examination

The pelvic examination should be carried out with great care and in a professional manner. It is important to use the right words. For example, the word *feel,* as in "feeling breasts," may arouse images of sexual exploitation, but the word *touch* or *palpate* is generally far less threatening. The physician must be concerned and gentle. The patient then feels free to indicate whether she feels pain and will answer questions (Fig. 2-2).

The examining physician should carefully observe the vulva, urethra, Bartholin's glands, and Skene's glands. It is important to palpate the texture of these structures. A small speculum or a Peterson vaginal speculum should be carefully inserted, holding the blades parallel to the introitus. The instrument should be turned slowly so that the posterior blade rests against the posterior wall of the vagina. Gentle downward pressure on the instrument opens the vagina without disturbing the sensitive organs anteriorly. It is important to explain to the patient what is

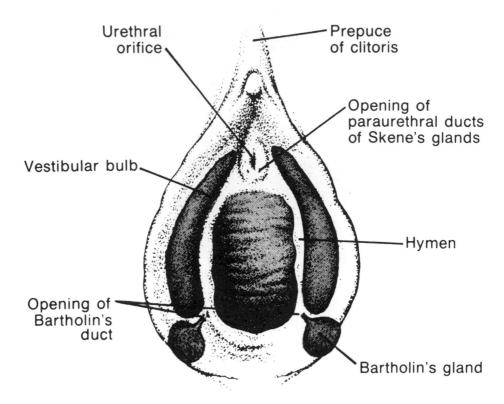

Figure 2-2. External anatomy.

being done. This serves two purposes: it distracts the patient and establishes confidence in the fact that she is being kept informed.

The cervix is identified and a vaginal secretion is removed. A careful Papanicolaou smear is taken from the cervical canal, if possible, and also from the posterior fornix. In the elderly patient, the cervix is often flush with the vagina and is difficult to identify. In addition, the upper vagina is often conical, especially in patients who have not delivered a baby vaginally. Although it is important to screen the endometrium, it is better to do this later in the examination or to schedule it as a separate procedure after a good physician–patient relationship has been established.

A careful one-finger examination of the entire length and breadth of the vagina, including the fornices, is ideally carried out first. Next, the uterus should be outlined in regard to size, shape, and mobility, and the adnexa should be examined. It is important to explain each step of the examination and to assure the patient that if there is any pain, the examination will be stopped immediately. At this point, the lubricated middle finger is inserted into the patient's rectum for a rectovaginal examination, providing an opportunity to explore the rectovaginal septum and cardinal ligaments, as well as the uterosacral ligaments. A careful rectal examination is a very important part of the examination, including a rectovaginal examination. A test for occult blood should be part of the rectal examination.

It is often necessary to have one or more attendants lift and position a patient for the gynecologic examination. The patient's breasts and abdo-

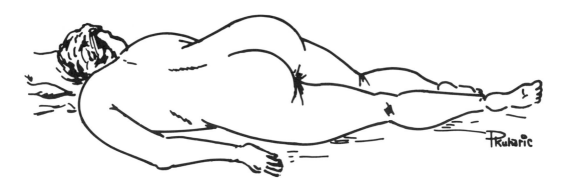

Figure 2-3. Sim's position.

men must be routinely palpated. In the presence of neurologic, neuromuscular, or skeletal disorders, the patient's legs may have to be supported by the attendants. If a severely disabled patient is brought on a stretcher for examination, it may be necessary to perform the examination on the stretcher in the left lateral (Sim's) position (Fig. 2-3). In this instance, a speculum examination may be difficult or even dangerous because of the severe atrophic vulvitis and vaginitis. The physician must decide whether the symptoms warrant speculum examination and whether a routine Papanicolaou smear is necessary in view of the low yield of cytologic abnormalities in an asymptomatic patient over 60 years of age. A rectal examination should be performed routinely in all such patients separately from the pelvic examination.

After the examination is completed, the patient is asked to dress and return to the physician's office for a full discussion of the findings. If she has any pathology, it should be carefully explained to her, with recommendations for treatment. Before the patient leaves, if the findings are normal, she should be urged to return for subsequent examinations at 6-month intervals.

SUMMARY

Taking a history from an aging female patient requires special sensitivity. It is important to create a comfortable environment, whether the assessment is being performed at a community center, at the hospital, in the home, or in the office. Many patients have poor eyesight, and it is important to use increased illumination that does not cause glare. The patient must have privacy, and if she appears to be uncomfortable with family members present, they are asked to leave the room. However, since they may be able to supply valuable information, they should be available if the physician elects to ask them questions.

It is important to begin the history by making general observations about the patient. Is she heavy, thin, or of average weight? Does she appear healthy and energetic, or is she ill, fatigued, and pale? Does the patient seem to be in pain, or is she uncomfortable or ill at ease? It is important to notice her grooming and gait.

The patient must be addressed in respectful terms—as "Mrs." or "Miss," rather than by her first name. However, having done this, the patient is asked her preference regarding the way she wants to be addressed.

It is important to have the patient seated directly in front of the physician so that if there is any difficulty in hearing, she will be able to read the physician's lips. The question should be phrased simply, and the patient should be given plenty of time to respond.

As the history progresses, the physician should notice the patient's facial expression, mood, speech, and orientation. One should remember that it is possible to mistake confusion, disorientation, memory loss, slowed reaction time, or anxiety due to drugs or alcohol for a physiologic or mental dysfunction.

The family history is important. The physician should ask about the patient's father, mother, siblings, children, and grandparents. The patient should identify the diseases they had and state the causes of death in members of her family and the age at which they died.

It is good medical care to obtain some basic statistics about the patient. She should be asked about her height, weight, date of birth, and education. It is important to inquire tactfully about her economic resources and financial management. During this time, an effort should be made to find out how she lives, whether she is alone or with her family, whether she has resided at her present residence for a short or long period of time, and the type of neighborhood or housing that she lives in. In determining her usual day's activity, it is possible to evaluate her ability to manage by herself or to determine whether she needs help. Certain areas of the patient's personal history deserve special attention. It is important to find out if there are any psychological problems, problems with alcohol, drug abuse, or sexual concerns.

The medication history is important, especially in the elderly. The physician should find out about each drug that she is taking, how she takes it, and in what dosage. Since the older patient metabolizes medication differently from the younger one, due to slowed metabolism and decreased liver or kidney function, she may be more vulnerable to drug reactions. Also, since the patient may be taking a number of drugs, she has a greater chance of developing adverse interactions. It is important to ask which over-the-counter drugs she is taking because she may not consider them to be drugs that would have any affect on her health.

It is important to discuss the patient's eating habits in some detail. The physician must decide whether the diet is well balanced, if the patient drinks enough water, and if there is any problem with chewing. It is important to ask about the bowel habits and whether the patient needs laxatives, suppositories, or enemas.

Urinary patterns must be explored with the aging patient. The physician must ask whether, when she urinates, she feels as though her bladder is completely empty or not. Does she have any burning, pain, or bleeding when urinating? Does she have urinary frequency? Does she get up at night to urinate? Has she ever had or does she have urinary tract infections?

It is important to go into the past medical history and to review the body systems carefully with the patient.

The physician must tactfully explore the aging patient's sexual needs must be discussed. These needs cover a wide range, from touching and closeness to actual intercourse. This should be explored in an objective manner, conveying to the patient the feeling of wanting to help her with any problems she may have. It has been shown that the aging woman may have intercourse until late in life. She should be encouraged to continue her sexual activities.

The physical examination of the aging woman must start at the top of her head and go literally to the soles of her feet. The gynecologist should pay special attention to the breasts, and the examination should be carried out in a systematic and unhurried manner. The pelvic examination must be carried out very carefully, and since the urinary system and the genital tract are so closely associated in many of their functions and pathology, they should be evaluated as a single unit. It is important to include in the pelvic examination a careful rectovaginal and rectal examination. The finger used to examine the rectum can be tested on one of the commercial preparations to determine if there is any blood present. If there is a positive blood reaction, the patient should be carefully evaluated. If hemorrhoids are evident, this is probably the cause, but further investigation is mandatory.

During the examination, the patient should be given an explanation of each step. This puts her at ease, makes her more cooperative, and permits the physician to do a much more thorough pelvic examination.

REFERENCES

Anderson, F. 1981. *Practical Management of the Elderly,* 3rd ed., Blackwell Scientific Publications. London.

Barber, H. R. K. 1986. Geriatric gynecology, in: *Clinical Geriatrics,* 3rd ed. (I Rossman, ed.), J. B. Lippincott Co., Philadelphia.

Becker, P., and H. Cohen. 1984. Functional approach to the care of the elderly. *J. Am. Geriatric Soc.* 32(12):923.

Eastwood, H. D. H. 1979. Urodynamic studies in the management of urinary incontinence in the elderly. *Age Ageing* 8:41.

Hoffman, J. W. 1982. Gynecologic disorders in the geriatric patient. Geriatric gynecology. *Postgrad. Med.* 71:38.

———. 1983. The diagnosis and treatment of gynecologic disorders in elderly patients. *Compr. Ther.* 9:54.

Iosif, C. S., and Z. Bekassy. 1984. Prevalence of genitourinary symptoms in late menopause. *Acta Obstet. Gynecol. Scand.* 63:257.

Kennie, D. C. 1984. Good health care for the aged. *JAMA* 249:770.

Masters, W. H., and V. E. Johnson. 1966. *Human Sexual Response,* Little Brown & Co., Boston.

McKeithen, W. S. 1975. Major gynecologic surgery in the elderly female. *Am. J. Obstet. Gynecol.* 59:63.

Mohr, D. M. 1983. Estimation of surgical risk in the elderly: A correlative review. *J. Am. Geriatric Soc.* 31:99.

Renshaw, D. 1985. Sex, age and values. *J. Am. Geriatric Soc.* 33(9):635.

Somers, A. 1985. Toward a female gerontocracy? in: Haug, M., Ford, A. and Shaefer, M. eds. *Current Social Trends in the Physical and Mental Health of Aged Women* (M. Haug, A. Ford, and M. Schaefer, eds.), Springer Publishing Co., New York, p. 16.

Steel, K. 1980. A clinical approach to communication with the elderly patient, in: *Language and Communication in the Elderly: Clinical, Therapeutic and Experimental Aspects* (L. Obler and M. Albert, eds.), D.C. Heath, Lexington, Mass., p. 133.

Stenkvist, B., R. Bergstrom, A. Eklund, et al. 1984. Papanicolaou smear screening and cervical cancer—what can you expect? *JAMA* 252:1423.

Stieglitz, E. J. 1954. Foundations of geriatric medicine, in: *Geriatric Medicine,* 3rd ed. (E. J. Stieglitz, ed.), J. B. Lippincott Co., Philadelphia, pp. 3–26.

U.S. Department of Health and Human Services Administration, Administration on Aging. 1980. *Facts About Older Americans, 1979,* Washington, D.C.

Wingate, M. B. 1982. Geriatric gynecology. *Primary Care* 9:53.

Winkler, M., and R. Stone. 1985. The feminization of poverty and older women. *Gerontologist* 25(4):351.

3

Theories of Aging

INTRODUCTION

Etiology of Aging

From time immemorial, humans have searched for an elixir or a method that would not only restore youth but make it perpetual. A search for the fountain of youth played a role in the early history of the United States. Juan Ponce de Leon was a Spanish explorer and discoverer who searched for it. The Indians talked about an island called Bimini, and there was a report about a fountain whose waters would guarantee youth. In 1513 de Leon set out to find Bimini, where he hoped to discover the miraculous spring. He sighted land on Easter Sunday, March 27, and named it Florida after the Spanish name Pascua Florida, meaning "flowery Easter." The spot at which he landed was just north of modern St. Augustine. Unfortunately, he did not find the fountain of youth.

Long before Ponce de Leon's search, ancient civilizations had initiated the eternal struggle to forestall death by prolonging youth. In the Greek pantheon, Aurora, the goddess of dawn, pleaded with Zeus for immortality for her husband but did not mention that she wanted him to remain eternally young. He grew old and decrepit and longed for death. The sorceress Medea claimed that she had a magic potion that would restore

31

eternal youth. She gave this to King Aeson, who promptly leaped from his sick bed, bursting with energy and vitality. The Old Testament related that restoring body heat is one way to prevent aging. It suggested placing young virgins in the bed of old men who wished to be revitalized, and King David was the recipient of this treatment. Greek physicians recommended good food and wine, massage, and exercise in order to restore body heat and youth. In the Middle Ages an ancient custom was revived whereby milk from the breast of young girls was taken by elderly men. Medieval scholars sought the imaginary philosopher's stone, thought to have the power of prolonging life, and alchemists worked in their laboratories trying to find the secret of long life. Transfusions from young, vigorous men into older men were tried, usually with fatal results. In the late 1800s, aging males had the testicles of monkeys grafted onto them for rejuvenation.

Still pursuing youth at a ripe 72 years of age, Dr. Charles Edouard Brown-Séquard performed numerous self-experiments while he was teaching at Harvard University in 1889. At one point, he gave himself 10 subcutaneous injections of a liquid containing a small quantity of water mixed with the three following ingredients: blood of the testicular vein, semen, and juice extracted from a testicle crushed immediately after it had been taken from a dog or a guinea pig. He described the change in strength in his limbs, his intellectual powers, and his increased vitality. Other researchers did not confirm his findings. However, later researchers noted that Brown-Séquard's trials were responsible for drawing attention to the juice internally secreted by ducts and other glands and reabsorbed into the circulation.

Contributions of the National Institute on Aging

On May 31, 1974, the Research on Aging Act was signed into law. This legislation authorized the establishment of the National Institute on Aging (NIA) for the conduct and support of biomedical, social, and behavioral research and training related to the aging process and the diseases and other special problems and needs of the aged. It was probably this act that launched a scientific approach to the problem of aging. Research scientists began by studying the basic unit of life, that is, the cell. The human body is made up of billions of cells. These cells live for varying amounts of time. Red blood cells, for example, live for about 120 days, while nerve cells can live for up to 100 years. Every minute about 3 billion body cells die; however, at the same time, about the same number of new cells are created through cell division. Molecular chemical research on intracellular changes caused by aging has led to several theories, including genetic, programmed aging, mutation theory, autoimmune, cross-linkage, and other theories. These cellular theories recognize a series of events within the cell that prevent an orderly process of growth and metabolism. No single theory of human aging is totally able to explain all of these biologic phenomena.

GENETICS AND HEREDITY FACTORS OF AGING

It is interesting to look at the maximum recorded life span of various species. These include the following: humans, 111 years; horse, 46; goat, 20;

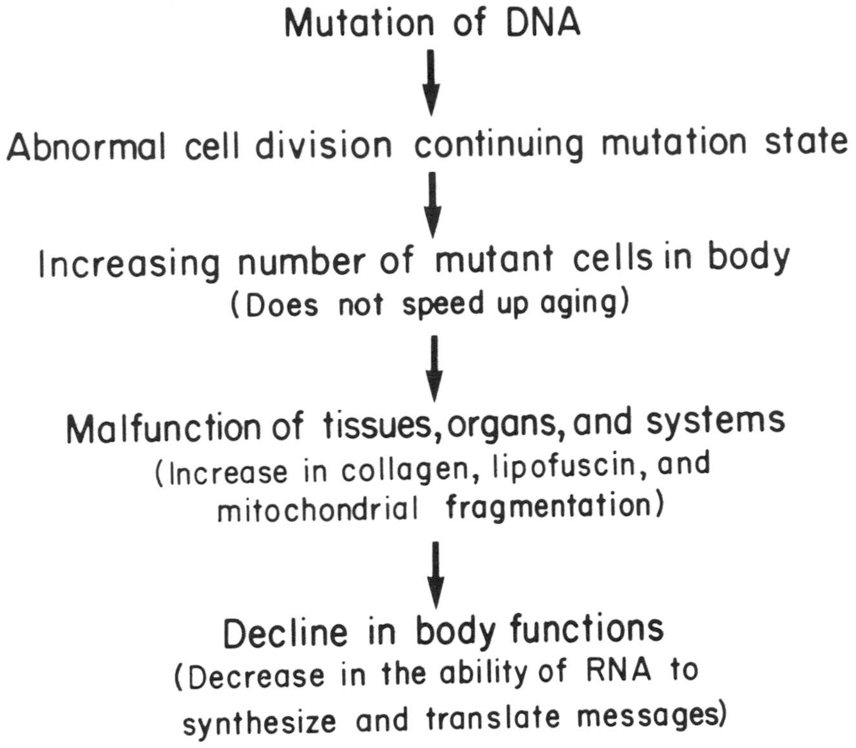

Mutation of DNA

↓

Abnormal cell division continuing mutation state

↓

Increasing number of mutant cells in body
(Does not speed up aging)

↓

Malfunction of tissues, organs, and systems
(Increase in collagen, lipofuscin, and mitochondrial fragmentation)

↓

Decline in body functions
(Decrease in the ability of RNA to synthesize and translate messages)

Figure 3-1. Genetic Factors. (Courtesy of Patricia Kuharic, Lenox Hill Hospital, Department of Medical Photography.)

guinea pig, 7.6; rat, 4.7; and mouse, 3.5. A mouse, no matter how healthy, cannot live for more than 3.5 years. This is because the genes that determine that a mouse squeaks, rather than talks, and uses four legs rather than two, also determine that the mouse lives for a maximum of 3.5 years rather than 20. Human genes determine that humans use language, walk on two legs, and live for a maximum of 111 years. It thus appears that genes that determine the nature of the species also determine its life span.

It is apparent that the genetics of aging involves the inheritance of longevity and inherited differences in patterns of aging. Some of the difference in the inherited life span of individuals might be explained by inheritance of age, as well as of associated diseases such as diabetes, arteriosclerosis, and atherosclerosis. However, the major need in this area is to understand the number and nature of the genes controlling aging and how they work. Progress is being made (Fig. 3-1).

From studies of identical twins, it is estimated that 60 to 80 percent of an individual's longevity is inherited. The incidence of age-related disorders differs among races; for example, hypertension is common among blacks. These disorders affect longevity and possibly aging. While there is little doubt that single-gene mutation can produce syndromes of many other features of aging, such as adult progeria, it is not clear how many genes determine normal longevity and how their actions are manifested. Another aspect of the genetics of aging is the effect of maternal and paternal age on diseases of the offspring. The best-known example is Down's syndrome, which occurs frequently among the offspring of older women. Several genetic diseases related to mutations associated with paternal aging have also been recognized.

Genetic determination provides everyone with a predetermined longevity and perhaps quality of life. Genetic expression is a result of preformed biologic conditioning. The genetic theory has remained viable for a long period of time because of the results of epidemiologic studies, life insurance actuarial research, intraspecies records, and longevity data on identical vs nonidentical twins. Statistical studies indicate that the primary basis for the longevity of an individual, strain, or species appears to be the genetic material incorporated in the fertilized egg at the climactic moment when the spermatozoon meets the unfertilized egg. Research to date has been limited. Some effort has been made in theoretic studies to delineate the effects of inheritance on the rate of aging, and in actuarial studies on the influence of parental longevity on the life span of offspring. It is interesting to note that maternal longevity has been found to be a significant correlate in the life span of human offspring. The variety of aging patterns in inbred strains of mice has been studied in detail. It is difficult to assess what variations and patterns of human aging are caused by diet, social and economic factors, and health care. The study of isolated, long-lived populations will probably not yield important information on the genetics of aging since populations, although geographically separated, are probably not genetic isolates.

Few Americans celebrate their 100th birthday, but many persons in other societies live well beyond that age. One group lives in a small village in Ecuador called Vilcabamba. Two others are in Asia; the Hunzukuts occupy the Karakoram range in Kashmir and the Abkhazians live in the autonomous Republic of Georgia in the southern Soviet Union. Unfortunately, their longevity remains a mystery. Many investigators believe that diet and genetics play a key role in prolonging life, but no concrete data are available to substantiate this conclusion. All three cultural groups share some characteristics, and perhaps these traits are significant. These centenarians all live in mountainous regions that are relatively isolated. Their cultures are primarily agrarian; physical activity is high in all three groups. Besides farming, the Abkhazians especially enjoy swimming and horseback riding. A strong sense of family exists in all three groups and the elderly are respected and honored, often governing their communities. In general, those who are married live longer than those who remain single, and surprisingly, women who bear many children seem to outlive those that do not.

Genetics gets a strong boost as an important aspect of longevity. In each of these groups, it has been shown that most of the old people are born of parents who lived to 100 years of age or more.

Research on the genetics of aging should focus on identifying the specific genes controlling aging, elucidating their effects, and correcting any biologic deficiencies that shorten the life span. Obviously, if it were possible to have colonies of suitable genetically controlled experimental animal models, this effect could be explored more readily. It is conceivable that the isolation of genes from people who live to be 100 could be genetically engineered to produce substances that might act as the elixir of youth.

Hereditary factors are both genetic and nongenetic, that is, some are transmitted by genes, while others occur within the chromosome. This, of course, complicates the role of genes in the aging process. The memory of how to survive rests within two complex molecules, deoxyribonucleic acid (DNA) and ribonucleic acid (RNA). DNA has greater stability and is more dominant. The DNA contained within a cell is really a vast library of instructions; its resources and information are called upon when a given cell requires certain material to be made. Although there are billions of different cells within a living body, they all contain identical DNA libraries. It is becoming apparent that cells contain controller genes that block or release resources stored within the DNA. It would be interesting to know how the controller gene functions in aging. The importance of errors inherent in DNA duplication and in other types of somatic mutations needs to be evaluated. Does mutation in a somatic cell depend on numbers of generations or on time (age)? When somatic mutations occur, are they randomized or do they grow out as clones? Can prevention or repair of nuclear damage be facilitated by chemicals or other agents? The question arises of how each step in DNA synthesis through transcription and translation can be improved. Furthermore, it must be asked whether there is any advantage in inhibiting stem cell proliferation in the immune system early in order to conserve accurate stem cells when one is older and needs them. It is obvious that this is a very complex problem. Most of the research must focus on how the flow of genetic information varies as a function of help in species of varying life spans. This may be vital in the understanding of biologic aging.

PROGRAMMING

The theories of genetic aging and cellular programming are inseparable, clearly illustrating that many theories of aging overlap. The programming of aging is the concept that within the cell itself the biochemical factors that occur genetically have been chemically programmed. This provides one mechanism for the genetics of aging. It is evident that changes occurring in the cytosol and the nucleus eventually lead to disintegration of the cell. Although not well understood, this process appears to operate on a pretimed basis. This theory has two advantages: it is more applicable than other theories, and it may provide a way to reverse the degenerative processes that accompany aging.

ERROR THEORY

The mutation, repair, and expression of genetic material, which have commonly been referred to collectively as the *error theory,* are receiving a great deal of attention. It is felt that aging may be the result of altered gene structure or gene action. Injury to DNA in somatic cells may be spontaneous or introduced by outside agents such as chemical and ionizing radiation. Long-lived animals appear to have a more efficient enzyme system for repairing the DNA that has been disrupted. Thus far, researchers focusing on genetic determinants have been unable to identify any gene responsible for extending the life span, but they have pinpointed defective genes that result in the shortening of life. It may be necessary to approach the problem from this point of view. In support of this conclusion, it has been shown that the maintenance of a correct phenotype in aging cells also depends on the ability of these cells to renew the proteins of their chromatin in order to copy the DNA accurately to RNA transcripts and to translate these transcripts with high predictability. This is bound up with their ability to control protein synthesis. Chromosomal aberrations have been found under some circumstances during aging and in persons with senile dementia. Thus chromosomal breakage and repair processes may be important in understanding aging.

SOMATIC MUTATIONS

Somatic mutations refers to environmental insults that affect the cells. These may range from radiation to drugs and stress. The theory is compatible with other approaches to aging. It is accepted that the organism is affected by many factors that influence cell activity. It is interesting that this theory may apply particularly to women. Ovarian tissue may undergo alterations that could result in mutations transmitted through reproductive activity. Unlike the male, the female gamete is present from birth, arrested in the first meiotic division. It is evident that agents in the external environment could bring about damage. There is convincing evidence that altered proteins, such as enzymes and connective tissue molecules, exist in aging organisms. Much of the current work has been inspired by error theories that have not been proved or denied conclusively. Age-dependent changes and the adaptive regulation of enzyme activity have been documented in a variety of tissues from several different species. It is not yet known conclusively whether these regulatory deficiencies are intrinsic to the tissues in which measurements were performed or instead reflect changes in neurologic control mechanisms, hormonal control mechanisms, or both. Although not germane to this particular part of the discussion, the concept of *free radicals* may play an important role at this point. Free radicals are found only in living substances but are not essential to biologic systems. As a product of normal metabolism, they are produced by such processes as autooxidation of lipids and by exposure to ionizing radiation and such chemical toxins as ozone and hydrogen peroxide. Free radicals are highly reactive because they contain an unpaired electron. They have the highest concentration in the mitochondria. Some free radicals effects, supposedly deleterious, are DNA mutations and the cross-linking of collagen, the body's most abundant protein. Other suspected deleterious effects concern the development of aging pigments, especially in myocardial neuron cells. Assuming that there is validity to the free radical theory of aging, it has been proposed that human or animal life spans might be increased by the intake of antioxidants that tie up free radicals and inactivate them. Vitamin E is one of the antioxidants. If the free radical theory of aging has merit and if vitamin E is an effective biologic antioxidant, then vitamin E's presence in adequate quantities is an important antiaging vitamin. This theory has to be pursued in more detail.

The somatic mutation theory of aging has advanced the notion that there is a progressive accumulation of mutations or other more general damage in the DNA that leads to the incapacitation of individual cells. This could explain why nondividing or postmitotic cells such as those of the brain and muscle may demonstrate a more rapid rate of deterioration; the regenerative potential is low in these tissues, and damaged cells cannot easily be replaced. There is lack of support for the somatic mutation theory. Mice subjected to radiation at levels sufficient to produce significant mutations have a shorter than average life span, but they do not appear to experience an acceleration in the true aging process. The same holds true for the survivors of the atomic bomb blast. On careful analysis of the data, it appears that there is an increasing number of mutations. These mutations may account for the rising number of pathologic foci that appear over time in vivo, but they cannot be the universal mechanism of aging.

Interesting work supported by the federal government is in progress. The fibroblasts from young and old donor groups have been compared. Fibroblastic cells are obtained by taking a skin biopsy (2 mm, or 1/10th of an inch, in diameter) from each subject's upper arm, in an area that receives little sunlight or other radiation exposure. These biopsy specimens are then placed in tissue culture. After 7 weeks, approximately 1 billion fibroblasts are obtained. Measurements of the cell cultures from young and old donors are compared with regard to (1) total proliferative ability, (2) population proliferation rate, (3) percentage of proliferating cells, and (4) proliferative behavior of individual cells.

The findings have shed some light on the process of aging. The total proliferative ability was considerably reduced in the cell cultures derived from the old donor group. The cell population doubling time was significantly longer in cultures from the old donor group. The percentage of proliferating cells was significantly lower than the cell cultures derived from old donors than in those from the young donors. In the experiments with individual cells, 60 percent of the young donor cells were able to proliferate eight or more times during a 2-week period, while only 2 percent of the old donor cells were able to do so.

Thus, the behavior of cells in culture was generally related to the chronologic age of the donor. It is likely that in a cross-sectional study such as this one, a relatively vigorous old population was selected, as less healthy subjects had died before age 65. Therefore, the results may underestimate the in vitro alterations that accompany in vivo aging.

AUTOIMMUNITY

The immunologic theory of aging has at least two different components. The first is related to the alteration in the immune defenses; the second focuses on the increase in the autoimmune autoaggressive processes.

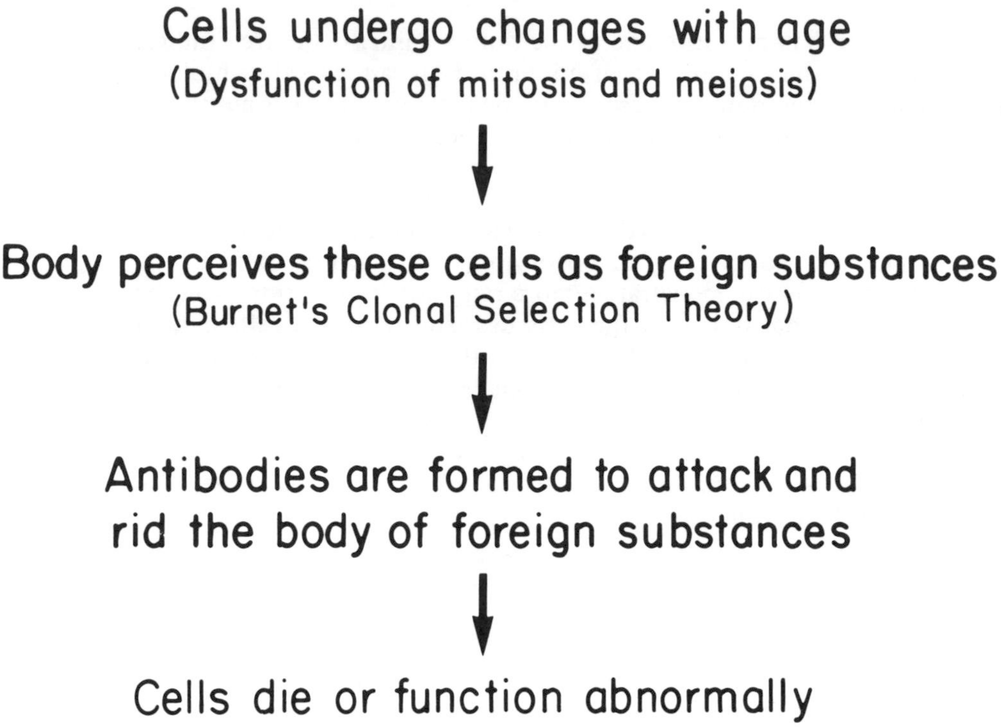

Cells undergo changes with age
(Dysfunction of mitosis and meiosis)

Body perceives these cells as foreign substances
(Burnet's Clonal Selection Theory)

Antibodies are formed to attack and rid the body of foreign substances

Cells die or function abnormally

Figure 3-2. Autoimmune theory. (Courtesy of Patricia Kuharic, Lenox Hill Hospital, Department of Medical Photography.)

It is evident that both affect longevity. It has been reported that autoimmune protection is reduced through loss with aging. The immune factors circulating throughout the body can then overwhelm the individual cells, causing cellular destruction. With aging there is a marked decline in both the availability and the activity of all of the immune systems. Thus there is a decrease in protection against infection, immune complex diseases, and carcinogenesis, which might contribute to an acceleration of the intracellular aging processes. The autoimmune reactions have been postulated to be responsible for aging because the host attacks its own kind. A reason advanced for this may be that the body perceives old, irregular cells as agents to attack (Fig. 3-2).

MAINTENANCE AND INTEGRITY OF CELLULAR ORGANELLES

Cell Membrane

The decreasing physiologic and biochemical function of the aging organism may result from the declining ability of cells to carry on normal functions or to respond to stress. It is known that cell membranes play a significant role in the overall vitality of the cell. Recent studies have focused on possible changes in the structure and function of membranes that might contribute to the overall deterioration of an aging organism. It is known that alterations in the electrical activity of the heart develop with increasing age; these changes affect the heart's responsiveness and sensitivity to drugs used to treat cardiac disorders.

Mitochondria

Many species have shown age-dependent changes in the structure of the mitochondria. There has been a decline in oxidation capacity, changes in enzyme composition, and accumulation of abnormal and degenerative forms. This subject—the mechanism by which the mitochondrial components are synthesized and organized into a functional structure—is an important area for further research. The effect of abnormalities on the physiology of the cell needs further study. Closely related to these questions is the topology of the different enzymes and the mitochondrial membrane; the role of the membrane in producing the energized state that, in turn, controls the rate of respiration in a cell; and the regulatory factors involved in mitochondrial functions.

Lysosomes

Lysosomes are structures found in all living cells and are characterized by the presence of distinct enzymes separated from external substrates by a membrane-like lipoprotein barrier. Lysosomes have a complete digestive system capable of breaking down all major cell constituents, including proteins, nucleic acid, carbohydrates, and lipids. The lysosomes are capable of generalized breakdown of material required for continuing renewal. Therefore, damage to the lysosome could jeopardize cell survival. The biochemical characterization and morphologic identification of lysosomes have opened up many new prospects for the study of cell pathology, particularly in relation to aging.

Intracellular accumulation materials called *lipofuscin pigment (age pigment)* is a predominant characteristic of nondividing cells, such as nerve cells, and all organisms. This age pigment is linked to lysosomes. Cells that cannot discharge the contents of their lysosomes into the outside medium by exocytosis must retain nonpermanent, undegradable materials inside their lysosomes indefinitely. The material most commonly found accumulating in lysosomes is lipofuscin. It is not known whether the accumulation of lipofuscin with age results in any significant change in cellular function. It has been shown that with age lysosomes become increasingly loaded with indigestible materials and that they definitely do age. In order to evaluate fully the role of lysosome overloading and cellular aging, the quantitative relationship between the proportion of total cytoplasmic volume occupied by lysosomes and the severity of the resulting cellular deficiencies must be determined. Important areas requiring study include characterization of the lipofuscin pigments, as well as analysis of their role in lysosome accumulation. Of primary importance is the effect of lysosome accumulation on functional impairment. Lipofuscin tends to accumulate in the liver, heart, ovaries, and neurons.

Ribosomes

The ribosomes and nucleoli have been studied in the aging process. Practically every aspect of the translational apparatus has been shown to be defective in the aging organism. General protein synthesis is impaired, and some proteins appear to be aberrant. In laboratory cultures, loss of the potential for cell division during aging is accompanied by decreased ribosome synthesis and function. Faulty protein synthesis has been studied in bacteria and is now being extensively studied in the cells of aging animals.

Nucleus

In the nucleus, age-associated alterations in chromatin composition had been noted in tissues of various ages. Accompanying these alterations is a decrease in transcriptional activity, which may result from changes in the number and types of genes being expressed.

Nuclear Cytoplasmic Interactions

Interactions between the cytoplasm and nuclei have been studied primarily through different methods of nuclear transplantation. In protozoa, this has been done surgically; in mammalian cells in culture, it has been done through cell hybridization.

CELL HYBRIDIZATION

This is an excellent means of investigating the age-related pathology of cellular organelles. Two types of hybrid have been derived from mammalian cells: heterokaryons, in which there are two or more nuclei in a common pool of cytoplasm; and synkaryons, in which there has been nuclear as well as cytoplasmic fusion. Eventually there is the possibility of developing cybrids—cells having cytoplasm from one parent and a nucleus from another. Evidence is now available from work with human cells that suggests that the cytoplasm may not play the primary role in the control of senescence: when young and old cells are fused, the senescent state dominates. Isolated nuclei of human cells can be fused to nucleated cells (cytoplasts), thus creating a cell that is capable of division. Viable cells are obtained when young nuclei are fused to either young or old cytoplasts. Thus, cell assembly techniques already possible with protozoa may be applied to mammalian cells in vitro and the import of aging cells examined. Mammalian embryonic cells and ova undoubtedly will be used to examine differences between short- and long-lived animals. Cells freshly derived from aging animals should be used in addition to cells that have aged in culture.

CELLULAR PROLIFERATION

Defects in the regulation of aging cells lead to alteration and decline in the ability of cells to proliferate. Whether these defects are genetically or nongenetically based is not well understood. Most likely both elements are operative. The work of Hayflick is applicable at this time. Hayflick demonstrated that normal human fibroblast cells have a limited capacity to multiply in tissue culture. These diploid cells maintain the genetically stable karyotype of 46 intact chromosomes, and perhaps for this reason appear to follow a well-defined intrinsic program of senescence. Following an initial period of vigorous proliferation, fibroblasts from therapeutically aborted fetuses display a gradual loss of mitotic potential, with ultimate death at about the 50th division. Cells from mature adults and elderly subjects achieve only 20 divisions prior to their demise. The validity of Hayflick's model of cellular aging has been substantiated by many other investigators. It has been shown that the faster the cells are driven to divide, the sooner these cells become senescent and develop pathology. It seems clear, therefore, that minimizing cellular turnover, particularly in vulnerable tissues such as the vascular tree and the epithelial surfaces, may delay the appearance of age-related diseases such as arteriosclerosis and cancer. Hayflick has pointed out that the maximum mitotic capability of diploid cells may be closely related to the longevity of species. For example, the mouse has a life span of approximately 3 years and produces culture cells that double only 12 times, in contrast to the cells of the chicken, which undergo about 25 divisions in the course of a 30-year lifetime. In humans it has been shown that the older the individual, the fewer the number of cell divisions achieved by a cell prior to in vitro senescence. It has also been shown that culture cells propagated from individuals with inherited disorders show premature senescence. This indicates that the physiologic rather than the chronologic age is the prime determinant of the cellular life span in vitro. It has been shown that older people who are vigorous will produce cultures that perform disproportionately well, while many patients with the early onset of a malignant or degenerative process will not survive long enough to be studied. It is evident that there are genetic as well as environmental factors at work.

HAYFLICK PHENOMENON

The Hayflick phenomenon has provided solid data that give some insight into the cellular changes that come with aging. Hayflick demonstrated that normal human fibroblast cells have a limited capacity to multiply in tissue cultures.

Organisms and cells age at different rates and have distinct species-specific life spans. This implies that cells from long-lived species should proceed through more population doublings than those from short-lived species if such phenomena reflect actual aging in vivo. Studies indicate that this is the case. Embryonic cells from the long-lived Galapagos tortoise (life span, 175 years) displayed 90 to 125 population doublings, while human (110 years) cells underwent 40 to 60 doublings, chicken cells (25 years) showed 15 to 35 doublings, and mouse cells (3.5 years) demonstrated 19 to 28 doublings. It is interesting to note that fibroblasts from a 9-year-old donor with a rare genetic disease, progeria, doubled only twice. The older the individual, the fewer cell divisions his culture cells achieve prior to in vitro senescence.

EXPERIMENTAL MODEL SYSTEMS

Experimental model systems have used mammals, metazoa, protozoa, *Tokophyra,* and amoeba.

The large majority of aging studies have been performed on animals such as rats, mice, and to a lesser extent, dogs, pigs, and nonhuman primates. Rodents are usually used because they have short life spans, can be genetically controlled, and are inexpensive to provide. Pedigreed dogs and thoroughbred horses have well-documented birth records and genetic backgrounds and may provide an invaluable source of information.

The use of metazoa in aging research has been limited almost entirely to insects, rotifers, and nematodes. Of these, nematodes are generally regarded as the most practical to use because they are morphologically similar throughout their life span, can be grown readily under pure and standard conditions, are reproduced in sufficient quantity for most biochemical measurements, and are amenable to genetic analysis. If it is assumed that the mechanism of aging is the same among various animal species, the advantage of studying aging in shorter-lived, lower forms of animals is obvious.

Aging studies on protozoa have focused principally on age-related changes during clonal senescence. The reason for using protozoa is that something as fundamental as aging is characteristic of all animals.

Tokophyra has been used for studies of the changes in unicellular digestive systems during aging and the accumulation of secondary lysosomes and residual bodies in old organisms. The amoeba lacks some of the advantages of the ciliates but has others. In addition to showing clonal senescence, the amoeba is large and has been used in studies of nuclear –cytoplasmic interactions. These studies involve surgical transfer of nuclei from one cell to another cell of a different age. Such studies are of fundamental importance, and the amoeba is one of the best models for this approach.

ESTROGEN AND AGING

Aging due to reduced responsiveness to estrogen has been studied fairly extensively. The studies were originally undertaken in an effort to understand the observation that the female reproductive system becomes less sensitive to estrogen as it ages.

The estrogen released by the ovaries of a female mammal controls the function of the hypothalamus or pituitary, depending on the species being studied. Ongoing release of estrogen during the maturation of follicles in the ovaries eventually leads to a burst of LH from the pituitary. The LH causes ovulation and starts the maturation of a new set of follicles, allowing the cycle to repeat. However, aged mammals are unresponsive to estrogen. If the ovaries are removed from an old mouse and replaced with a set from a young mouse, the normal ovulation cycle continues. However, if young ovaries are transplanted into an aged mouse that has not been ovulating for some time, cycling is not reinitiated.

It has been stated that loss of responsiveness to estrogen in old rodents is associated with the ovaries themselves. If the ovaries are removed from a young rodent that is then allowed to age, implantation of a young set of ovaries into the aged experimental animal results in the reestablishment of the ovulatory cycle.

Studies have shown that removal of a rat's ovaries slows hypothalamic aging by a number of criteria. Morphologically, the hypothalamus of the animal that has had its ovaries removed appears to be less active. Glial cells remove damaged neurons, and they normally become abundant in the hypothalamus just when the ability to ovulate is lost. It is interesting to note that oophorectomy also blocks the formation of nonmalignant, prolactin-secreting pituitary tumors that appear in 10 to 20 percent of test mammals. It may be that estrogen causes damage and changes in the hypothalamus and the pituitary. At present, it can be stated that, under some conditions, estrogens interact with brain and pituitary aging and that, in some individuals, estrogen may be a cause of disease. This has not been confirmed in human research.

There are many unknown factors in the environment that influence the life span. One environmental factor that has been studied in some depth is metals—elements such as iron, copper, zinc, manganese, molybdenun, cobalt, and metals that, in minute quantities, are essential for an organism's growth and development. Other metals, such as calcium, sodium, magnesium, and potassium, are essential in larger amounts. Several diseases can result if there is too much or too little of these metals. A well-known example is anemia caused by iron deficiency. At birth, a healthy infant has all of the necessary metals in the needed quantities. In addition, metals from the environment pass into cells. The environment thus helps to supply the organism with the essential quantities of metals.

Research has showed that there is an increase in the concentration of certain metal irons in cells aged in tissue culture. But the effect of this increased concentration of metals is still unknown. It has been found that if the activating metal iron in RNA synthesis is magnesium or cobalt, there is only ribonucleotide incorporation and essentially no deoxynucleotide incorporation. But if the activating metal iron is manganese, there is substantial deoxynucleotide incorporation; this could produce an RNA with molecular abnormalities, leading to deterioration of the cells. It appears that abnormal RNA may result if there is an excess of manganese in the environment. Another study has shown that as the concentration of magnesium iron is raised, there is an error in transmitting genetic information. That is, RNA does not function properly, resulting in abnormalities in making a protein. Such abnormalities may cause diseases such as sickle cell anemia.

SUMMARY

Environmental effects of aging may be responsible for the variations in the life span of organisms with similar genetic potential, that is, organisms from the same species. The study of the environment—a secondary cause of aging—is therefore of great importance, since the possibility of controlling it is greater than that of controlling the primary cause, the genes.

Life begins with a cell. In animals, cells begin to divide after the fertilization of the egg cell by a sperm cell; the body of a mature man and woman contains billions of cells. At or near the cell's center is the nucleus, filled with a substance named for the nucleus known as *nucleic acid;* the cytoplasm is the fluid surrounding the nucleus. Within the nucleus are chromosomes, known as *chromatin* in an early state; the chromosomes are tiny, thread-like bodies that contain the genes. The genes, in turn, are sections of nucleic acid known as *deoxyribonucleic acid (DNA);* DNA controls the organism's development process by (1) making copies of itself each time a cell divides and (2) carrying the information necessary to make proteins, the substances that form the body's structural materials. DNA is the basic material of life.

Environmental effects of aging may be responsible for variations in the life span of organisms with similar genetic potential, that is, organisms from the same species. The study of the environment—a secondary cause of aging—is therefore of great importance, since the possibility of controlling it is greater than that of controlling the primary cause, the genes.

It is difficult to determine which human cells should be selected for the study of cell senescence. Numerous studies clearly show that senescence involves a wide variety of cells and tissues, rather than the failure of one cell or tissue type. There are two basic types of cells: proliferating (replaceable) and nonproliferating (irreplaceable) cells; most body cells belong to the latter class. Both types of cells are equally important to the aging process. However, proliferating cells are easier to obtain and simpler to use experimentally; in addition, the key cell function of proliferation itself can be examined. This cell function plays a crucial role in the survival of the organism, as well as in age-related disabilities and diseases.

Among proliferating cells, fibroblasts found in connective tissue because of their sustained growth and short life span in vitro are especially suitable for growth in tissue culture. They can proliferate rapidly in vitro for a number of divisions, usually about 40. The fibroblasts then enter a period of declining cell proliferation and finally, after a certain number of divisions (usually 50), stop proliferating. In aging studies, early-passage cells (cells in the rapid growth phase) have been used as young cells and senescent-phase cells as old cells.

Fibroblast cells were obtained by taking a skin biopsy specimen (2 mm, or 1/10th of an inch in diameter) from each subject's upper arm, an area that receives little sunlight or other radiation exposure. These specimens were then placed in tissue culture. After 7 weeks, approximately 1 billion fibroblast cells were obtained.

The researchers wanted to determine if the in vitro aging of cells is influenced by the age of the donor. Measurements of these cell cultures from the young and old donors were compared with regard to (1) total proliferative activity, (2) cell population proliferation rate, (3) percentage of proliferating cells, and (4) proliferative behavior of individual cells.

This careful study revealed some interesting results: (1) the total proliferative ability was considerably reduced in the cell cultures derived from the old donor group; (2) cell population doubling time was significantly longer in the cultures from the old donor group than in those from the young donor group; (3) the percentage of proliferating cells was significantly lower in the cell cultures derived from old donors than in those from young donors; (4) in the experiments with individual cells, 60 percent of the young donor cells were able to proliferate eight or more times during a 2-week period, while only 2 percent of the old donor cells were able to do so.

Aging still remains an enigma. Scientists continue to learn more about the process, but generally the information is simply descriptive, at times disputed, and invariably difficult to fit into a coherent interpretable pattern. However, there are some bright spots. There has been an enormous advance in biology in the past three decades, which offers a method for probing the fundamental aspects of aging. For example, current knowledge of the structure of genes and protein synthesis, the complexities and workings of the immunologic system, and the role of the cell membrane in regulating the function of cells is contributing to an understanding of the central questions related to biologic aging: What is it? What controls its rate? What tempers its impact? New work in molecular biology, genetic engineering, and recombinant DNA technology, as well as the use of DNA probes, will undoubtedly supply some answers to the question of the aging process.

REFERENCES

Adelman, R. C. 1971. Age-dependent effect in enzyme induction—a biochemical expression of aging. *Exp. Gerontol.* 6:75.

Adelman, R. C. 1977. Macromolecular metabolism during aging, in: *Handbook of the Biology of Aging* (C. E. Finch, and L. Hayflick, eds.), Van Nostrand Reinhold, New York.

Albertini, R. J., and R. DeMars. 1973. Detection and quantification of x-ray induced mutation in cultured diploid fibroblasts. *Mutat. Res.* 18:199.

Alexander, P., and D. Cornell. 1960. Shortening of the life-span of mice by irradiation with x-ray and treatment with radiomimetic chemicals. *Radiat. Res.* 12:38.

Anderson, W. F., and T. G. Judge (eds.). 1974. *Geriatric Medicine,* Academic Press, New York.

Armstrong, D. 1984. Free radical involvement in the formation of lipopigments, in: *Free Radicals in Molecular Biology. Aging and Disease* (D. Armstrong, R. S. Sobal, R. G. Cutler, and T. F. Slater, eds.), Raven Press, New York.

Bellamy, D. 1967. Hormonal effects in relation to aging in mammals. In Bellamy, D. (ed): *Aspects of the Biology of Aging* (D. Bellamy, ed.), Academic Press, New York, p. 428.

Birren, J. E., R. N. Butler, S. W. Greenhouse, L. Sokoloff, and M. R. Yarrow. 1963. *Human Aging: A Biological and Behavioral Study.* U.S. Government Printing Office, Washington, D.C. U.S. Government (reprinted 1974).

Boutliere, F. 1964. The comparative biology of aging. A physiological approach, in: *Ciba Foundation Colloquia on Aging,* vol. 3 (G. E. W. Welstenholme and M. O'Connor, eds.), Little Brown & Co., Boston.

Brody, H. D. Harman, and M. Ordy. 1975. *Clinical, Morphological and Neurochemical Aspects of Aging,* Raven Press, New York.

Bullough, W. S. 1971. Aging of mammals. *Nature* 229:608.

Burnet, M. 1974. *A Genetic Approach to Aging.* Medical and Technical Publishing, Lancaster, England.

Comfort, A. 1974. *The Process of Aging.* New American Library, New York.

Comfort, A. 1966. The prevention of aging in cells. *Lancet* 2:1325.

Comfort, A. 1979. *The Biology of Senescence.* Elsevier-North Holland, New York.

Cristofalo, V. 1972. Animal cell cultures as a model system for the study of aging, in: *Advances in Gerontological Research,* vol. IV, (B. L. Strehler, ed.), Academic Press, New York.

Cristofalo, V. J., J. Roberts, and R. C. Adelman (eds.). 1975. *Explorations in Aging.* Plenum Publishing Co., New York.

Cutler, R. G. 1975. Evolution of human longevity and the genetic complexity governing aging rate. *Proc. Natl. Acad. Sci. USA* 72:4664.

Finch, C. E. 1971. Comparative biology of senescence. Some evolutionary and developmental considerations, in: *Animal Models for Biomedical Research,* vol. 4, National Academy of Sciences, Washington, D.C.

Finch, C. E., L. S. Felicio, K. Flurkey, et al. 1980. Studies on ovarian-hypothalamic-pituitary interactions during reproductive aging in C57BL/6J mice. *Peptides* (Fayetteville) 1 (suppl.):163.

Goldfisher, S., and J. Bernstein. 1969. Lipofuscin (aging) pigment granules of the newborn human liver. *J. Cell. Biol.* 42:253.

Goldstein, S. 1971. The biology of aging. *N. Engl. J. Med.* 285:1120.

Harley, C. B., and S. Goldstein. 1978. Cultured human fibroblasts; distribution of cell generations and a critical limit. *J. Cell. Physiol.* 97:509.

Hayflick, L. 1965. The limited in vitro lifetime of human diploid cell strains. *Exp. Cell Res.* 37:614.

Hayflick, L. 1977. The cellular basis for biological aging, in: *Handbook of the Biology of Aging* (C. E. Finch and L. Hayflick, eds.), Van Nostrand Reinhold, New York, p. 159.

Hayflick, L. 1980. The cell biology of human aging. *Sci. Am.* 242:58.

Hayflick, L., and P. Moorhead. 1961. The serial cultivation of human diploid cell strains. *Exp. Cell Res.* 25:585.

Holeckova, E., and V. J. Crostofalo. 1970. *Aging in Cell and Tissue Culture.* Plenum Publishing Co., New York.

Kirkwood, T. B. L. 1977. Evolution of aging. *Nature* 270:301.

Kohn, R. R. 1963. Human aging and disease. *J. Chronic Dis.* 16:6.

Landfield, P. W., R. K. Baskin, and T. A. Pitler. 1981. Brain aging correlates; retardation by hormonal-pharmacological treatment. *Science* 214:581.

Makinodan, T. 1977. Immunity and aging, in: *Handbook of the Biology of Aging.* (C. E. Finch and L. Hayflick, eds.), Von Nostrand Reinhold, New York.

Maletta, G. J. (ed.). 1972. *Survey Report on the Aging Nervous System.* U.S. Government Printing Office, Washington, D.C. (reprinted 1977).

Meredith, R., A. L. Taylor, and F. M. Ansi. 1978. High risk of Down's syndrome at advanced maternal age. *Lancet* 1:564.

Orgel, L. E. 1973. Aging of clones of mammalian cells. *Nature* 243:441.

Ostfeld, A. M., and D. C. Gibson (eds.). 1972. *Epidemiology of Aging.* U.S. Government Printing Office, Washington, D.C. (reprinted 1977).

Price, G., S. Modak, and T. Makinodan. 1971. Age-associated changes in the DNA of mouse tissue. *Science* 171:917.

Reichel, W. 1966. The biology of aging. *J. Am. Geriatric Soc.* 14:431.

Reichel, W. 1968. Lipofuscin pigment accumulation and distribution of five rat organs as a function of age. *J. Gerontol.* 23:145.

Reichel, W., J. Hollander, J. H. Clark, and B. L. Strehler. 1968. Lipofuscin pigment accumulation as a function of age and distribution in rodent brain. *J. Gerontol.* 23:71.

Rockstein, M. et al. 1974. *Theoretical Aspects of Aging.* Academic Press, New York.

Schipper, H., J. R. Brawer, J. F. Nelson, et al. 1981. The role of the gonads in the histologic aging of the hypothalamic arcuate nucleus. *Biol. Reprod.* 25:413.

Strehler, B. L. 1971. Aging at the cellular level, in: *Clinical Geriatrics* (I. Rossman, ed.), J. B. Lippincott Co., Philadelphia.

Strehler, B. L. 1977. *Time, Cells and Aging,* 2nd ed. Academic Press, New York.

Szilard, L. 1959. On the nature of the aging process. *Proc. Natl. Acad. Sci. USA* 45:30.

Terry, R. D., and S. Gershon (eds.). 1974. *Neurobiology of Aging.* Raven Press, New York.

Thorbecke, G. J. (ed.). 1975. *Biology of Aging and Development.* FASEB Monographs, vol. 3, Plenum Publishing Co., New York.

Walford, R. L. 1969. *The Immunologic Theory of Aging.* Ejnar Munksgaard, Copenhagen.

Walford, R. L. 1974. The immunologic theory of aging. Current status. *Fed. Proc.* 33:2020.

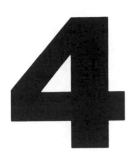

4

Anatomic Changes in the Genitourinary Tract and Breast With Aging

INTRODUCTION

There are certain changes in the genital tract and breast that have been traditionally identified with the aging process. However, women of any age deprived of estrogen can develop similar changes. Therefore, it is concluded that there are probably changes that are directly related to the aging process and that these changes are accentuated by estrogen deprivation.

The one major and almost constant change that is seen in the reproductive system in the menopausal and geriatric patient is atrophy. The tissue shows progressive avascularity, and at the microscopic level, collagenous fibers tend to swell, fuse together, and become hyalinized. Elastic fibers undergo fragmentation. There is increasing density of nuclear chromatin resembling pyknosis, and cell cytoplasmic volume decreases.

There is an increase in the amount of collagen and a loss of ground substance with age. Collagen becomes cross-linked, rigid; and less permeable. The higher density of the connective tissue may reduce the rate at which nutrients are deposited and wastes removed; leading to deterioration of collagen and the consequent slowing of bodily processes.

VULVA

In many postmenopausal and geriatric patients, the aging process in the vulvar area is often more marked than it is in other areas of the body. On inspection of the vulva, it is not uncommon to find excess folds of loose skin, with a prominent clitoris and a urethra that is unprotected by the vulvae, which are often gaping. The pubic hair may become gray at the time of menopause and becomes scanty after the menopause.

The external genitals are of ectodermal origin and resemble the skin. They include the labia majora and minora, the clitoris, the vestibule and its glands, and the mons veneris or mons pubis. The vulvar tissue contains mucus-secreting and apocrine sweat glands, the erectile tissue, wolffian duct remnants, and the insertion of the round ligament with its accompanying pelvic peritoneum. Some women have many more sweat glands than oil glands in this area compared to other women, with variations according to race. Blacks have a large number of sweat and oil glands in this area. The vulvar tissue is comparable to the sex skin of the higher primates and is similarly subjected to influences of the steroid hormones.

LABIA MAJORA

The labia majora are two large folds containing sebaceous and sweat glands embedded in fat and fibrous tissue and covered by skin. They form the lateral boundaries of the vulval cleft and are the homologues of the scrotum. Anteriorly, the two folds are united at the mons pubis or mons veneris, an elevation produced by an extra deposition of adipose tissue over the symphysis pubis. Posteriorly, the folds are united by the posterior commissure. At puberty the lateral aspects of the labia majora and adjacent mons pubis become covered with coarse hair. The distribution of the pubic hair differs in the two sexes. In the female it has a sharply defined horizontal upper border, while in the male it is carried irregularly toward the umbilicus. Sebaceous glands are found on both surfaces of the labia majora, although the pubic hairs are confined to the lateral aspects. As the patient enters the postmenopausal and geriatric age group, fat begins to atrophy and the amount of connective tissue increases. This often gives the appearance of sagging skin. In some elderly women, the fat over the pubis and the mons pubis remains quite prominent and gives the appearance of a mass over the pubic area. The oil and sweat glands become atrophic. As atrophy increases in this area, it is not uncommon to see small blood vessels near the surface; these are called *telangiectasia.* Following a very hot bath these blood vessels become engorged, and when the patient uses a bath towel, bleeding may occur. Needless to say, it is a most traumatic event for the patient, who believes that she must have a malignancy.

LABIA MINORA

The labia minora are two flat connective tissue folds free of fat tissue. They lie between the labia majora. They are covered by skin on the lateral aspect and to a varying extent on the medial aspect, but there the epithelium changes to stratified squamous tissue of the mucous membrane variety. After the age of 5 years, sebaceous glands are numerous on both aspects below the epidermis. The cleft between the labia minora is known as the *vestibule*. Into this vestibule the vagina, the urethra with the paraurethral ducts of Skene, and the ducts of the greater vestibular (Bartholin's) glands open. Anteriorly, the labia minora split into two parts, one stretching over the clitoris, forming a prepuce for that organ, and the other passing beneath the clitoris to form a frenulum. The labia fuse posteriorly, forming the fourchette, a structure that is present only in the nulliparous patient.

The labia minora are more prominent in children than in adults because the labia majora are not well developed. After the menopause, the labia majora atrophy to the point where the labia minora are again prominent. As the patient passes from the menopausal to the geriatric age group, the labia minora are very much in evidence. In some elderly women, there is actual gaping at the introitus.

CLITORIS

The clitoris is the homologue of the penis and contains erectile tissue. It consists of two cylindrical bodies called the *corpora cavernosum* of the clitoris, which has a gland at the end. The clitoris, with vascular erectile tissue, lacks the male corpus spongiosum, which is represented by the venous congeries of the vestibulovaginal bulbs. This stricture becomes smaller as the reproductive era ends. At about age 70, there is a decrease in the sensation of the clitoris, which is probably secondary to diminution of the blood supply and to an increased amount of connective tissue in the clitoris.

HYMEN

The hymen, a double-plated mucosa lined with a stratified squamous epithelium supported by rather firm connective tissue and a fairly rich vasculature, is found in some elderly virginal women. It is often very tough, and insertion of a pediatric speculum is almost impossible. However, in some nonvirginal elderly women, remnants of the hymen are seen and are referred to as the *carunculae myrtiformis*. Occasionally, these remnants become hyalinized. If inflamed, they present as a hard nodule that may be mistaken for a neoplasm.

VESTIBULAR BULBS

The bulbs of the vestibule consist of two flask-shaped masses of erectile tissue that lie on either side of the distal portion of the vagina. They are the homologues of the urethral bulb in the male and are incorporated within the bulbocavernosus muscle. Although they are greatly atrophied in the elderly woman, injury may result in a significant hematoma in this region.

BARTHOLIN'S GLANDS

In the base of the bulb on either side of the vagina are the greater vestibular glands of Bartholin, the ducts of which open into the vestibule, between the labia minora and the attached margin of the hymen. These are mucus-secreting glands. However, as the patient enters the postmenopausal and geriatric age group, these glands become very atrophic and have a great deal of connective tissue deposited in them. It is very rare for them to secrete and provide lubrication at the introitus.

BLOOD SUPPLY TO THE VULVA

The external genitalia are vascular, and are supplied by branches of the internal pudendal arteries from the internal iliac artery and by the external pudendal arteries from the femoral artery. During the reproductive period, the veins of the vulva form a large venous plexus that becomes enormously dilated in pregnancy. However, as the patient grows older, the size of the veins decreases markedly.

NERVE SUPPLY

The anterior superior part of the vulva is supplied by cutaneous branches of the ilioinguinal nerve, and the posterior inferior part by the pudendal branches from the posterior femoral cutaneous nerve. Between these two groups of nerves, the vulva is supplied by the posterior labial and perineal branches of the pudendal nerve.

LYMPHATIC DRAINAGE

The lymphatic drainage is into the superficial inguinal nodes in the groin. Some lymphatic vessels are described as crossing the midline. Thus, in malignant disease of the vulva, it is usually necessary to remove the glands on both sides of the body.

URETHRA

The female urethra extends from the neck of the bladder to the external urethral orifice. Its length is given as 3 to 5.5 cm, with an average of 4.1 cm. The most important feature of the adult female urethra is the ease with which it can be dilated, sometimes to a diameter of 10 mm. The mucous membrane of the meatus, which is the narrowest part of the canal, may, however, split before this limit is reached.

It has been shown that the vulva, vagina, cervix, corpus uteri, fallopian tube, urethra, and trigone in the bladder all have large numbers of estrogen receptors and are sensitive to a decrease in available estrogen. Estrogen deprivation often results in atrophic changes that may become quite marked, especially in the urethra. There is often a weakness of the paraurethral musculature that predisposes to an ectropion of the mucous membrane of the urethra, giving the appearance of a urethral caruncle. As women pass into the geriatric age group and the estrogen deficiency becomes very marked, they often develop an atrophic distal urethritis that results in a thickened, nondistensible distal urethra with partial bladder outlet obstruction. These patients often have nonbacterial urethritis, and no matter how much antibiotic or sulfa drug is given, the condition recurs. However, the judicious use of local estrogen cream and/or combined with systemic estrogen corrects the problem.

The upper part of the urethra is separated from the anterior vaginal wall by connective tissue, but the lower half is actually adherent to the musculature of the vaginal wall. The urethra pierces both layers of the urogenital diaphragm, where it is surrounded by the sphincter urethra membranaceous. The urethra is surrounded by a number of rudimentary glands of the compound racemose variety. These glands open into the paraurethral ducts of Skene, which descend in the wall of the urethra and open into the interior nearest termination. The paraurethral glands are believed to be the homologues of the prostrate gland. In the postmenopausal and geriatric patient, Skene's glands undergo marked atrophy. However, if there is any inspissated material in them, they occasionally form small nodules lateral to the urethra.

VAGINA

The vagina is a tube averaging about 3 inches in length from the vulva to the uterus. In the natural condition of the parts, the cavity of the vagina is only a potential space, its walls lying in close contact; in cross section it appears as an H-shaped slit. This shape allows it to expand when required. The wall of the vagina is thick and strong. It can be dissected into two layers. The outer layer of the wall is a strong musculofibrous layer. The fascial part is continuous above with the superficial layer of the uterus, forming a continuous tube, the uterovaginal fascia. Laterally, the strong fascial layer is continuous with the fibrous sheath of the structures related to the vagina. The vagina is lined with mucous membrane that is covered with a stratified squamous epithelium; the mucous membrane is not smooth but is thrown into a series of transverse folds called *rugae.*

As the menopause progresses and estrogen deprivation becomes more marked, the rugae of the vagina become less prominent and the vaginal wall becomes pale because of a decrease in the underlying vascularity. In women who have not had children or who had a cesarean section, the vagina and its upper part often become conical, inelastic, and quite narrow. This interferes with an adequate pelvic examination and makes it almost impossible to attain good placement of colpostats when radiation is being used to treat cancer of the cervix. The elastic fibers in the submucosa are progressively replaced with collagen. In women who are sexually active, this process seems to be delayed.

Vaginal secretions diminish, resulting in a predisposition to poor lubrication. Vaginal cytology at the menopause shows a great number of parabasal and intermediate cells. In the geriatric patient there is usually a total absence of hormonal activity, and only basal cells are seen. These are often undergoing autolysis, and chromatin filaments are present. The protective effect of Doderlein's bacillus is lost, and the vaginal pH rises from an acid pH of 4.5 to a pH of 6 to 8. This alkaline environment predisposes the vagina to a multitude of bacterial pathogens, and the incidence of vaginitis increases in the postmenopausal woman. Whenever there are recurrent bouts of *Monilia* infection on the vulva or in the vagina, the patient should be tested for a carbohydrate imbalance.

CERVIX

The cervix projects into the vagina, where it forms the external os of the uterus. This is a region of great histologic and clinical interest. Somewhere near the os but usually still inside the cervical canal, the lining columnar epithelium joins a stratified squamous epithelium on the vaginal mucous membrane. This covers the vaginal aspect of the cervix and is reflected onto the vaginal wall. The point of junction of the two epithelia varies greatly. The area between the columnar and squamous epithelium is known as the *squamocolumnar junction.* Distal to this region for a short distance is a intermingling of columnar and squamous epithelium termed the *transformation zone.* Within this zone, most of the cancers of the cervix originate. As the patient enters the geriatric age group, the squamocolumnar junction moves higher in the endocervical canal and may reach almost as high as the internal os. In doing a Papanicolaou smear, it is therefore important to enter the endocervical canal to obtain cytology samples.

In the postmenopausal patient, atrophic changes occur in the cervix. Atrophy gradually becomes marked, and both the internal and external os may become stenotic. The marked atrophic changes often make it difficult to do endometrial aspirations or biopsies as an office procedure. With those patients in whom the staining and spotting cannot be easily identified and the external and internal os cannot be bypassed, it is important to admit the patient for a dilatation and curettage. The cervix often shrinks and retracts, and, with the fornices, becomes flush with the vaginal wall. In these patients, it is very difficult to identify the cervix as a separate specimen. Again, it is difficult to biopsy the cervix in these patients.

UTERUS

The uterus is a muscular organ. This is its outstanding characteristic, and it is upon this property that its function is based. It is designated by nature as a site for the development of the fertilized ovum into the mature fetus. At the completion of this process it must expel its contents to the outer world and, therefore, is mainly muscular in structure.

The walls of the uterus are composed of involuntary muscle. They enclose a cavity that conforms to the general shape of the body. This cavity is continuous below, through the internal os, with the canal of the cervix; above, at each cornu, is continuous with the lumen of the corresponding uterine tube. It is lined with mucous membrane that is smooth and soft, covered by columnar ciliated epithelium, and containing many glands. It undergoes marked changes during menstruation and pregnancy.

At the time of menopause, marked changes take place in the uterus and endometrium. These changes are usually markedly atrophic. The endometrium becomes thin and atrophic, and contains only scattered and inactive glands in the stroma. There may be cystic hyperplasia in an inactive endometrium. There are abnormal changes that will be described later.

The myometrium shrinks markedly. It may be for this reason that the elderly women who develop carcinoma of the endometrium do poorly. A small amount of penetration into the myometrium brings the cancer close to the lymphatics on the serosa because of the atrophy of the myometrium. The myometrial vessels thicken and the interstitial fibrous content of tissue increases. The uterine fundus decreases in size, and the uterus usually becomes much smaller than during the reproductive years.

FALLOPIAN TUBE

Attached to the uterus at each cornu is a uterine tube. As its name implies, it is a hollow structure with a lumen. Immediately this lumen opens directly into the cavity of the uterus; laterally it opens through its abdominal ostium into the peritoneal cavity. Thus, through the vagina, the cervical canal, the cavity of the uterus, and the lumen of the uterine tube, there is a direct pathway between the exterior of the body and the peritoneal cavity.

The uterine tube is described as consisting of four parts: (1) the interstitial portion, (2) the isthmus, (3) the ampullary portion, and (4) the infundibular portion. During the postmenopausal period there is a progressive reduction of secretion, but the ciliated epithelium and tubal peristalsis are preserved. However, as the patient moves into the geriatric age group, there is flattening of the epithelium and loss of ciliated cells. Since the fallopian tubes are mullerian structures, estrogen deprivation causes marked atrophy of the tubes. There is a decrease in internal motility, and later the tube becomes quite atrophic.

OVARY

The menopause is the most striking feature of the climacteric. The dramatic decline in circulating estrogen concentrations that accompanies ovarian failure is the most clinically significant endocrine alteration of the menopause. The principal circulating estrogen of the premenopausal woman is 17-beta-estradiol.

Oogenesis begins in the ovary at around the third week of gestation. Primordial germ cells appear in the yolk sac of the embryo and by the fifth week migrate to the germinal ridge, where they undergo successive mitotic cellular divisions to give rise to oogonia that eventually give rise to oocytes. It has been estimated that the fetal ovary contains approximately 7 million oogonia at 20 weeks' gestation. From then until the menopause, there is a reduction in the number of germ cells. After 7 months' gestation no new oocytes are formed. At birth, there are approximately 2 million oocytes, and by puberty this number has been reduced to 300,000. Nearly all oocytes vanish by the time of atresia, with only 400 to 500 actually being ovulated. The menopause apparently occurs in the human female because of two processes. First, oocytes responsive to gonadotropins disappear from the ovary. Second, the few remaining oocytes do not respond to gonadotropins.

The ovaries are solid, slightly nodular, pink-gray bodies with the approximate proportions of unshelled almonds. They are situated on either side of the uterus, behind and below the uterine tubes. The human ovary undergoes marked changes in size, shape, and position in its lifetime, in addition to the histologic changes brought about by various endocrine stimuli. It is important to appreciate the changes in size, shape, and consistency that occur in the ovary in different age groups, as well as within any given menstrual cycle. The ovaries are usually not symmetric, and the right ovary is often larger than the left.

The ovary of the newborn is an elongated structure approximately 1.5 cm long and 0.5 cm wide, and varies from 1.5 to 3.5 mm in thickness. The ovarian surface is pinkish white, smooth, and glistening. It weighs about 0.3 to 0.4 g. The ovary gradually grows larger and changes shape and position between birth and puberty. It is developed between the 10th and 12th segments on the posterior wall near the kidney, slowly moves into the true pelvis, and enlarges to a size of about 3 × 1.8 × 1.2 cm. The weight of both ovaries at puberty is between 4 and 7 g.

The premenopausal ovary measures 3.5 × 2 × 1.5 cm. The menopausal ovary tends to atrophy and shrink when the graafian follicles and ova disappear. The ovary eventually becomes an inert residue that consists of connective tissue and clings to the posterior leaf of the broad ligament. Its pink color becomes pure white. It shrinks to 2 × 1.5 × 0.5 cm, and in some women it may be as small as 1.5 × 0.75 × 0.5 cm. Its wrinkled surface resembles the gyri and sulci of the cerebrum. At this point, it is almost impossible to palpate on examination.

Postmenopausal ovaries exhibit an increase in connective tissue and a decrease in germinal elements. Follicles are rarely seen, and when they are, they appear to be undergoing atresia and the cells lining these follicles are in regression. It is conceivable that activity at a reduced level may be present in some cells. The thick internal cells from atrophic follicles differentiate into stromal or interstitial cells. An abundance of stromal cells is seen in postmenopausal ovaries, and in vitro experiments indicate that these cells are the source of androgens. A dramatic decline in circulating estrogen, particularly estradiol, is probably the most marked clinically significant endocrine change of the menopause. This occurs with the reduced number of ovarian follicles needed to synthesize estradiol.

BREAST

The breast has always been the ultimate symbol of femininity. The great painters of the Renaissance often painted the breast, with or without a child nursing. Some of these paintings have been commercialized. Botticelli's "Birth of Venus" is used to sell bras.

The breast is part of the upper genital tract of the woman, which includes the endometrium, ovary, and breast. These organs resemble each other in their epidemiology and in whatever hormonal relationships exist among them.

In the female the breasts are two large, hemispherical eminences lying in superficial fascia and situated on the front and sides of the chest; each breast extends from the second rib above, from the sixth rib below, and from the side of the sternum to near the midaxillary line. Their weight and dimensions differ at different periods of life and in different individuals. Before puberty, they are small in size, but they enlarge as the genitalia become more completely developed. They increase during pregnancy and especially after delivery, and become atrophied in old age. The mammary papilla, or nipple, is a cylindrical or conical eminence situated above the level of the fourth intercostal space. It is capable of undergoing a type of erection from mechanical excitement, a change due mainly to the contraction of its muscular fibers. It is of a pink or brownish hue, its surface wrinkled and provided with secondary papilla. It is perforated by 15 to 20 orifices, the apertures of the lactiferous ducts. The base of the mammary papilla is surrounded by an areola.

After the menopause, the breasts begin to atrophy and droop. The skin often becomes loose and the breasts show signs of aging. Estrogen deprivation is probably the main cause of the changes in the breast. However, it cannot be the only main reason because estrogen replacement does not reverse these changes.

On examination the breasts arc softer, there is usually less fat, the breast tissue itself is decreased, and the usual nodularity and cystic areas found in the breast at the height of the reproductive period are missing.

The main histologic changes include flattening of the ductal epithelium, with thinning of the ducts and a decrease in areolar size. The reduction in the proportion of glandular tissues is accompanied by an increase in the proportion of subcutaneous fat. The breasts usually become flaccid and are smaller after the menopause.

Some women maintain normal-appearing breasts even into the geriatric period. A small proportion of women even report that their breasts became larger after the menopause, and they complain of tenderness. There is no adequate explanation for this change from the usual atrophic condition that is found.

SUMMARY

The menopause and the geriatric changes that occur in tissue are due to the process of aging and the cessation of ovarian function. There is a strong interplay between these two processes, and until more is known about the theory and therapeutics of aging, it will be difficult to know the exact role each plays. The changes in the ovary have been fairly well documented. The ultimate exhaustion of primary primordial follicles has been blamed for the phenomena of menopause. Invariably, however, at least some primordial follicles can be found in the ovaries of postmenopausal women. However, they are usually undergoing atresia or have been so altered that they do not respond to pituitary stimulation. Although follicular development is almost completely eliminated after the menopause, the stroma continucs to function and is stimulated by the LH to produce androgenic substances. These androgenic substances may account for some of the hair growth and atrophy that take place. It is a contributing factor to the aromatization of androgenic substances that takes place in the peripheral fat to produce estrone. Cancer of the genitalia or breast can occur at any age after the menopause, and the incidence of cancer of the ovary peaks at about age 77.

Many gerontology patients recognize that they have atrophic vaginal and vulvar tissue and that an examination may be painful; therefore, they are inclined to avoid routine examinations. It is thus important that the patient receive as little discomfort and pain as possible during the examination.

A one-finger vaginal examination should first be carried out, and the finger should be carefully swept around the entire length and breadth of the vagina, as well as to explore the fornices. Once this has been done, the uterus should be outlined in regard to size, shape, and mobility and the adnexal area carefully examined. It is important to explain to the patient each step of the examination and to assure the patient that if there is any pain, the examination will stop immediately. At this point, the middle finger is lubricated and inserted into the rectum for a rectovaginal examination, exploring the rectovaginal septum and cardinal ligaments, as well as the uterosacral ligaments. Following this a careful rectal examination should be carried out and any blood on the finger identified; in those patients in which blood is not identified one of the tests for occult blood should be carried out.

Having completed the routine examination, the physician must decide whether to attempt an endometrial aspiration at this time or have the patient return. Whatever decision is made, the patient should have a careful explanation of what is being done.

REFERENCES

Barber, H. R. K. 1986. Geriatric gynecology, in: *Clinical Geriatrics,* 3rd ed. (I. Rossman, ed.), J. B. Lippincott Co., Philadelphia, p. 364.

Costoff, A. 1974. An ultrastructural study of ovarian changes in the menopause, in: *The Menopausal Syndrome* (R. B. Greenblatt, V. B. Mahech, and P. G. McDonough, eds.), Medcon Press, New York, p. 12.

Hendrickson, M. R. 1980. Embryology and anatomy, in: *Surgical Pathology of the Uterine Corpus* (R. L. Kempson, ed.), W. B. Saunders, Philadelphia, p. 1.

Krouse, T. B. 1980. Menopausal pathology, in: *The Menopause. Comprehensive Management* (B. A. Eskin, ed.), Masson Publishing USA, Paris, p. 3.

Nolelovitz, M. 1978. Gynecologic problems of menopausal women: Part 3, Changes in extragenital tissues and sexuality. *Geriatrics* 33:51.

Rossman, I. 1986. The anatomy of aging, in: *Clinical Geriatrics,* 3rd ed. (I. Rossman, ed.), J. B. Lippincott Co., Philadelphia, p. 3.

Siiteri, P. K., and P. C. MacDonald. 1973. Role of extraglandular estrogen in human endocrinology. In Greep, R. O. and Astwood, E. (eds.). *Handbook of Physiology: Endocrinology.* America Physiological Society, Washington, D. C., vol. 2, part 1, p. 615.

Neuroendocrinology in the Perimenopausal and Geriatric Patient

5

INTRODUCTION

The most common endocrinologic change in the menopause is an increase in follicle stimulating hormone (FSH) concentration that results in the loss of the negative feedback inhibition of estradiol E_2 and, possibly, of inhibin. FSH serum values of 40 mIU/mL or more are generally associated with failure of ovarian function, and values greater than 100 mIU/mL indicate menopause with relative certainty. Luteininzing hormone (LH) is a less sensitive indicator of the gonadotropic changes of menopause than is FSH. Concentrations of LH in postmenopausal women are not generally increased as much as those of FSH.

Endocrine regulation is altered with age. Changes in hormone secretory rate, patterns of secretion, and responses to physiologic and pharmacologic stimuli have been demonstrated. Target tissue sensitivity to hormones appears to be age related and involve hormone receptor mechanisms, enzymatic responses, and carrier proteins. A wide variation is found among various women in this age group and is probably related to many factors including genetic, environmental, and general overall lifestyle.

FSH and LH concentrations increase in the perimenopausal and postmenopausal years. LH does not show the same correlation with the menopause as FSH. LH levels may reach levels that are comparable to the premenopausal woman with severe polycystic ovarian disease or hyperandrogenism, or during the preovulatory LH surge.

In order to appreciate the changes in the perimenopausal and geriatric age groups it is important to review basic and clinical aspects of the neuroendocrine system during the reproductive years.

HYPOTHALAMUS

The hypothalamus lies in the lower part of the lateral wall of the third ventricle. Its boundaries are:

anteriorly—the optic chiasma

posteriorly—the mammillary bodies

laterally—it extends for a distance of about 1 cm on each side of the third ventricle

superiorly—the thalamus

inferiorly—tuber cinereum which, is formed by the converging walls of the third ventricle

Role of the Hypothalamus

The endocrine system meets the nervous system at the hypothalamic –pituitary interface. The hypothalamus regulates pituitary activity through two pathways. Neural pathways extend from the hypothalamus, where two hormones—antidiuretic hormone (ADH) and oxytocin—are synthesized, to the posterior pituitary lobe, where the hormones are stored and secreted. Portal venous pathways, which connect the hypothalamus to the anterior pituitary lobe, carry hypothalamic releasing and inhibiting hormones, as well as most of the lobe's blood supply.

Functions

The hypothalamus produces pituitary regulating hormones, which pass down the pituitary portal system to regulate the production of pituitary trophic hormones by the anterior pituitary. In addition, vasopressin and oxytocin are elaborated in the supraoptic and paraventricular nuclei once they pass down the axons of the nerves connecting these structures to the posterior pituitary, where the two hormones are stored. (Fig. 5-1).

Reference is frequently made to tonic and cyclic control in the hypothalamus. The tonic control is regarded as responsible for the day to day constant production of gonadotropins, while the cyclic control accounts for the surges of LH and FSH activity that lead to ovulation. Tonic control is mainly under negative feedback control, whereas the cyclic control is under positive feedback control. In postmenopausal women, pulses of both LH and FSH occur at a frequency of approximately 1 to 2 hours. This pulsatile fluctuation is superimposed on the extremely rapid and noncoincidental oscillations in the release of both gonadotropins, which recur at 1- to 3-minute intervals.

FUNCTIONAL ANATOMY OF THE HYPOTHALAMUS AND PITUITARY

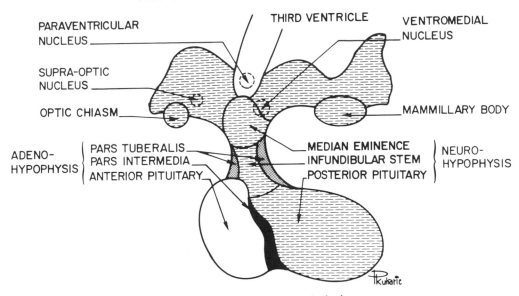

Figure 5-1. Functional anatomy of the hypothalamus and pituitary.

The increase of concentrations of gonadotropins that occur during the normal climacteric is generally gradual and episodic. Throughout the menopause, the FSH/LH ratio is almost invariably greater than 1. Peak concentrations of FSH and LH are reached by 2 to 3 years after the menopause. Gonadotropin concentrations of the next decades remain stable or may actually decrease.

By its connections with its limbic system, the hypothalamus functions as a center in which external stimuli reaching the body are converted into the appropriate emotional response such as rage, fear, anger, temperature regulation, feeding and behavior.

Regulating Hormones. The hypothalamic regulation hormones are: luteinizing hormone releasing hormone (LH-RH), also known as gonadotropin releasing hormone (GnRH); the corticotropin releasing hormone (CRH); growth hormone release-inhibiting hormone—somatostatin; thyrotropic hormone releasing hormone (TRH); prolactin inhibiting factor (PIF) (dopamine). LH-RH is a decapeptide, and somastatin is a tetradecapeptide. TRH is a tripeptide. Recently, CRH and GH-RH have been isolated as larger peptides (41 and 44 amino acids, respectively).

Mode of Production of Regulating Hormones. The mode of production of the regulating hormones is a neurosecretory one. The hypothalamic nerve cells act as both neurons and endocrine cells. The hormones are synthesized in the cytoplasm of the neuron, and are then passed along the nerve axon to the nerve terminal. From there, they are released into the hypophyseal portal vessels, where they pass to the anterior pituitary.

61

PITUITARY GLAND

The pituitary gland is also known as the *hypophysis.* The pituitary gland is about 1 cm in diameter and weighs 0.5 to 0.75 g. It lies in a cavity of bone at the base of the skull (the sella turcica) and is connected to the hypothalamus by the pituitary stalk. The pituitary has two distinct parts: an anterior lobe (adenohypophysis) and a posterior lobe (neurohypophysis). The anterior lobe constitutes most of the gland.

Hormones of the Anterior Pituitary

The anterior pituitary produces a number of important trophic hormones: follicle stimulating hormone (FSH); luteininzing hormone (LH); prolactin (PRL); adrenocorticotropic hormone (ACTH); thyroid stimulating hormone (TSH), which is sometimes called thyrotropin; and growth hormone (GH).

All are proteins or complex associations of sugars and polypeptides (glycoproteins). The molecular weights are on the order of 20,000 to 40,000 daltons.

FSH and LH. These hormones have an important combined action on the ovary. FSH is responsible for early development of the graffian follicle. LH may contribute to follicular growth and estrogen production, but its principal actions are to cause ovulation and to convert the ruptured graffian follicle to a corpus luteum. In the menopause and postmenopausal period, there is an increase in FSH concentrations that results from loss of the negative feedback inhibition of E_2 and possibly of inhibin. LH is a less sensitive indicator of gonadotropin changes of the menopause than is FSH.

In a postmenopausal patient, the adenohypophysis continues to maintain a normal content of GH, ACTH, and TSH. The reduction in the sensitivity of the pituitary to the hypothalamic releasing hormones may explain the findings of a decrease in circulating GH concentrations in an elderly subject and a diminished TSH response to TRH.

In the aging patient, there is a slight diminution in circulating concentrations of GH despite maintenance of normal pituitary content. This probably is a response to the normal sequela of pituitary aging.

TSH

TSH, which is also known as thyrotropin, is secreted upon stimulation by TRH from the hypothalamus and causes the thyroid gland to release thyroxin (T4) and triiodothyronine (T3). Elevated circulating T4 and T3 levels exert a negative feedback effect on TSH secretion from the pituitary. Plasma TSH values remain relatively constant throughout the lifespan. There is a slight decrease in radioactive iodine uptake in the thyroid gland of an elderly patient. Concentrations of total and free thyroxin are unchanged with age, despite a slight decrease in concentrations of thyroid binding globulin, which is due to diminished serum concentrations of estrogen or protein. In persons older than 50, concentrations of triiodothyronine are diminished by 25 to 40 percent. Although the exact reason for the decrease is unclear, diminished peripheral conversion of thyroxin to triiodothyronine is suspected to account for most of it.

ACTH

ACTH, also known as corticotropin, stimulates the production of aldosterone, cortisol, and other glucocorticoids. Plasma cortisol levels largely control ACTH secretion through a negative feedback mechanism. For example, high cortisol levels act directly on the corticotropic cells in the pituitary to suppress ACTH secretion.

ACTH concentrations are apparently undiminished in the elderly patient. The aging adrenal gland appears to maintain a relatively normal response to ACTH stimulation; however, the rate of adrenocorticosteroid secretion decreased by 30 percent during the entire adult lifespan. Serum aldosterone concentrations decrease by 50 percent in the elderly, causing a blunted response to sodium restriction in 30 to 40 percent of adults. Approximately one third of women older than 70 have low plasma renin contractions.

PRL

PRL is similar in chemical structure to GH. It stimulates milk production in the mammary glands once they have been prepared by the influence of other hormones, including GH, estrogen, progesterone, T4, parathyroid hormone, insulin, and corticosteroids. PRL synthesis and secretion is reduced by prolactin inhibiting factor (PIF).

The existence of PRL was suspected for many years before it became a reality. It is a protein hormone that possesses 190 amino acid residues and has a molecular weight of about 22,000 daltons. Its similarity to growth hormone has been reported; 80 percent of its amino acid residues are shared with human placental lactogen and 20 percent with GH.

PRL is produced by cells of the anterior pituitary. By using special staining techniques, it can be shown that PRL arises from different alpha cells than does GH. These PRL-secreting cells are present in comparatively small numbers in the nonpregnant patient, but increase markedly during pregnancy.

The secretion of PRL by the pituitary is the result of a reduction in the amount of PIF, which the hypothalamus uses to keep the hormone in a state of tonic inhibition. It is known, however, that TRH can increase prolactin secretion. This has lead to speculation that there may be a PRL-releasing hormone that is similar to, or even the same as, TRH. There is no confirmation of such a releasing hormone at present.

A wide variety of stimuli influence PRL production. Suckling is a powerful stimulant. Other events that may increase production significantly are general anesthetic, a surgical operation, coitus, and physical exercise. Several drugs raise PRL production by interfering with dopamine function; these include reserpine, antihistamines, diazepam, tricyclic-antidepressants, and haloperidol. Estrogens, natural and synthetic, also stimulate PRL production.

The substances that inhibit PRL production include L-dopa and dopamine agonists of which the most important are drugs of the ergot group.

Basal serum levels of PRL decline in normal women over the lifespan reflecting, at least in part, the age-dependent decline in estrogen secretion. The physiologic role of PRL in men and in elderly subjects remains to be elucidated. PRL is secreted in response to administration of TRH, but aging has no effect on this response.

The symptomatic climacteric woman, in contrast to her asymptomatic counterpart, has been characterized in a recent study by Gonnendecker et al. by high FSH and LH and low PRL values. The symptomatic women in this study were described as having anxiety and depression of various kinds, whereas the asymptomatic women had high FSH, lower LH and estrogen values, and higher PRL levels. It has been hypothesized that postmenopausal dysphoria may occur when high PRL levels are associated with low estrogens, whereas postmenopausal irritability may occur when high PRL levels are associated with low progesterone. Direct clinical testing of this idea has not been performed. Although little work has been done on prolactin in geriatric patients, it should be emphasized that estrogens, natural and synthetic, also stimulate PRL production.

POSTERIOR PITUITARY

The posterior pituitary (neurohypophysis) is a neurosecretory gland. The cell bodies lie in the hypothalamus, and the axon and axon terminals make up the stalk and the gland itself. The axon terminals are closely associated with capillaries as a neurohemal organ.

The main physiologic action of ADH is to increase the permeability of the renal collecting system to water; in the absence of vasopressin there is an inability to concentrate the urine (diabetes insipidus). Secretion is controlled by the osmotic pressure of extracellular fluids via osmoreceptors in the hypothalamus. It is stimulated by nicotine and inhibited by alcohol. The pressor effect of vasopressin is of no significance under normal circumstances, but substantial elevations may be seen in acute events, such as hemorrhage and anoxia. The supraoptic and paraventricular nuclei of the hypothalamus show distinct age-specific cytologic changes. Circulating ADH concentrations in the elderly are normal or increased, presumably because of a decreased sensitivity of the distal renal tubules.

Although the posterior pituitary does not secrete hormones, it is connected to the hypothalamus by terminal nerve endings. These nerve endings store oxytocin and antidiuretic hormone, which are produced in the hypothalamus.

Oxytocin production is mainly limited to the reproductive years, and, therefore, has not been studied in perimenopausal and geriatric patients.

Antidiuretic Hormone

The antidiuretic hormone (ADH), which is known as vasopressin, regulates fluid balance by making the collecting ducts in distal renal tubules more permeable to water. Osmoreceptor cells in the hypothalamus control the secretion of ADH into the circulation. In a dehydrated patient, the osmolality of extracellular fluid increases, drawing water across an osmotic gradient from body cells. As a result, the cell volume of osmoreceptors decreases, causing them to stimulate release of ADH. Conversely, excessive circulating water reduces extracellular fluid osmolality, and water flows into body cells. This increases receptor cell volume and inhibits ADH release.

The ADH is produced primarily in the supraoptic and paraventricular nuclei of the hypothalamus, and is released from the posterior lobe of the pituitary. Although these hypothalamic areas show distinct age-specific cytologic changes, circulating ADH concentrations in the elderly are normal or increased, presumably because of the decreased sensitivity of the distal renal tubule.

It has been shown that osmoreceptor sensitivity is enhanced over the lifespan and that secretion of ADH is increased in elderly women in order to maintain normal plasma osmolality. These changes are secondary to increased distal renal tubular resistance to ADH effect in older individuals. This resistance explains the impaired urine concentrating ability seen in elderly women. Urine diluting ability is relatively intact in older women. Clinical consequences of these changes are not yet apparent.

Ovarian Hormone

The ovary continues to secrete substantial quantities of androgens, principally testosterone, after the menopause, but it secretes little or no estradiol. The serum of androstenedione in the menopausal woman approaches the low levels found in the premenopausal woman after ovarian ablation. There is also a decrease in ovarian adrostenedione production, even though some secretion continues. The postmenopausal ovaries secrete higher quantities of testosterone than they do premenopausally, but the serum level of testosterone is usually unchanged because the portion of the premenopausal woman's testosterone was formed by conversion from androstenedione, and the decrease in androstenedione leads to a reduced amount that is converted to testosterone. The excess in levels of pituitary gonadotropins, which is due to the reduction of circulating estrogens, stimulates the ovarian stroma to increase its secretion of testosterone.

The neuroendocrinology in the perimenopausal and geriatric patient is mainly concerned with the hypothalamus and the pituitary gland, including the anterior and posterior lobes. The ovary, therefore, has been covered in greater detail in other chapters, 3 and 6, as has been the classic contribution by Finch.

The dramatic decline of circulating estrogen concentration that accompanies ovarian failure is the most clinically significant endocrine alteration of the menopause. The principal circulating estrogen of the premenopausal woman is 17β-estradiol. Estradiol E_2 is produced both by direct ovarian secretion and by peripheral conversion of testosterone and estrone. E_2 accounts for the greatest amount of estrogen in the premenopausal patient and estrone accounts for most of the circulating estrogen in the postmenopausal woman. The production rate in the circulating concentration of estrone in the postmenopausal patient are two and four times those of E_2. As in the case of E_2, virtually no estrone is produced by the postmenopausal ovary or adrenal gland. Most, if not all, of the estrone is formed by the peripheral conversion of androstenedione. This extraglandular aromatization has been identified in adipose tissue, the liver, and specific hypothalamic nuclei. The conversion rate of androstenedione to estrone is significantly correlated with obesity. It also seems to increase with age, rising twofold in postmenopausal women. Although influenced by age and obesity, estrone concentrations are apparently determined mainly by the circulating concentrations of androstenedione.

Clinically, in the perimenopausal years, there is very often a progressive shortening of the total cycling, which gets more pronounced as the patient moves into the menopausal and geriatric years. The increase in FSH in the perimenopausal and geriatric years remains until the seventh or eighth decade, when FSH slowly decreases as part of the aging process.

It has been shown that elevated FSH does not influence vasomotor symptomatology. It has been reported that after a series of experiments in humans that LH showed pulsatile activity closely associated with the occurrence of symptoms and skin temperature increases during hot flushes. This association suggests that factors concerned with pulsatile release of LH may be involved in the pathophysiology of hot flushes.

SUMMARY

As the pituitary ages, various changes occur. After the age of 50, the weight of the pituitary decreases significantly—its size is decreased by as much as 20 percent by the ninth decade of life. The blood supply of the pituitary gland is also reduced measurably after the age of 60. In spite of these changes, the adenohypophysis (the anterior and posterior lobes of the pituitary) continues to maintain a normal content of growth hormone (GH), adenocorticotropic hormone (ACTH), and thryoid-stimulating hormone (TSH).

The decreased responsiveness of the pituitary to its physiologic stimuli has been reported. The aging pituitary fails to respond to stress with as rapid an increase of adrenocorticotropic hormone (ACTH) synthesis or release as it does in the premenopausal patient. This may be a protective mechanism because with the aging of target tissues, a change in the hormonal environment that is too rapid could have a deleterious effect.

There is a modest diminution in circulating concentrations of GH with advancing age, despite maintenance of normal pituitary content. It probably represents a normal sequela of pituitary aging and does not denote decreased GH reserves.

Plasma TSH values remain relatively constant throughout the lifespan. It is interesting to note that TSH response to TRH infusion in elderly women is characteristically entirely normal.

The aging adrenal gland exhibits some morphologic alterations that include increased pigment deposition in collagen content, as well as vasucular dilation and hemorrhage within both the cortex and the medulla.

It has been reported that the aging adrenal gland maintains a relatively normal response to ACTH stimulation, and the rate of adrenal corticosteroid secretion decreases by 30 percent during the entire adult lifespan.

Serum aldosterone concentrations decrease by 50 percent in the elderly, causing a diminished response to sodium restriction in 30 to 40 percent of the adults. One third of women older than 70 have low plasma renin concentrations.

Basal serum levels of prolactin (PRL) decline in normal women over the lifespan reflecting, at least in part, the age-dependent decline in estrogen secretion. The physiologic role of PRL in aging women remains to be elucidated. PRL is secreted in response to the administration of thyrotropin-releasing hormone (TRH), but aging has no effect on this response. Estrogen, natural and synthetic, also stimulates PRL production. The substances that inhibit PRL production include L-dopa and dopamine agonists, of which the most important are drugs of the ergot group.

REFERENCES

Amos, M., R. Burgus, Blackwell, and R. Guillemin, 1971. Purification, amino acid composition and terminus of the hypothalmic luteinizing hormone releasing factor (LRF) of ovine origin. *Biochem. Biophys. Res. Commun.* 44:205.

Belchetz, P. E., T. M. Plant, Y. Nakai, E. J. Keogh, and E. Knobil. 1978. Hypophyseal responses to continuous and intermittent delivery of hypothallamic gonadotrophin-releasing hormone. *Science* 202(4368):631.

Blackwell, R. E., and R. Guillemin. 1973. Hypothalamic control of adenohypophyseal secretions. *Ann. Rev. Phyiol.* 35:357.

Casper, R. F., S. S. C. Yen, and M. M. Wilkes. 1979. Menopausal flushes: A neuroendocrine link with pulsatile luteinizing hormone secretion. *Science* 205:823.

Felicio, L. S., J. F. Nelson, R. F. Gosden, et al. 1983. Restorations of ovulatory cycles by graphs in aging mice; Potentiation by long-term ovarectomy decreases with age. *Proc. Natl. Acad. Sci. USA* 80:6076.

Finch, C. E., 1971. Comparative biology of senescence: Some evolutionary and development considerations, in: *Animal Models for Biomedical Research*, Vol. 4, National Academy of Sciences, Washington, D.C.

Finch, C.E. 1976. The regulation of physiological changes during mammalian aging. *Q. Rev. Biol.* 51:49.

Finch, C. E. 1975. Aging and the regulation of hormones: A view in October 1974, in: *Advances in Experimental Medicine and Biology.* Plenum Press, New York.

Finch, C. E., L. S. Felicio, K. Flurhey, et al. 1980. Studies in ovarian–hypothalamus –pituitary interactions during reproductive aging in C57BL/6 mice. *Peptides* (Fayetteville) 1 (suppl):163.

Gonnendecker, E.W.W., E.S. Polakow, and L. Gerdes. 1981. Psycho-endocrine difference and correlations in symptomatic and asymptomatic climacteric women—the possible role of prolactin. *SAMED J* 60:661.

Judd, H. L. 1984. Menopause and postmenopause, In: *Current Obstetric and Gynecologic Diagnosis and Treatment,* 5th edition (R. L. Benson, ed.), Lange Medical Publishers, Los Angeles.

Knobil, E. 1980. The neuroendocrine control of the menstrual cycle. *Rect. Prog. Horm. Res.* 36:53.

MacDonald, P. C., J. M. Grodin, and P. K. Suteri. 1969. The utilization of plasma androstenedione for estrone production in women, in: *Progress in Endocrinology. Proceedings of the Third International Congress of Endocrinology.* Amsterdam Excerpta Medica International Congress Series 184:770.

Mildrum, D. R., I. M. Shamouki, M. Frumar, et al. 1979. Elevations of skin temperature of the finger as an objective index of postmenopausal hot flashes: Standardization of the technique. *Am. J. Obstet. Gynecol.* 135:713.

Miller, D. S., R. R. Reid, N. S. Cetel, R. W. Rebar, and S. S. Yen. Pulsatile administration of low-dose gonadotropin releasing hormone. *JAMA* 250:2937.

Research on the menopause. 1981. WHO Techinical Report Series 670:1.

Schally, A. V., and J. Kasting. 1971. Isolation and properties of FSH and LH releasing hormone. *Biochem. Biophys. Res. Commun.* 43:393.

Schally, A. V., and A. J. Kastin. 1971. Stimulation and inhibition of fertility through hypothalamic agents. *Prog. Ther. Bull. 1:29.*

Schipper, H., J. R. Braver, J. F. Nelson, et al. 1981. The role of the gonads in the histologic aging of the hypothalamic arcuate nucleus. *Biol. Reprod.* 25:413.

Upton, G. V. 1982. The perimenopause: Physiologic correlates and clinical management. *J. Reprod. Med.* 27:1.

Yen, S. S. C. 1977. The biology of menopause. *J. Reprod. Med.* 18:287.

Yen, S. S. C., L. A. LLevana, B. H. Pearson, and A. S. Littell. 1970. Disappearance rates of endogenous follicle stimulating hormone in serum following surgical hypophysectomy in man, *J. Clin. Endocrinol.* 30:325.

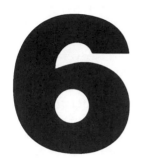

Age and the Endocrine Changes Occurring With Aging

INTRODUCTION

A gland is a structure that produces and secretes certain chemical substances that are necessary for the functioning of the body's organs. There are two kinds of glands: exocrine and endocrine.

Exocrine glands have ducts through which their secretions pass directly to the area of the body that needs them, such as lacrimal glands, salivary glands, mammary glands, intestinal glands, and sebaceous glands.

Endocrine glands, on the other hand, are ductless; their secretions are discharged directly into the blood or lymph. The major endocrine glands are the adrenals, gonads, pancreas, parathyroid, pituitary, and thyroid.

With aging there is a decline in the number of hormone receptors, specialized parts of cells that control the cell's ability to respond to specific hormones and other body chemicals. The loss of these receptors may be responsible for the decreased ability of the body to respond to hormones with age. Adrenal or stress hormones may be responsible for some of the gradual changes in the brain during aging. It is interesting to contemplate the relationship between aging and the endocrine system and how one affects the other. From time immemorial, scientists have tried to establish a method for preserving youth indefinitely. Charles Edouard Brown-Sequard carried out classic self-experiments in 1889.

The word *hormone* means to urge or arouse or set into motion. Although Hippocrates used the word in the fourth century B.C., it wasn't until early in the twentieth century that the word came to be used commonly in medical circles to denote the then newly discovered body secretions. These are substances produced by a gland that are secreted into the blood stream and affects another part of the body. *Hormones* are secreted by the endocrine glands. One of the first hormones understood was thyroid hormone, produced by the thyroid gland. It was initially extracted from animal sources for treatment of human metabolic illnesses. Then came the discovery of insulin, the hormone secreted from the islets of the pancreas that regulate the way the body controls sugar. This knowledge made the treatment and control of diabetes possible. Cortisone, discovered later, is one of the hormones produced by the adrenal gland. The endocrine glands secrete hormones directly into the bloodstream to regulate various body functions. In addition to the usual endocrine glands, the gastrointestinal mucosa and the placenta also secrete hormones.

PRODUCTION AND RELEASE OF HORMONES

Endocrine cells manufacture and release their hormone products in several ways. Many endocrine cells possess receptors on their cell membranes that respond to stimuli, such as abnormal extracellular ion levels, or hormones from other glands, or impulses from neurons impinging on the membrane. The pancreas has been studied in depth. It has been shown that neurostimulation of the pancreatic beta cells synthesizes the hormone precursor preproinsulin and converts it to proinsulin in bead-like ribosomes located on the endoplasmic reticulum. Proinsulin is transferred to the Golgi complex, which collects it into secretory granules. Insulin is formed on the Golgi complex and the secretory granules. These granules move to the cell wall, where they fuse with the plasma membrane and release insulin into the bloodstream. Hormonal release by membrane fusion is called *exocytosis.*

The thyroid decreases in weight, and the follicles become smaller and stain less intensely with advancing age. In general, thyroid cells store a hormone precursor, colloidal iodinated thyroglobulin, which contains iodine and thyroglobulin. When stimulated by TSH, a follicular cell takes up some of the stored thyroglobulin by *endocytosis,* which is the reverse of exocytosis. The cell membrane extends finger-like projections into the colloid and then pulls portions back into the cell. Lysosomes in the cell fuse with colloid, which is then degraded by protolysis into triiodothyronine (T_3) and thyroxin (T_4), which are released into the circulation and lymphatic system by exocytosis.

As the pituitary ages, various changes occur. Interstitial fibrosis occurs and adenomas form. The anterior and posterior secretions are controlled by hypothalamic signals. As an example, the hypothalamic neuron produces antidiuretic hormone (ADH), which travels down the axon and is stored in secretory granules in nerve endings in the posterior pituitary. When the axon membrane is depolarized, calcium ions flow into the axon, the hormone granules fuse with the membrane of the terminal bulb, and the hormone is released.

The anterior pituitary is stimulated to produce its many hormones. A hypothalamic neuron manufactures hormone-releasing factors and secretes them into a capillary of the portal system. These factors travel down the pituitary stalk to the anterior pituitary. There they cause the release of many pituitary hormones, including adrenocorticotropine hormone (ACTH), thyroid stimulating hormone (TSH), growth hormone (GH), follicle stimulating hormone (FSH), luteinizing hormone (LH), and prolactin (PRL).

STEROID AND THYROID HORMONE ACTION

Steroid hormones combine with steroids in the cytoplasm, whereas thyroid hormones enter the nucleus before combining with receptors. These activated receptors bind to the DNA and chromatin, where they modulate the transcription of specific genes to form messenger RNA (mRNA). The mRNA enters the cytoplasm and promotes the formation of new proteins in the ribosomes, which then mediate the appropriate response to the hormone. This will be discussed in the chapter on breast tumors in the aging (Chap. 11).

Endocrine disorders are usually classified as hyperfunctional or hypofunctional. The dysfunction may originate in the hypothalamic–pituitary unit, the hormone-producing gland, the target organ, or possibly a tumor.

THYROID GLAND

The thyroid gland consists of two lateral lobes connected by an isthmus. The lobes partially envelop the anterior and lateral surfaces of the trachea, just below the cricoid cartilage. The gland is composed of follicular cells containing an iodinated colloidal protein, thyroglobulin. This globulin acts as a reservoir for thyroid hormone precursors and for iodide. The gland actively concentrates iodide from ingested food and water. The TSH causes the follicular cells to synthesize T_3 and its suspected precursor, T_4, from thyroglobulin and to release them directly into the bloodstream. From 50 to 90 percent of T_3 is thought to be derived from T_4. The remaining 10 percent or more is secreted directly by the thyroid gland.

Most circulating T_3 and T_4 is bound to a serum protein, thyroxin-binding globulin (TBG), leaving a minute amount of hormone free to exert its effects. The plasma level of free thyroid hormones mediates a complex negative feedback system based on TSH secretion from the anterior pituitary. The thyroid hormones increase the metabolic activities of all body tissues.

Calcitonin is a hypocalcemic hormone secreted predominantly by thyroid parafollicular cells in response to hypercalcemia. The exact role of calcitonin in normal human physiology is not fully understood. Its principal effect is to inhibit bone resorption.

Normally, a negative feedback system regulates hormonal balance. TSH secreted by the pituitary in response to low levels of T_4 and T_3 stimulates the production and secretion of T_4 and T_3. As the levels of these hormones rise, the pituitary stops secreting TSH.

Thyroid disorders strike up to 20 percent of the population and profoundly affect virtually every body system. Because of their widespread and sometimes nonspecific effects, thyroid disorders may initially be mistaken for disorders of the body systems. Thyrotoxicosis can cause significant cardiovascular abnormalities, such as tachycardia and widened pulse pressure. This explains why detection of thyroid disorders requires a sound knowledge of thyroid pathophysiology and a complete assessment of all body systems. Most important, timely detection and treatment of these disorders can help forestall potentially life-threatening complications, such as thyroid storm and myxedema coma. Hypothyroidism is not uncommon in the aging female.

In Graves' disease, thyroid-stimulating immunoglobulin (TSI) acts like TSH, causing excessive T_4 and T_3 secretion in response to elevated T_4 and T_3 levels. TSH secretion decreases, but TSI secretion continues. In hypothyroidism due to increased thyroid tissue mass, insufficient production of T_4 and T_3 causes increased TSH secretion. The elderly patient also exhibits progressive fibrosis and nodularity. This may be the result of less need for thyroid hormone by target tissues.

Little evidence is available to indicate that thyroid activity per se decreases with aging. There may be a small diminution in thyroid hormone secretion, but this may be due to secondary diminished metabolic disposal of thyroid hormone and to primary glandular failure. The basal metabolic rate of the geriatric patient decreases, but this may be secondary to a decrease in body mass. Oxygen consumption per unit of body mass does not change. TSH remains fairly constant, although a small change in serum TSH concentration may occur. In men, but not women, a progressive fall in the sensitivity of pituitary TSH secretion (not prolactin release) to TRH occurs with age. The physiologic significance of this observation is unknown at this time. Most elderly patients remain euthyroid unless they have an intrinsic thyroid disease. In general, adequate thyroid hormone reserve is maintained throughout the geriatric period, as tested by TSH.

Most aged thyrotoxic patients present with sufficiently classic findings of hyperthyroidism to permit a correct diagnosis of that disorder. However, a thyroid disorder that is diagnosed in a youthful patient may go unrecognized in an elderly patient because the same disorder will produce different symptoms. An elderly patient with hyperthyroidism frequently presents with cardiovascular symptomatology such as paroxysmal, irregular tachycardia or congestive heart failure. Hypermetabolic symptoms (nervousness, sweating, frequent bowel movements) may be lacking or inconspicuous. After the diagnosis is made, the best form of therapy—the administration of radioactive iodine—must be used cautiously. Correcting the thyroid hormone excess too rapidly may lead to cardiovascular collapse. Surgical management is recommended only for those patients who have a goiter large enough to compromise the airway.

Thyroid disorders develop from the effects of excess or insufficient thyroid hormones on peripheral tissues, from pathologic changes in the thyroid gland itself, or both. Thyroid disorders affect up to 20 percent of the population and occur more commonly in women than in men. Graves' disease, an immunogenetic disorder caused by an abnormal thyroid stimulator, is the most common cause of thyrotoxicosis. Reduced thyroid tissue mass or interference with thyroid hormone synthesis or release causes hypothyroidism. In the elderly, it is most important to make an accurate diagnosis because either hyper- or hypothyroidism may mimic other diseases and may be mistaken for organic brain disorders.

Hypothyroidism has similar presentations in young and elderly patients. Older patients, however, are more tolerant of the symptoms and signs of thyroid hypofunction and, as a result, may present with far advanced disease. Hypothyroidism may present with a slowing of mentation, edema, reflex and skin changes, or constipation. It may go undiagnosed by the clinician. Clinicians attribute these symptoms to old age or arteriosclerosis. Myxedema coma seldom occurs under age 50.

The diagnosis of hypothyroidism rests upon the findings of (1) an elevated serum TSH concentration and (2) a low circulating level of thyroid hormone (total serum T_4 content). Serum TBG in hypothyroid patients is estimated by measuring resin T_3 uptake. If the patient is found to have a low serum T_4 level, low resin T_3 uptake, and a normal or low serum TSH level, pituitary hypothyroidism is present, and radiographic evaluation of the sella turcica and measurement of the plasma cortisol level are mandatory. In the geriatric patient, measurement of other pituitary trophic hormones to confirm the presence of panhypothyroidism is unnecessary. Hypothyroidism is usually associated with elevated serum cholesterol. Serum creatinine phosphokinase (CPK) activity is usually elevated in hypothyroidism. It begins to decline within several days after initiation of low-dose thyroid hormone replacement. Macrocytic anemia frequently accompanies hypothyroidism. It is important to differentiate this condition from pernicious anemia. Ventilatory failure may not be obvious in a hypothyroid patient; measurement of arterial blood pH, ($PaCO_2$) and arterial oxygen pressure (PaO_2) is indicated in newly diagnosed, untreated hypothyroid subjects. Both hypoxic and hypercapnic ventilatory drives are suppressed in severe myxedema. Overweight hypothyroid patients seem particularly susceptible to hypercarbia. It is important to treat unrelated nonthyroidal illnesses during the treatment of hypothyroidism. Superimposed infections or cardiovascular catastrophe may acutely worsen the hypothyroid state.

In the average person, oral thyroid hormone is given in a larger dosage. The initial thyroid hormone replacement should consist of 0.025 mg (25 ug of L-T_4 daily. After 2 to 4 weeks, this dose may be increased to 0.050 mg/day and thereafter to 0.075–0.125 mg/day. The total daily replacement dosage in patients over age 60 may be only 0.075–0.125 mg. It is important to follow the patient very closely and determine the dosage that is needed.

PARATHYROID GLANDS

Four small parathyroid glands are normally located beside the thyroid, embedded in the dorsal surface of each upper and lower pole. Composed mainly of granular chief cells and large glandular oxyphil cells, these glands secrete parathyroid hormone (PTH), which regulates calcium and phosphorus metabolism.

PTH stimulates reabsorption of calcium and phosphate from the bone by activating bone-removing osteoclast cells and temporarily depressing bone-renewing osteoblast cells. In the kidneys, this hormone acts on the renal tubules to cause excretion of phosphate and reabsorption of calcium and magnesium. It also increases calcium and phosphate absorption in the intestine. Vitamin D, after it is activated to its most potent metabolite, 1-alpha-dihydroxyvitamin D_3, enhances the absorption of calcium and phosphate from the intestinal tract. The control of PTH largely depends on extracellular calcium levels. Decreased calcium levels increase PTH secretion and elevated calcium levels suppress it. Calcitonin opposes the effects of PTH, reducing serum calcium levels.

Many elderly people have normal blood calcium, phosphorus, and electrolyte levels, but abnormal values are not uncommon. The most striking pathologic change in the parathyroid in the elderly is an increase in the number of eosinophils. The significance of this finding is unknown, since the secretion of PTH appears to be within the normal range. However, with more sophisticated techniques, a reevaluation of calcium abnormalities is taking place. With the use of automated biochemical screening procedures, detection of hypercalcemia has led to increasing recognition of nonendocrine neoplasms and primary hyperparathyroidism. With declining sex steroid levels, normal PTH levels can lead to the skeleton's demineralization. This explains why the osteoporosis of aging and hyperparathyroidism are identical radiologically and symptomatically. Demineralization of the skeletal system and its consequences are now being detected.

The symptoms of hypercalcemia are nonspecific and very often difficult to identify. Many of them are found in fairly normal geriatric patients. The earliest manifestations of hypercalcemia include polyuria, nocturia, anorexia, nausea, constipation, lethargy, weakness, dry mouth, kidney stones, and psychosis. These symptoms can lead to severe dehydration, azotemia, mental confusion, coma, cardiovascular collapse, and even death.

Hypoparathyroidism in the elderly is almost always due to thyroid surgery. In geriatric patients this condition is rare and is managed by administering high oral doses of an alkaline form of calcium, along with a vitamin D supplement.

Calcium absorption from the gastrointestinal tract has been reported to be decreased in many older subjects. Basal plasma calcitonin levels decline progressively with age in both men and women. As noted earlier, calcitonin is a hormone secreted by the thyroid glands that regulates serum calcium levels. Because the primary biologic effect of calcitonin is inhibition of bone resorption, decreasing circulating levels of this hormone throughout life could predispose the individual to demineralization bone disease. Since it has been shown that calcitonin levels decline and PTH levels increase, these changes may work synergistically to increase bone calcium loss. The response of calcitonin to calcium infusion (a stress that results in calcitonin secretion) is decreased with aging, more dramatically in women than in men.

Primary hyperparathyroidism is usually revealed by findings of hypercalcemia, hypophosphatemia, and hyperchloremic acidosis. In terms of specific studies to separate hyperthyroidism from other hypercalcemic disorders, determination of the nephrogenous component of urinary cyclic adenosine monophosphate (AMP) is superior to PTH radioimmunoassay.

However, in the final analysis, definitive diagnosis and therapy rest on surgical identification and removal of adenomatous, hyperplastic parathyroid tissue.

In addition to the studies discussed, examination of the neck with ultrasound helps identify small parathyroid lesions, except in the mediastinal area. Mediastinal parathyroid, however, lesions may be detected by CT scan. If a lesion is found, thyroid arteriography may confirm the diagnosis.

Parathyroid disorders result in abnormal secretion of or response to PTH. These disorders may be revealed by only subtle physical and psychologic signs, and they may mimic a variety of other conditions. High or low serum levels of calcium may be the only indication of abnormality. Severe hypercalcemia, a medical emergency, requires saline diuresis to speed calcium excretion.

Calcium gluconate may be needed to treat tetany and prevent the seizures of acute hypoparathyroidism. In this disease, the physical examination may reveal the pathology more accurately than the serum calcium level.

ADRENAL GLANDS

The adrenal glands lie on the superior pole of the kidneys and weigh about 4 to 5 g each. They are composed of two morphologically and physiologically distinct parts: an outer cortex and an inner medulla. The cortex constitutes 90 percent of the glands and is divided into three distinct cellular zones: the zona glomerulosa, a thin outer layer making up about 15 percent of the cortex and secreting aldosterone, which is under angiotensin stimulation amineralocorticoid; the zona fasciculata, or middle layer, constituting about 75 percent of the cortex; and the zona reticularis, constituting the rest. The last two zones secrete glutocorticoids and androgen precursors, respectively.

Many endocrine glands are studied in relation to the aging process, and studies of adrenal function are second only to those of the gonads. The senescent adrenal gland exhibits morphologic alterations including increased pigment deposition and increased collagen content, as well as vascular dilatation and hemorrhage in both the cortex and the medulla. The adrenal response to ACTH stimulus decreases slightly with age. Thyroid hormone and gonadal steroids tend to temper the catabolic action of cortisol. This represents a physiologic response to decreased body needs for cortisol. Although ACTH stimulus of the adrenal decreases only slightly with age, the rate of adrenal corticoid secretion decreases by 30 percent throughout adult life.

Plasma cortisol concentration appears to remain in the same range at all ages, but the secretion rate decreases by about 30 percent in the aged. This is probably due to a decrease in the metabolic clearance of the products of age-related enzymatic reactions and hepatic steroid matabolism. Urinary 17-hydroxysteroids and urinary 17-ketosteroids show an age-related decrease. This indicates the decreasing production of adrenal androgens such as androsterone and dchydroepiandrosterone with advancing age.

Aldosterone secretion in response to stress decreases with normal aging. In the geriatric patient, aldosterone secretion in response to sodium restriction and upright posture is decreased, as is the response of plasma renin activity to the same stimuli. A decrease in circulating renin, with parallel lowering of plasma aldosterone concentrations, has been seen with age. In addition, low renin essential hypertension has been described more commonly in older than in younger adults, and the syndrome of hyporeninemic hypoaldosteronism has been described almost exclusively in patients over 50 years of age.

In 1942 Albright introduced the concept of *adrenopause,* to which he attributed the observable age-related decrease in adrenal hormone production. Dehydroepiandrosterone sulfate (DHEA-S) and dehydroepiandrosterone (DHEA), the main adrenal androgens, are produced almost entirely (95 and 75 percent, respectively) in the adrenal gland. In the postmenopausal patient, the concentration of DHEA-S decreases by 20 percent and that of DHEA by 40 percent. Estrogen replacement produces a twofold increase in DHEA-S values; therefore, the diminished concentrations are probably due to estrogen deprivation.

Adrenal hypersecretion can result in Cushing's syndrome, hyperaldosteronism, or virilization. Adrenal cortical insufficiency, also known as *Addison's disease,* occurs in primary and secondary forms. A patient with adrenal insufficiency requires lifelong hormone replacement and should wear a medical alert bracelet. This is particularly important in the elderly. Acute adrenal insufficiency constitutes an adrenal crisis, a medical emergency requiring rapid glucocorticoid and saline solution administration.

Adrenal cortical disease is uncommon in elderly patients. The clinical findings characteristic of hypoadrenolcorticism are unchanged over the life span. Adrenal cortical replacement doses for the treatment of Addison's disease are also unaltered in older patients.

Most cases of Addison's disease are thought to be due to an autoimmune phenomenon. In many of these cases antibodies are produced against other endocrine gland secretions, so that ovarian or thyroid failure may accompany Addison's disease. When evaluating a patient whose symptoms or signs are suggestive of adrenal failure, it is important to remember the normal sluggish adrenal response to ACTH and to extend the usual stimulation studies accordingly. If the diagnosis of Addison's disease is established, replacement therapy with cortisone acetate or its equivalent should be carried out. Mineralcorticoids may also be needed. Other endocrine systems should also be evaluated, since there may be multiple gland failure from the autoimmune involvement.

Cushing's syndrome may occur in elderly patients. The disorder may be due to loss of the hypothalamic–pituitary regulatory mechanism or ACTH secretion; pituitary tumor; adrenal tumor; nonendocrine tumors that produce an ACTH-like substance; or nonendocrine tumors such as neoplastic lesions of the bronchi, gallbladder, and thymus, which produce a substance that acts on the hypothalamus to stimulate the ACTH-releasing factor.

The diagnosis is made by finding clinical signs of cortisol excess, along with laboratory evidence of cortisol hypersecretion. Elevated ketogenic urinary steroids that are not suppressed with large doses of dexamethasone are characteristic of adrenal or extraadrenal tumors.

Therapy depends upon the cause of the disease and consists of surgically removing the tumor; if bilateral hyperplasia is present, the surgeon performs a bilateral adrenalectomy. Regardless of the etiology of Cushing's disease, adrenal steroid replacement must follow treatment. This is because removal of one adrenal is often associated with hypofunction from suppression of a high level of cortisone in the opposite adrenal, which may persist for a long period of time.

PANCREAS

The pancreas is composed of both endocrine and exocrine tissue. It lies transversely across the posterior abdominal wall in the epigastric and hypochondriac regions of the body. It is about 13-cm long and weighs about 70 g. In its exocrine function, it secretes digestive enzymes via ducts that empty into duodenum.

The endocrine function of the pancreas is carried out by the islets of Langerhans, which are composed of beta, alpha, and delta secretory cells. The beta cells secrete insulin, which directly regulate glucose metabolism and the processes necessary for intermediary metabolism of fats, carbohydrates, and proteins. The alpha cells secrete glucagon, which counters the action of insulin. The delta cells secrete the hormone somatostatin, the function of which is under investigation.

Beta cell degeneration is a normal consequence of aging and carbohydrate tolerance gradually decreases with aging. Although 50 percent of patients 65-years old and older have chemically abnormal responses to the glucose tolerance test, frank diabetes mellitus is clinically evident in only 7 percent.

Diabetes mellitus is the most common endocrine disorder. It afflicts more than 10 million persons and is diagnosed at a rate of approximately 600,000 each year. After heart disease and cancer, diabetes is the third largest cause of death by disease in the United States. Diabetes more than doubles the risk of coronary heart disease and stroke, is associated with an almost 40-fold higher amputation rate, accounts for nearly 20 percent of all patients with end-stage renal disease entering dialysis, and causes most new cases of blindness. Diabetes is not a single disease but a cluster of disorders related to abnormal glucose metabolism.

The term *old-age diabetes* is often used in describing changes that may occur in geriatric patients. The change in glucose tolerance that accompanies normal aging is not dramatic but is of consequence, lest the diagnosis of diabetes mellitus be applied incorrectly to elderly subjects, in whom glucose tolerance differs from that in younger normal subjects. Although changes in glucose tolerance occur with age, the fasting blood sugar level does not rise concomitantly. An elevated fasting blood sugar value, then, indicates the presence of disordered glucose metabolism, regardless of the patient's age.

As the pancreas age, accompanying regressive changes in the islets cells and decreased functional capacity for insulin synthesis and release are sometimes found. All elderly patients will show varying degrees of carbohydrate intolerance when subjected to the usual glucose tolerance test. An aged pancreas can maintain carbohydrate metabolism at normal levels if it is not presented with unusual demands.

Beta cell degeneration is a normal consequence of aging, and carbohydrate tolerance gradually decreases with age. Although 50 percent or more of patients aged 65 or older have chemically abnormal responses to glucose tolerance, frank diabetes is clinically evident in only 7 percent. Increasing age has no apparent effect on peripheral tissue sensitivity to insulin or on the metabolic clearance rate or the secretion rate of insulin.

Physicians can manage elderly patients by outlining proper dietary intake. Hyperglycemic agents and insulin therapy are usually not required. When patients require these forms of therapy, the dosages will be lower than those administered to younger patients. Glucose may be spilled more rapidly in many older persons because of a decrease in renal function. Therefore, blood sugar levels are the only reliable criteria in monitoring glucose control in such patients.

Potential physical findings with diabetes may occur in the cardiovascular system and may include hypo- or hypertension, tachycardia, and other cardiac dysrhythmias, as well as hypobulemia. There may be respiratory problems such as abnormal breathing sounds, which are decreased, or the rhythm may be increased under stress, or there may be dyspnea. Renal problems may occur, and urinary output may be characterized by polyuria, anuria, or oligouria. Glucose or acetone is found in the urine, and there is an altered specific gravity. The urine is often infected and, as a result, may be cloudy or malodorous. The central nervous system may be affected, and there may be headache, drowsiness, nervousness, depression, anxiety, stupor, or coma. Sensorimotor disturbances may be present and there may be depressed muscle tone, depressed reflexes, blurred vision, or altered responses to stimuli. The skin, head, and neck may be affected. The skin may appear to be dry, flaky, or shiny; there may be hair loss, thickened toenails, or brown spots on the skin of the lower extremities. Since infection is often present, the lymph nodes may be enlarged. There may be irritation at the site of injections, xanthomas may be present.

Diabetes mellitus obviously affects nearly every body system. The etiology of type 1 diabetes is thought to involve genes, viruses, or autoimmunity. The etiology of type 2 diabetes is thought to be predominantly hereditary. It is known that the hyperglycemia and hyperlipidemia secondary to a diabetic state can cause vascular diseases such as microangiopathy and macroangiopathy.

Home blood glucose monitoring and a variant of hemoglobin A, known as HbA_{1c} ($HgbA_{1c}$) testing illustrate the advances made in monitoring blood glucose levels. New developments have also occurred in insulin therapy, such as genetically engineered human insulin and insulin infusion pumps.

Since the elderly are inclined to have a glucose imbalance, it is important to check for this problem and very important to educate the patient. This is essential to ensure compliance with the diabetic treatment regimen.

ADRENAL MEDULLA

The medulla of the adrenal gland is composed mostly of chromatin cells and acts as a functional extension of the sympathetic nervous system. After sympathetic stimulation, the medulla secretes catecholamines, primarily epinephrine and norepinephrine; their effects on target organs persist about 10 times longer than those of direct nervous stimulation. Both catecholamines work with the sympathetic nervous system to produce a physiologic response to stress—the fight-or-flight response—that increases heart rate, increases cardiac output, dilates the pupils, constricts blood vessels in the skin, elevates serum glucose and fatty acid levels, and induces an aroused mental state.

Neuroendocrinologic Controls—Catecholamines

Recent work, mostly from animal studies, suggests that there is an interplay between hormones and brain catecholamines or other hormonally sensitive substances that modulate the aging process. Work in progress suggests that a deficiency of catecholamines in certain brain regions underlies the cessation of cyclic gonadotropin production. It has long been known that drugs that alter brain catecholamines also modify pituitary hormone secretion. Plasma norepinephrine levels increase throughout adult life, primarily as a result of decreased catecholamine clearance. Increases of a magnitude which could have a biologic risk in a cardiovascular system or may increase sympathetic nervous system tone could cause a serious problem. Fortunately, it has been shown that the presence of catecholamine-responsive enzymes indicates a decreased sensitivity of monoamine oxidase (MAO) to norepinephrine in cells from elderly subjects. This may provide a protective mechanism for the vascular systems of the aged. It may be concluded that aging involves a hyperadrenergic state. However, there are no hard data to support this statement.

POSTERIOR PITUITARY

The posterior pituitary does not secrete hormones, but upon proper hypothalamic stimulation oxytocin and antidiuretic hormone (ADH) are released from their axonic end bulbs, found in the posterior pituitary.

Oxytocin is present in the male but it has no known function. In the female, oxytocin exerts its effect primarily during labor and lactation.

ADH, also known as *vasopressin* regulates fluid balance by making the collecting ducts and distal renal tubules more permeable to water. Osmoreceptor cells in the hypothalamus control the secretion of ADH into the circulation. In a dehydrated patient, the osmolality of extracellular fluid increases, drawing water across an osmotic gradient from body cells. As a result, the cell volume of osmoreceptors decreases, causing them to stimulate release of the ADH. Conversely, excessive circulating water reduces extracellular fluid osmolality, and water flows into the body's cells. This increases receptor cell volume and inhibits ADH release.

Antidiuretic Hormone

Studies have shown that osmoreceptor sensitivity is enhanced over the life span and secretion of ADH is increased in elderly subjects in order to maintain normal plasma osmolality. ADH is produced primarily in the supraoptic and paraventricular nuclei of the hypothalamus and is released from the posterior lobe of the pituitary. Circulating ADH concentrations in the elderly are normal or increased, presumably because of the decreased sensitivity of the distal renal tubule. This may explain the impaired urine-concentrating ability seen in elderly patients. Urine-diluting ability is relatively intact in older subjects.

GROWTH HORMONE (GH)

GH secretion is decreased in the aged. This decrease is seen and is maintained in the face of stress and even when there is dopaminergic stimulation. A biologic action of GH is mediated by proteins termed *somatomedins.* The level of GH falls throughout life in normal subjects. The overall effect of this decrease is not known, but it may contribute to the loss of bone mass.

ANTERIOR PITUITARY GLAND

The pituitary gland is as known as the *hypophysis.* It is about 1 cm in diameter and weighs about 0.5 to 0.7 g. It lies in a cavity of bone at the base of the skull (the sella turcica) and is connected to the hypothalamus by the pituitary stalk. The pituitary has two distinct parts: an anterior lobe (adenohypophysis) and a posterior lobe (neurohypophysis). The anterior lobe constitutes most of the gland.

As the pituitary ages, various changes occur. Interstitial fibrosis occurs and adenomas form. The weight of the pituitary progressively decreases after age 50, and is reduced as much as 20 percent by the ninth decade of life. The blood supply to the pituitary is also reduced. However, even though the pituitary undergoes interstitial fibrosis and a decrease in its blood supply, it continues to maintain a decreased content of GH, but a relatively normal ACTH, TSH, and prolactin.

Autopsy reports show that 25 percent of pituitaries contain adenomas, most of which are clinically inapparent pituitary microadenomas. Despite the presence of adenomas, however, hypersecretion syndromes originating in later life are very rare.

Decreased responsiveness of the pituitary to physiologic stimuli has been noted. The aging pituitary fails to respond to stress with as rapid an increase in ACTH synthesis or release as the younger organ. It should be noted that a slower response to stimuli is very important in evaluating endocrine disorders in elderly patients. Therefore, sluggish responses to the usual stimulation tests of endocrine organ function should be considered normal and interpreted properly. The slower response may be a protective one, since with aging of target tissues, too rapid a change in the hormonal environment could be disastrous. A reduction in the sensitivity of the pituitary to hypothalamic-releasing factors explains the decrease in circulating GH concentrations and the diminished TSH response to thyrotropin-releasing hormone (TRH) infusion in the elderly.

Aging affects virtually every physiologic aspect of life, certain ones, such as hormone synthesis and release, seem little affected. Some studies indicate elevated gonadotropin secretion up to the sixth or seventh decade.

There is a modest diminution in circulating concentrations of GH with advancing age, despite the maintenance of normal pituitary content. In the elderly, GH surges such as those occurring in the younger patient during deep sleep are absent. The GH response to hypoglycemia or arginine infusion is also blunted. About 20 percent of geriatric patients have a greatly diminished GH response to insulin-induced hypoglycemia. This decreased response is probably a normal sequela of pituitary aging and does not denote decreased GH reserve secondary to a neoplastic or degenerative process.

Little is known about ACTH and prolactin levels in older persons. Increasing age does not appear to alter the hormone level appreciably, and presumptive evidence of continued TSH activity is present, as thyroid hormone values remain unchanged. Plasma TSH values remain relatively constant throughout life. Unlike the reaction in men, the TSH response to TRH infusion in elderly women is characteristically normal.

GASTROINTESTINAL MUCOSA

The gastrointestinal hormones are secreted into the bloodstream by endocrine cells scattered throughout the wall of the stomach and intestines rather than clustered in discrete structures or glands. These endocrine cells contain secretory granules that respond to stimuli such as ingested food, blood factors, or neural stimulation.

The known gastrointestinal hormones are gastrin, secretin, and cholecystokinin, as well as several others that have been less well studied. Gastrin, found in the antrum in the first part of the duodenum, stimulates the release of gastric acid and pepsin and promotes the growth of acid-secreting mucosa. Secretin and cholecystokinin are distributed throughout the small bowel. Both hormones act on pancreatic acinar cells, promoting secretion of bicarbonate and water. Cholecystokinin also stimulates pancreatic enzyme secretion and gallbladder contraction.

As persons age, they are less inclined to absorb calcium from the intestine and may develop a lactose imbalance. The motility of the bowel is decreased, and the aging patient has more gastrointestinal disorders than the younger person.

OVARY

The contrast between the premenopausal and the postmenopausal ovary is striking. Whereas the normal premenopausal ovary measures 3.5 × 2 × 1.5 cm the menopausal ovary tends to atrophy and shrink when the graafian follicles and ova disappear. The tunica albugenia becomes very dense and causes the surface of the ovary to become scarred and shrunken. The cortex is marked by increased thinning, as well as numerous corpora fibrosa and corpora albugenia with areas of dense fibrosis and hyalinization. The ovary shows varying degrees of avascularity. Eventually the ovary becomes an inert residue that consists of connective tissue and clings to the posterior leaf of the broad ligament. Its pink color becomes pure white. It shrinks to $2 \times 1.5 \times 0.5$ cm, and in some cases may be as small as $1.5 \times 0.75 \times 0.5$ cm. Its wrinkled surface resembles the gyri and sulci of the cerebrum. At this point it cannot be palpated.

LYSIDS IN THE AGING

Cholesterol and triglyceride concentrations increase with age, and there is an augmented risk of coronary disease associated with cholesterol concentrations greater than 120 to 250 mg/dl. An increase in cholesterol values is associated with increased concentrations of low-density lipoprotein cholesterol (LDL-C), whereas a rise in triglyceride values is associated with increased concentrations of very-low-density lipoprotein cholesterol (VLDL-C). High-density lipoprotein cholesterol (HDL-C), which consists of about 20 percent of the total cholesterol, seems to protect against the development of atherosclerosis. It has been shown that a low HDL-C concentration is a more potent risk factor than a high concentration of LDL-C.

It is interesting that HDL concentrations are decreased with smoking and increased with regular exercise or alcohol intake. Recently, it has been shown that the addition of a nonandrogenic progestational agent such as medroxyprogesterone (Provera) augments the effect of estrogen in increasing the HDL-C level.

SUMMARY

The endocrine system acts together with the nervous system to maintain homeostasis. The endocrine glands include the pituitary, thyroid, parathyroid, adrenals, islet cells of the pancreas, and ovaries. The endocrine glands release hormones directly into the bloodstream. A hormone is a potent chemical messenger that exerts a physiologic effect on specific target cells and tissues. Excessive or diminished hormone secretion cause most endocrine disorders.

A volume of research has shown that the endocrine system ages in much the same way as the remainder of the body. In some instances, it demonstrates a remarkable ability to adjust to the changing needs of an older person. Frequently, adaptive endocrine changes are both helpful and deleterious. Female reproductive capacity ceases when childbearing is dangerous to the cardiovascular and renal systems, but cessation of gonadal steroid production leads to distressing symptoms and frequently disabling metabolic sequelae. Although there is a striking variation in the susceptibility of individuals to atherosclerosis, one of the most important factors is the concentration of circulating lipids.

When target tissues age, a less intense response to stress results, preventing an overload of the target organ. This decreased response unfortunately leads frequently to a less than optimal endocrine milieu. This paradox presents considerable problems in both diagnosis and therapy. Correcting a hormone lack in one system may cause a temporary imbalance in another system. A control feedback mechanism is necessary for the optimal functioning of the endocrine system. More life-threatening symptoms may result from the therapy than from the disease if one is not careful to allow sufficient time for sluggish responses to catch up with changing hormone levels. The gynecologist who is dealing with geriatric patients must consider the endocrine system in its entirety. Focusing only on one system may produce unfavorable results.

Since elderly persons with hormone imbalances are often thought to have organic brain disease, it is important to make an accurate diagnosis. Diagnostic studies are essential in determining endocrine dysfunction. Radioimmunoassay techniques have made direct measurement of most hormones possible. Provocative tests assess glandular responsiveness to stimuli. It is important for the gynecologist caring for the perimenopausal and geriatric patient to know about these tests and be able to interpret them.

The pituitary gland exhibits age-related changes. After the age of 50, the weight of the pituitary decreases significantly, and its size decreases by as much as 20 percent by the ninth decade of life. Interstitial fibrosis and adenoma form. Although it has been reported that 25 percent of the pituitaries examined at autopsy contain adenomas, there are practically no hypersecretion syndromes originating in the aging. The blood supply of the pituitary is also reduced measurably after 60 years of age. The aging pituitary fails to respond to stress with as rapid an increase in ACTH or release as happens before the age of 60. This may only be a protective response because too rapid a change in the hormonal environment upon an aging target tissue could be deleterious.

The posterior pituitary also undergoes certain changes. ADH is produced primarily in the supraoptic and paraventricular nuclei of the hypothalamus and is released from the posterior lobe of the pituitary. Although these hypothalamic areas show distinct age-specific cytologic changes, circulating ADH concentrations in the elderly remain normal or are increased, presumably because of decreased sensitivity of the distal renal tubule.

The thyroid decreases in weight and the follicles become smaller and stain less intensely with advancing age. This would appear to be the result of less need by target tissues for thyroid hormone. Because of decreased body mass, the basal metabolic rate of the older patient also decreases; oxygen consumption per unit of body mass does not change. There is a slight decrease in the radioactive iodine uptake in the thyroid gland of the elderly subject. Concentrations of total and free thyroxin are unchanged with age despite a slight decrease in the concentration of thyroid-binding globulin, which may be secondary to diminished serum concentration of estrogen or protein. In persons older than 50 concentrations of triiodothyronine are diminished by 25 to 40 percent. Although the exact reason for the decrease is unclear, diminished peripheral conversion of thyroxin to triiodothyronine is a suspected cause for most of it. In general, the aging patient without intrinsic thyroid disease remains clinically euthyroid and her TSH values remain within the normal range, consistent with adequate thyroid hormone function.

The most striking pathologic change in parathyroid as a result of aging is an increase in the number of eosinophils. The significance of this is unknown because the secretion of parahormone appears little changed. Recent studies show, however, that the sex steroids temper parahormone action on calcium metabolism in bone. With declining sex steroid levels, therefore, normal parahormone levels can lead to demineralization of the skeleton. This explains why the osteoporosis of aging and hyperparathyroidism are radiologically and symptomatically identical.

Many endocrine glands are studied in relation to the aging process, and the studies of the adrenal function are second only to those of the gonads (fibrosis and decreased secretory activity may be demonstrated in sections of the aged adrenal). It has been demonstrated that some decrease in 17 keto and ketogenic steroid production occurs in older individuals, with the former decreasing more than the latter. It has also been shown that the adrenal response to ACTH stimulus decreases with age. The thyroid hormone and the gonadal steroids tend to temper the catabolic action of cortisol, an action that appears to be a physiologic response to decreased body needs for cortisol. The aging adrenal gland exhibits some morphologic alterations, including increased pigment deposition and collagen content, as well as vascular dilation and hemorrhage within both the cortex and medulla. Electron microscopic studies have also revealed mitochondrial fragmentation.

The aging pancreas is often accompanied by regressive changes in the islets cells and a decreased functional capacity for insulin synthesis and release. Beta cell degeneration is a normal consequence of aging, and carbohydrate tolerance gradually decreases with age. Although 50 percent of patients aged 65 years and older have chemically abnormal responses to the glucose tolerance test, frank diabetes mellitus is clinically evident in only 7 percent.

The adrenal medulla is part of the sympathetic nervous system derived from the neuroectoderm. Two catecholamines are present in the adrenal medulla, adrenalin and noradrenalin, in the ratio of about 4:1. These are synthesized from the amino acid thyrosine by the following sequence reaction: thyrosine— dihydroxyphenylalanine (DOPA)— dopamine— noradrenalin— adrenalin. The catecholamines are metabolized by two enzyme mechanisms: the monamine oxydase and the catechol-o-methyl-transferase (COMT). One of the principal metabolites is vanillylmandelic acid (VMA); other metabolites are known collectively as metanephrines. The aging process of the adrenal medulla includes pigment deposition and collagen content, as well as vascular dilation and hemorrhage.

The pineal gland is still poorly understood after decades of research. The pineal gland serves a neuroendocrine function since it responds to neural stimuli rather than hormones secreted by other glands. It is similar to the adrenal medulla in this respect. Although there is evidence that the pineal gland does function in timing puberty in humans, there is no concrete evidence that it serves any function in the aging.

When the primordial germ cells degenerate, two of the three compartments of steroidogenesis, the follicle and corpus luteum, are no longer active, and the ovary's reproductive capacity ceases. The aging ovary presents a typical wrinkled, prunelike appearance and that reveals a characteristic absence of primary follicles on microscopic examination. A follicle will be found occasionally, however, but it does not function and usually does not regress. The third ovarian compartment for steroid synthesis, the stroma, may continue to be active, and hormone production can continue for some time until the latter decades of life. The stroma secretes an androgenic substance that may produce some hirsutism on the upper lip of the aging woman. This androgen can be converted in the peripheral fat into an estrogenic substance.

REFERENCES

Asch, R. H., and R. B. Greenblatt. 1978. The aging ovary: Morphologic and endocrine correlations, in: *Geriatric Endocrinology* (R. B. Greenblatt, ed.), vol. 5, Raven Press; New York, p. 141.

Andres, R., 1971. Aging and diabetes. *Med. Clin. North Am.* 55:835.

Armstrong, D. T., A. K. Goff, and J. H. Dorrington. 1978. Regulation of follicular oestrogen biosynthesis, in: *Ovarian Follicular Development and Function* (A. R. Midgley and W. A. Sadler, eds.), Raven Press, New York, p. 169.

Barber, H. R. K., 1982. *Ovarian Carcinoma: Etiology, Diagnosis and Treatment,* 2nd ed., Masson Publishing USA, New York.

Barber, H. R. K., and E. A. Graber. 1971. The PMPO syndrome (postmenopausal ovary syndrome). *Obstet. Gynecol.* 38:921.

Burrow, G. N., G. Wortzman, N. B. Rewcastle, R. C. Holgate, and K. Kovacs. 1981. Microadenomas of the pituitary and abnormal sellar tomograms in an unselected autopsy series. *N. Engl. J. Med.* 304:156.

Chang, R. J., and Judd, H. L. 1981. The ovary after menopause. *Clin. Obstet. Gynecol.* 24:181.

Davis, F. B., R. S. LaMantia, S. W. Spaulding, R. E. Wehmann, and P. J. Davis. 1984. Estimation of a physiologic replacement dose of levothyroxine in elderly patients with hypothyroidism. *Arch. Intern. Med.* 144:1752.

Davis, P. J., and F. B. Davis. 1974. Hyperthyroidism in patients over the age of 60 years. *Medicine* 53:161.

Davis, P. J., and F. B. Davis. 1982. Management of thyroid disease in the elderly, in: *Drug Treatment in the Elderly* (R. E. Vestal, ed.), ADIS Press, New York.

Dilman, V. M. 1979. Hypothalamic mechanisms of aging and of specific age pathology. V. A model for the mechanism of human specific age pathology and natural death. *Exp. Gerontol.* 14:287.

Grodin, J. M., P. K. Siteri, and P. C. MacDonald. 1973. Source of estrogen production in postmenopausal women. *J. Clin. Endocrinol. Metab.* 36:207.

Heber, D., and R. S. Swerdloff. 1981. Down regulation of pituitary gonadotropin serum in postmenopausal females by continuous GnRH administration. *J. Clin. Endocrinol. Metab.* 52:176.

Ingbar, S. H., and K. A. Woeber. 1981. The thyroid gland, in: *Textbook of Endocrinology* (R. H. Williams, ed.), W. B. Saunders Co., Philadelphia, p. 187.

Judd, H. L. 1976. Hormonal dynamics associated with the menopause. *Clin. Obstet. Gynecol.* 19:775.

Longrope, C., R. Hunter, and C. Franz. 1980. Steroid secretion by the postmenopausal ovary. *Am. J. Obstet. Gynecol* 130:564.

Rakoff, A. E., and K. Nowroozi. 1978. The female climacteric, in: *Geriatric Endocrinology,* vol. 5, (R. B. Greenblatt, ed.), Raven Press, New York, p. 165.

Scholz, D. A., and D. C. Purnell. 1981. Asymptomatic primary hyperparathyroidism: 10 year prospective study. *Mayo Clin. Proc.* 56:473.

Snyder, P. J., and R. D. Utiger. 1972. Thyrotropin response to thyrotropin releasing hormone in normal females over forty. *J. Clin. Endocrinol. Metab.* 34:1096.

Swanson, J. W., J. J. Kelly, Jr., and W. M. McConahey. 1981. Neurologic thyroid dysfunction. *Mayo Clin. Proc.* 56:504.

Vekemans, M., and C. Roby. 1975. Influence of age on serum prolactin levels in women and men. *Br. Med. J.* 4:738.

Vermeulen, A. 1978. The hormonal activity of the postmenopausal ovary. *J. Clin. Endocrinol. Metab.* 42:247.

Vermeulen, A., and L. Verdonck. 1978. Sex hormone concentrations in postmenopausal women. *Clin. Endocrinol.* 9:39.

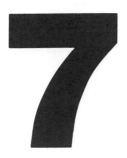

7 **Vulvovaginitis**

INTRODUCTION

The most common vaginitis seen in the postmenopausal and geriatric patient is atrophic vaginitis. It is not uncommon to have this condition complicated by another type of infection. Trichomonas and monilia vaginitis occur at all ages. The relation of vulvovaginal infections in the elderly is based upon the lessened resistance of the genital tract and so these two conditions are fairly common. Adhesive vaginitis, a little mentioned disorder, may also occur. This fibrosis, along with the adherence of adjacent mucosa, may actually close off the upper vagina.

The postmenopausal and geriatric patient can develop a vaginitis of the same type seen during the reproductive years. With current changes in lifestyle and a more liberal approach to their sexuality, women are engaging in intercourse at older ages and with multiple partners. They are therefore candidates for any of the sexually transmitted diseases. This should not be overlooked when evaluating a patient with vaginitis.

ATROPHIC VAGINITIS

In the postmenopausal and geriatric patient, the structural effacement of the vagina becomes manifest. The rugae of the wall gradually disappear, the wall becomes smooth, and the vaginal color fades from the moist, ruddy pink to bluish-red to a pale pink hue. Lubrication diminishes and the vagina loses its elasticity.

The clinical manifestations become pronounced with the withdrawal of estrogen. The vaginal epithelium becomes thin, and the amount of glycogen is decreased. The pH becomes alkaline. The vagina is often reddened, with punctate, hemorrhagic spots throughout the vaginal wall.

Diagnosis

The diagnosis is usually highly suspect in any patient in this geriatric age group who complains of leukorrhea, pruritis, burning, tenderness, and dyspareunia. It is suggested by the history and by evidence of vaginal atrophy on examination. Cytologic smears reveal leukocyts, erythrocytes, bacteria, and basal or intermediate epithelial cells. Cultures usually show a mixture of many organisms and are rarely of value. A wet preparation should be included to exclude an associated vaginal infection.

Trichomonas vaginalis thrives in an alkaline milieu, whereas *Candida albicans* is inhibited. It is important to determine the pH of the vagina.

Treatment

Although estrogen given by mouth is effective, topical administration of a vaginal cream containing estrogen is the treatment of choice. There is a higher local absorption rate. It can cause a reversal of the symptoms within 1 week of treatment. The vaginal tissue begins to thicken and the pruritis disappears. A maintenance dose, usually consisting of a weekly application of the cream, is enough to keep the vagina healthy. It is also in the patient's best interest to suggest that once a week the estrogen cream be applied around the introitus, particularly along the posterior part of the fourchette and introitus. The patient should be advised never to use more than half an applicator of cream. If more cream is applied, it tends to mix with the vaginal secretion and escape from the introitus. This often causes irritation around the entrance to the vagina and on the medial side of the vulvae. In addition it is a waste of the estrogenic cream.

CANDIDIASIS

The etiologic agent of this infection is the yeast (fungi) organism *Candida albicans* or *Monilia. Torulopsis glabrata* is the second most common fungal pathogen found in the human vagina. It is now called *Candida glabrata.* However, in North America, it makes up only 5 percent of the cases of fungal vaginitis. *Candida glabrata* causes a relatively mild inflammation of the mucosa, with no appreciable discharge. The patient may complain of burning.

Clinical Presentation

The infection may be asymptomatic; usually there is a minimal discharge externally, but the patient complains of intense vaginal and vulval itching and soreness. It is interesting to note that small numbers of *Candida* organisms are frequently present in the normal vagina, but their growth is checked by the competitive metabolism of the lactobacilli and corynebacteria, as well as by the specific fungal inhibitory factors they produce. Therefore, many candidal infections are not dependent on introduction from an external source. The organisms are opportunistic, requiring only the lack of competitive inhibition by the normal flora to gain the upper hand. Vulvovaginal candidiasis is rarely a sexually transmitted disease. In more than 85 percent of the cases, the source of the organisms is of endogenous origin. In less than 5 to 10 percent, sexual intercourse is the probable mode of dissemination.

Vulvovaginal candidiasis is a vulvitis rather than a vaginitis. The presence of a characteristic brown discharge should alert one to the probability that the disease is due to *T. vaginalis* and not *C. albicans.* When a discharge indicative of significant concomitant vaginitis is present, it tends to be relatively sparse in quantity and has a characteristic cottage cheese–like appearance. Vaginitis predominating over vulvitis is more characteristic of antibiotic-induced disease. Candida vulvovaginitis presents with pruritis. The discharge is sparse and curd-like (cottage cheese appearance) and has a pH of 4.0 to 4.5. On the potassium hydroxide (KOH) wet mount, branching filaments and blastospheres are seen.

By the use of KOH wet mounts, it is often possible to identify the exact fungus. *C. albicans* shows the presence of both spores (candida) and filaments (hyphae); *T. glabrata* shows only spores, and *Trichophyton* species demonstrate only filamentous forms.

T. glabrata may be a constituent of the biologic flora of the human skin, oral pharynx, genitourinary tract, and gastrointestinal tract. It grows preferentially in the presence of air, and in so doing produces blastospheres rather than pseudo- or ascospores. Certain conditions have been found in association with the pathogenic expression of the organism. These include previous antibiotic therapy, the use of an indwelling intravenous catheter and/or hyperalimentation, radiotherapy, chemotherapy, immunosuppressive therapy including steroids, and diabetes mellitus.

In stubborn, resistant, or recurring cases of candidal vaginitis, many factors may be responsible. Orogenital contact accounts for some of them. In all patients with recurrent infections, diabetes should be suspected and ruled out by appropriate tests. The immune system plays a definite role in candidal infection. Intermittent immune deficiencies can be produced by a variety of factors, including stress. This can be studied by obtaining an immunological profile.

On speculum examination the unique cheesy, yellowish-white discharge is seen, as well as a variable degree of vaginal erythema and swelling. The classic patches of thrush adherent to the mucosa are pathognomonic of *C. albicans* infection, but usually the discharge is more diffuse, with a less dramatic but definitely three-dimensional appearance, confined to the vaginal walls, and moderately adherent. It is relatively thick and dry, and may be scraped off the surface with a speculum blade or Papanicolaou smear spatula. The beefy red color seen on introduction of the speculum usually indicates the diagnosis. In all cases of recurrent and resistant candidal infections, it is important to test for diabetes.

Diagnosis

The Papanicolaou smear examination often reveals *Candida* organisms. However, this condition does not need treatment unless symptoms are present. The diagnosis of candida vaginitis involves the demonstration of yeast by microscopic examination and the testing of vaginal secretions in 10 percent KOH. This preparation will lyse the vaginal epithelial cells, inflammatory leukocytes, and debris. Against this clear background, the branched and budding pseudohyphae of the fungus will stand out clearly. It is important to examine many fields unless hyphae and spores are seen on the first field examination. If plated onto Nickerson's medium, brownish-black colonies will appear. The disadvantage of using Nickerson's medium is that the diagnosis takes at least 48 hours when the patient wants treatment and help immediately.

Treatment

The vagina should first be cleaned with a mucolytic solution. A mouthwash alkalol serves this purpose. After careful cleansing of all the rugal, the application of 1 percent aqueous gentian violet gives rapid relief. It is equally effective against *C. albicans* and *C. glabrata.* It is important to paint every part of the vagina, including the cervix and the vaginal fornices. Gentian violet can also be applied to the vulva to provide rapid relief from itching. The patient must be warned that gentian violet can stain and should be given a perineal pad to protect her clothing. The imidazole drugs are extremely effective in treating *C. albicans.* In resistant cases, the use of oral nystatin (500,000 units) three times a day for 2 weeks may be required. If the medication is not systemically absorbed, it does nothing for the vaginal infection directly. However, by eliminating fungal colonies within the intestine, the inoculum of organisms present on the anal skin after defecation is appreciably reduced. Many women, particularly elderly ones, with candidal vaginitis are not aware that wiping the anus from back to front can carry candidal organisms to the vagina. In some very resistant cases, a 3-month course of oral nystatin three times a day must be given, along with proper instruction about hygiene. Predisposing factors such as diabetes and chronic antibiotic use should be assessed. Weight reduction is useful because of the reduced sugar intake and the eventual improvement in air circulation in the vulval area. Ketozonazole is a potent antifungal drug, given orally and absorbed systemically. However, it is toxic to the liver and should not be used in the treatment of simple vaginal infections.

TRICHOMONAS VAGINALIS

During the reproductive years, the production of glycogen-enriched superficial cells supports the presence of Doderlein's bacilli and keeps the vaginal pH between 4.0 and 5.5. As ovarian function begins to wane, this maturational process is lost. Doderlein's bacilli are lost, and the vaginal pH increases to 6.0 to 8.0. These changes lead to a higher incidence of vaginitis.

Trichomonas vaginalis is probably present in one in five American women who have had intercourse. The causative organisms are flagellated protozoa that may live quietly in the paraurethral glands, and from this nidus of infestation cause overt infection in the susceptible vagina. *T. vaginalis* may also involve the urethra, as well as the periurethral glands. Almost 70 to 80 percent of the male partners of the affected patient harbor this organism; thus, trichomonas should be considered a venereal disease. *T. vaginalis* can survive in tap water as well as in hot tubs, chlorinated swimming pools, and even dilute soap solutions. However, the usual etiologic sequence begins with the deposit of a large inoculum of organisms contained in the buffered alkaline medium of the semen at the time of sexual intercourse. *T. vaginalis* thrives in an alkaline milieu, whereas *C. albicans* is inhibited.

The primary complaint is usually a perfuse watery discharge that varies in color from gray to yellow-green. There is often a characteristic odor. Pruritis may be present but is not as prominent as with candidal infections.

Clinical Presentation

On speculum examination, the discharge often appears frothy. This is due to the numerous small bubbles of carbon dioxide gas formed by the organism. The classic strawberry appearance of the vaginal and cervical epithelium is a rare finding. This appearance is due to small subepithelial abscesses that stand out as bright red granules or islets in the sea of thin discharge.

Diagnosis

A saline wet smear will show numerous multiorganisms that have a ovoid or teardrop shape and move independently of the fluid flow beneath the cover slip. The diagnosis can be made under low-power magnification.

Determination of the pH is one of the most important diagnostic aids. A pH of less than 4.9 effectively excludes *Neisseria gonorrhoeae, Gardnerella vaginalis, Hemophilus influenzae,* and *T. vaginalis.*

The principal organisms associated with an acid pH are *C. albicans* or group A or B hemolytic streptococcus (which usually functions with a member of the Enterobacteriaceae).

A small number of trichomonads survive a vaginal pH of 3.8 to 4.2, appearing as a small, ball-like group of organisms and immobile spheres. This form of *T. vaginalis* has no clinical significance unless the pH is changed.

Treatment

In the past, the standard treatment was the use of a vinegar douche. However, this produces only a transient alteration in vaginal pH. Aci-gel has had some benefit. Monitoring of the vaginal pH may be helpful in following the patient's response. Specific treatment is necessary and metronidazole (Flagyl), 600 to 1000 mg/day for 4 to 7 days, has been the major therapy for this infection. The patient must be aware that occasionally nausea will occur and that no alcohol should be used during the medication period. Recurrent cases require more intensive and longer treatment with metronidazole. Hygiene should be emphasized, and the patient's sexual partner must also be treated.

When the Papanicolaou smear is used as the only diagnostic method for *Trichomonas,* both false-positive and false-negative results occur. The error rate is nearly 50 percent.

GARDNERELLA VAGINALIS

Vaginitis caused by this organism was once designated as *nonspecific vaginitis.* However, through the work of Gardner, it has now been identified as a sexually transmitted disease that produces a characteristic odor often described as "fishy." The odor is probably due to the presence of amines produced by anaerobic bacteria and released under alkaline conditions. The odor is often first noted during coitus, when buffered alkaline semen contacts the amines present in the vaginal pool. The same phenomenon may be noted by the clinician when a *Gardnerella* discharge is mixed with KOH for a wet smear preparation.

Since *G. vaginalis* is a facultative anaerobe, many clinicians question its role as the primary organism in the production of vaginitis.

Clinical Presentation

The discharge is grayish-white and commonly malodorous. Pruritis may also be present. The infection is often associated with an alkaline pH. However, the most common vaginal pH found in the presence of *G. vaginalis* is between 5 and 6.

Diagnosis

The finding of *clue cells* and a gray discharge with a pH of 5 to 6 from a malodorous patient is usually sufficient to make the diagnosis. The clinical presentation is usually without irritative signs or symptoms. There is an amine-like, fishy odor and a white-gray, frequently frothy or foamy discharge with a pH of 5.0 to 5.5. Many bacterial clue cells, and little evidence of an inflammatory response is seen in the classical *Gardnerella* vulvovaginitis.

Treatment

Metronidazole, 500 mg, twice daily for 1 week, is usually sufficient to control the infection. Ampicillin, 500 mg, every 6 hours for a week, has also been used successfully in controlling *G. vaginalis.* Since it is very sensitive to KOH, a dilute solution of KOH as a douche is often very useful.

TRAUMATIC VAGINITIS

Traumatic vaginitis is usually the result of injury, chemical irritation, or the use of a variety of pessaries to correct a prolapse.

Treatment

Vaginitis secondary to the use of pessaries can be quickly corrected by removing the pessary and starting the patient on a vaginal cream. Since there is infection and atrophy combined, it is useful to alternate a sulfa cream (unless the patient has an allergy to sulfa drugs) with an estrogen cream. The patient usually responds quickly, and within 2 weeks the pessary can be reinserted. From this point on, it is important for the patient to insert estrogen cream at least once a week to keep the vagina healthy and make it resistant to the trauma from the pessary.

MISCELLANEOUS CONDITIONS

The new lifestyle adopted not only by women in the reproductive years but also in the postmenopausal and geriatric periods has increased the number of sexually transmitted diseases that heretofore were rarely seen in these age groups.

Vulvar and vaginal warts are now seen with increasing frequency among postmenopausal patients. The human papilloma virus (HPV) causes condylomata acuminata. The diagnosis is usually made on the basis of the characteristic appearance of the condylomata. However, before treatment is started, the patient should have a biopsy to rule out a more serious condition. Condyloma acuminata are associated with increasing frequency with vulvar carcinoma-in-situ, and occur in up to 31 percent of these cases. Any form of cauterization is usually effective. Laser therapy is particularly useful in the management of vaginal condylomata.

Herpes Simplex

Herpes genitalis is a widespread venereal disease. Most cases that occur on the vulva, in the vagina, and in the cervix are of the herpes virus hominis type 2. Heretofore, this lesion was almost never found in the postmenopausal patient. However, it is now seen occasionally in both postmenopausal and geriatric patients.

The clinical presentation is usually the appearance of a small, blister-like lesion that occurs approximately 3 to 7 days after intercourse. The symptoms consist of burning, itching, hyperesthesia, and occasionally pain. Lymphadenopathy is almost always present. The vesicles usually rupture rapidly and lead to a small ulcer formation. Occasionally they coalesce, forming a bulla with a fairly large ulceration.

The diagnosis should be suspected in the presence of superficial ulceration of the vaginal tissue. The Papanicolaou smear is often able to aid in the accurate diagnosis of a herpes infection. The virus may be recovered by rubbing the base of the ulcer with a cotton swab and culturing it in Eagle's medium containing 5 percent fetal calf serum.

With the use of acyclovir, an antiviral drug, the symptoms can usually be rapidly alleviated. Since the virus often travels along nerves, application of the local ointment is not always effective. Patients who appear ill, with elevated temperature, marked tenderness of the nodes, and large lesions should be treated with acyclovir by mouth. Again, this drug may not be curative, but it relieves the symptoms and reduces the systemic reactions. Sitz baths, witch hazel, wet dressings, analgesics, and ice bags may offer some symptomatic relief.

Chlamydia Trachomatis

Chlamydia trachomatis infection has reached epidemic proportions in the United States. Women who are sexually active at any age, particularly if they have more than one partner, often harbor a chlamydia infection.

On inspection of the vagina and cervix, there may be an erosion or a follicular inflammation. There is often a thick discharge around the cervix. Microabscesses and loss of epithelium are typical of severe infection. Although chlamydia is a bacterium, it acts very much like a virus. It can be accompanied by systemic reactions. Parahepatitis may occur with this infection, as with gonorrhea; typically there is acute pain in the right upper quadrant. These patients are often diagnosed as having cholecystitis or pancreatitis.

The treatment is tetracycline as the drug of first choice.

SUMMARY

The postmenopausal and geriatric patient can develop a vaginitis of the same type seen during the reproductive years. With current changes in lifestyle and a more liberal approach to their sexuality, women are engaging in intercourse at older ages and with multiple partners. They are therefore candidates for any of the sexually transmitted diseases. This should not be overlooked when evaluating a patient with vaginitis.

The patient should be taught vulvar hygiene. Some organisms do well on dry surfaces, while others require moist conditions. The quantitative microbiology of the vulva depends upon these factors. Diphtheroids, *Staphylococcus aureus,* and micrococci abound in numbers that exceed the rates known for other sites. Yeasts and gram-negative rods are also present in significant quantities. For these reasons, the vulva requires special hygienic attention, both for routine purposes and during episodes of disease, and should be kept as dry as possible. Obese women find it difficult to carry out good vulvar hygiene. The geriatric patient, in addition, often has stress incontinence, which results in a diaper rash. Rinsing with clear water after voiding, the use of corn starch during the day, and the avoidance of tight-fitting underclothing during the day and at night can do much to avoid many of the simple skin irritations caused by lack of air circulation and constant moisture. When thorough drying is essential, the patient may lie down on the bed, floor, or couch, with the heels together and the knees drawn up so that the vulva is exposed. A small fan or a portable hair dryer on a cool setting will serve to dry the vulva.

Nonabsorbent materials act to keep the vulva moist and the vaginal irritations in more or less continuous contact with the vulva surface. The patient should wear cotton underclothing instead of rayon or nylon. White underclothing is preferred because some dyes cause irritation. Detergents contain arsenicals that may act as topical irritants. The patient should use baby soap or Neutrogena. The underclothes should be washed in pure soap solution and carefully rinsed. Vaginal deodorants, perfumed soaps, and hygiene sprays serve absolutely no physiologic purpose. In addition, they may produce sensitivity reactions. When irritation of the vulva has resulted from the use of these materials, plain mineral oil should be used as a vulvar cleanser for a while until the irritation subsides.

REFERENCES

Balsdon, M. J. 1981. A comparison of miconazole-coated tampons with clotrimazole vaginal tablets in the treatment of vaginal candidosis. *Br. J. Venereal Dis.* 57:275.

Gardner, H. L., and C. D. Dukes. 1955. *Haemophilus vaginalis* vaginitis. *Am. J. Obstet. Gynecol.* 69:962.

Hafez, E. S. E., and T. N. Evans. 1978. *The Human Vagina.* North-Holland Publishing Co., Amsterdam.

Hare, M. J., D. Taylor-Robinson, and P. Cooper. 1982. Evidence for an association between *Chlamydia trachomatis* and cervical intraepithelial neoplasia. *Br. J. Obstet. Gynecol.* 89:489.

Hughes, D., and T. Kriedman. 1984. Treatment of vulvovaginal candidiasis with 500 mg vaginal table of clotrimazole. *Clin. Ther.* 6:662.

Kuo, C. C., S. P. Wang, and J. T. Grayson. 1977. Antimicrobial activity of several antibiotics and a sulfonamide against *Chlamydia trachomatis* organism in cell culture. *Antimicrobial Agents Chemother.* 12:80.

Ledger, W. J., and S. S. Witkin. 1985. Update on chronic vaginal candidiasis. *Perspectives Problems Obstet. Gynecol.* 3:6.

McLellan, R., M. R. Spence, M. Brockman, et al. 1982. The clinical diagnosis of trichomonas. *Obstet. Gynecol.* 60:30.

Roy, M., A. Meisels, M. Fortier, M., et al. 1981. Vaginal condylomata; A human papillomavirus infection. *Clin. Obstet. Gynecol.* 24:461.

Saral, R., et al. 1981. Acyclovir prophylaxis of herpes simplex virus infections: A randomized double-blind controlled trial in bone marrow transplant recipients. *N. Engl. J. Med.* 305:63.

Sobel, J. 1984. Vulvovaginal candidiasis—what we do and do not know. *Ann. Intern. Med.* 101:390.

Stamm, W. E., K. F. Wagner, R. Amsel, et al. 1980. Causes of the acute urethral syndrome in women. *N. Engl. J. Med.* 303:409.

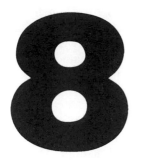

8

Disorders of Pelvic Support

INTRODUCTION: MORPHOLOGY OF THE PELVIC FLOOR

One of the characteristics that distinguishes humans from lower animals and other primates is that they walk upright on two legs. This trait has been identified with some of the marked progress that humans have made. On the other hand, it may have given rise to some of the disorders of pelvic support.

In reviewing the morphology of the pelvic floor, it must be noted that in fishes there is a cartilaginous bar placed transversely in front of the cloaca, and the pelvic floor occurs in its most primitive form. There are two muscular strands that pass from the tail muscles, encircle the cloaca, and are then inserted into the pelvic plate. These strands represent an attempt to form a pelvic floor. In the amphibians, there is progress in that the pelvic plate fuses with the lower ends of the vertebral column, forming a sacroiliac union. The caudopelvic strands are separated from the lateral muscles of the trunk and form distinct muscles. In the reptiles, evolution continues with the formation of an ischium and a pubis. Some reptiles have a definite symphysis. The pelvis is connected with the sacrum either by a mobile joint or by a bony union. It would appear that the conditions found in fish, amphibians, and reptiles suggest an increasing need for the production of a varying internal visceral pressure that is necessary not only for the functioning of the posterior end of the body but also for the repeated act of expiration and as an accessory circulatory mechanism. Among these three groups, there has been a gradual evolution of the bony pelvis and its muscular floor.

In quadruped mammals that walk with the body approximately horizontal, the pelvic floor is formed by the pubis. The pelvic outlet is guarded by the caudal muscles and lies at right angles to the bony pelvic floor. Thus, variations in intraabdominal pressure are countered by the pelvic musculature, while the weight of the pelvic organs is sustained by a bony shelf. The action of caudal muscles in lower animals moves the tail but also, by their contraction, increases intraabdominal pressure and closes sphincters.

The caudal muscles in quadrupeds that walk with the body horizontal consist of the pubococcygeus, the iliococcygeus and the ischiococcygeus. All of these muscles are inserted into the tail of the coccyx, and while the pubococcygeus and iliococcygeus are depressors of the tail, the ischiococcygeus is the tail wagger or lateral flexor.

When mammals assumed the upright position, these caudal muscles now had other duties to perform. They support the pelvic viscera, since the bony shelf that is the pubis symphysis, which was largely responsible for this important function when the body was horizontal, is now part of the abdominal wall. The pelvic floor is formed by the caudal muscles that previously wagged the tail. These muscles must now support the pelvic viscera, for this axial rotation has placed the pelvic organs in a precarious position. Not only gravity but especially changes in intraabdominal pressure tend to cause them to herniate through the gaps in the pelvic diaphragm.

The pubococcygeus and ischiococcygeus retain their primitive origins, but the iliococcygeus loses its attachment to the pelvic brim and gains its new origin from the parietal layer of the pelvic fascia on the lateral pelvic wall at the arcus tendineus. The caudal muscles gain extensive new insertions into the pelvic floor while still maintaining their primitive insertion into the coccyx. The pelvic floor is composed of the pubococcygeus, the iliococcygeus, and the ischiococcygeus. The pubococcygeus is the most important component of the pelvic floor and the best developed. It is a single, centrally situated muscle that arises from the pelvic aspect of the body of the pubis and from the part of the white line of the pelvic fascia that lies in front of the obturator canal. From this origin on either side of the body, its fibers swing backward and form three bands. The most medial fibers skirt the urethra, blending with its intrinsic muscular coat. They then form a U-shaped loop around the vagina and are inserted into its lateral and posterior walls and into the central point of the perineum. These fibers of the pubococcygeus constitute the pubovaginalis and can be plainly felt to contract per vaginum.

The pelvic floor helps to maintain intraabdominal pressure. In addition, during labor, it is possible to cause medial rotation of the presenting part and to direct it downward and forward along the birth canal. The pubococcygeus, which is the best developed of the pelvic floor muscles, lies in the midline and therefore is very vulnerable during parturition. It is this part of the pelvic floor that is perforated by the urethra and vagina at the hiatus urogenitalis and by the rectum at the hiatus rectus. It is evident that tearing or even overstretching of the pubococcygeus muscle may so weaken the visceral supports that prolapse of one or more organs may occur. When the presenting part reaches a certain point during the second stage of labor, the muscular mass forming the central point of the perineum becomes markedly attenuated and bulges downward, and the levator ani is drawn up over the advancing head. Failure of the levator ani to relax at the crucial moment may result in extensive damage to the perineal floor. This may not become apparent until the perimenopausal, postmenopausal, or geriatric age has been reached. It must be reemphasized that even though the levator ani may not have been torn, it is always widely dilated and stretched at childbirth.

GENITOURINARY SYSTEM

The genital and urinary systems are intimately related both embryologically and anatomically. Therefore, it is difficult to discuss one without discussing the other. As an example, a cystocele or prolapse of the uterus may also be complicated by a rectocele and/or enterocele.

It is accepted that the support of the pelvic structures depends on the endopelvic fascia, the uterosacral and cardinal ligaments, and the levator muscle. This intact musculofascial system, with its attachments to the vaginal fornices in the upper two-thirds of the lateral vagina, provides a well-supported vaginal tube, which in turn is the most important supporting structure for the uterus and vaginal wall. In uterovaginal prolapse, there is damage to or weakness of the structures that support the pelvic organs, so that some of these organs descend from their normal position and finally herniate through the vaginal opening.

PELVIC MUSCLES, LIGAMENTS, AND FASCIA

Perineum (Fig. 8-1)

The perineum is bounded by the levator ani above, by the vulva and anus below, and by the pubic outlet (subpubic angle, ischiopubic rami, ischiotuberosities, sacrotuberous ligaments, and coccyx) laterally. It is divided into a urogenital triangle anteriorly and an anal triangle posteriorly. There is a superficial fascia of fat and a deeper membranous fascia (Colles') that extends over the pubis as the fascia of Scarpa.

The muscles of the perineum consist of the following: The ischiocavernosus compresses the crus of the clitoris during sexual excitement to produce erection by venous congestion. The bulbocavernosus conceals the vestibular bulb and Bartholin's glands. Its function is to stretch the vaginal orifice during coitus. The transverse perinel superficialis is a feeble muscle

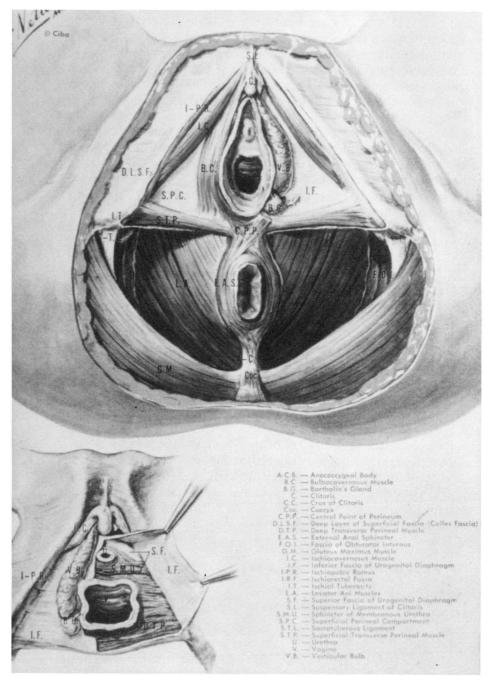

Figure 8-1. The female perineum and the urogenital diaphragm.

that helps to fix the perineal body. The sphincter ani externus normally is in a state of contraction to keep the anus closed. It also helps to fix the perineal body.

The perineal body is a fibromuscular structure between the anus and the vagina with attachments to eight muscles: (1) the sphincter ani, (2) one bulbospongiosus, (3) two transverse perinei superficialis, (4) two transverse perinei profundi, and (5) two levator ani muscles.

This area is the one gynecologists refer to when they talk about the perineum. If it is damaged during parturition and not properly repaired and healed, it will not function properly and the efficiency of the whole pelvic diaphragm may be impaired.

Urogenital Triangle

The urogenital triangle contains the termination of the vagina and urethra, the crura of the clitoris surrounded by ischiocavernosus muscles, the vestibule surrounded by the bulbocavernosus muscles, Bartholin's glands, the urogenital diaphragm, and the superficial and deep perineal pouches.

Urogenital Diaphragm (Triangular Ligament)

The urogenital diaphragm is a sheath of muscles encased between two triangular fascial membranes. The muscle is formed by the deep transverse perineal muscle and fibers from the sphincter urethra. The superior layer is the thin fascia bridging the gap between the anterior portions of the levator ani. The inferior fascia layer is tough and fibrous. The space between the fasciae is sometimes called the *deep perineal pouch.*

Superficial Perineal Pouch

This is a potential space between the inferior fascia of the urogenital diaphragm and the fascia of Colles'. It contains Bartholin's glands and superficial transverse perineal muscles.

Deep Perineal Pouch

This is a potential space between the two fascial layers of the urogenital diaphragm. It contains the membranous urethra surrounded by the external sphincter and deep transverse perineal muscles.

Levator Ani Muscles (Pelvic Diaphragm) (Fig. 8-2)

The pelvic diaphragm consists of the levator ani and coccygeus muscles. The obturator internus and piriformis muscles are also found in the pelvis but are not part of the pelvic diaphragm.

The levator ani arises from the back of the pubis, the obturator fascia (by a tendinous arch or white line), and the ischial spine. The fibers pass back and medial to be inserted into the vaginal wall, the perineal body, the anal wall, the anal coccygeal raphe, and the coccygeus. The nerve supply is from the third and fourth sacral nerves.

The most medial portion of the levator ani, the pubococcygeus, inserts in front of the rectum. The next portion is the puborectalis, which inserts into the rectum and the first of the raphes behind the rectum. The most posterior portion is the iliococcygeus, which inserts into the anococcygeal raphe and the coccyx.

The levator ani muscles form the funnel-shaped pelvic diaphragm. Contractions of the abdominal wall, as in straining or coughing, relax the levator ani muscles, diminishing the angle between the rectum and the anus.

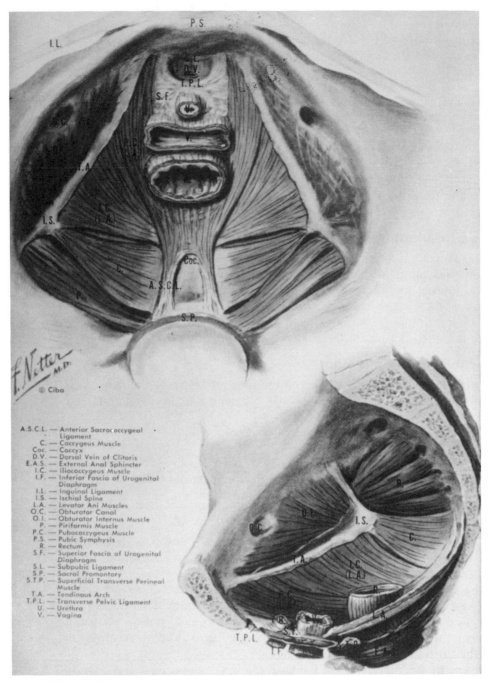

A.S.C.L. — Anterior Sacrococcygeal
      Ligament
   C. — Coccygeus Muscle
Coc. — Coccyx
D.V. — Dorsal Vein of Clitoris
E.A.S. — External Anal Sphincter
I.C. — Iliococcygeus Muscle
I.F. — Inferior Fascia of Urogenital
      Diaphragm
I.L. — Inguinal Ligament
I.S. — Ischial Spine
L.A. — Levator Ani Muscles
O.C. — Obturator Canal
O.I. — Obturator Internus Muscle
P. — Piriformis Muscle
P.C. — Pubococcygeus Muscle
P.S. — Pubic Symphysis
R. — Rectum
S.F. — Superior Fascia of Urogenital
      Diaphragm
S.L. — Subpubic Ligament
S.P. — Sacral Promontory
S.T.P. — Superficial Transverse Perineal
      Muscle
T.A. — Tendinous Arch
T.P.L. — Transverse Pelvic Ligament
U. — Urethra
V. — Vagina

Figure 8-2. The pelvic diaphragm.

     The coccygeus is a triangular muscle partly replaced by the sacrotuberous ligament. It arises from the ischial spine and fans out into an insertion on the sides of the sacrum and coccyx. The nerve supply is from sacral 4 and the anal coccygeal nerve (sacral 5).

     Two other muscles are also present in the pelvis. The obturator internus

102

arises from the anterior lateral wall of the pelvis (an obturator membrane) and passes backward through the lesser sciatic foramen to be inserted into the trochanter of the femur. It is supplied by nerves L5, S1, and S2. The piriformis arises from the front of the sacrum and passes through the greater sciatic foramen to be inserted into the trochanter femur. It is supplied by nerves from S1 and S2. These two muscles are primarily lateral rotators of the hip and postural muscles.

The main function of the pelvic diaphragm, apart from helping to fix the perineal body and assist the vaginal and anal sphincters, is to support the pelvic viscera.

THE PELVIC PERITONEUM

The peritoneum is reflected from the lateral borders of the uterus to form on either side a double fold of peritoneum known as the *broad ligament.* This is not a ligament but a peritoneal fold, and it does not support the uterus. The fallopian tube runs in the upper free edge of the broad ligament as far as the point at which the tube opens into the peritoneal cavity; the part of the broad ligament that is lateral to the opening is called the *infundibulopelvic fold,* and in it the ovarian vessels and nerves pass from the side wall of the pelvis to lie between the two layers of the broad ligament. The portion of the broad ligament that lies above the ovary is known as the *mesosalpinx,* and between its layers many wolffian remnants may be present. Below the ovary, the base of the broad ligament widens out and contains a considerable amount of loose connective tissue called the *parametrium.* The ureter is attached to the posterior leaf of the broad ligament at this point.

The ovary is attached to the posterior layer of the broad ligament by a short mesentery (meso-ovarian) through which the ovarian vessels and nerves enter the hilum.

It will be noted that while the vagina does not have any peritoneal covering in front, behind it is in contact with the rectovaginal pouch for about 2 cm, where the vagina is separated from the abdominal cavity only by the peritoneum and thin fascia. The peritoneal cavity can be opened by posterior colpotomy at this point.

The ovarian ligament lies beneath the posterior layer of the broad ligament and passes from the medial pole of the ovary to the uterus just below the point of entry of the fallopian tube.

The round ligament is a continuation of the same structure and runs forward under the anterior leaf of the peritoneum to enter the inguinal canal, ending in the subcutaneous tissue of the labium majora. Together, the ovarian and round ligaments are homologous with the gubernaculum testis of the male. The round ligament is seldom tense enough to prevent the uterus from becoming retroverted; it has no other supporting function.

PELVIC CONNECTIVE TISSUE OR PELVIC FASCIA

The fascia of the body consists of superficial and deep layers. The superficial layer lies beneath the skin and consists of the areolar tissue impregnated with fat.

The deep layers consist of a tough, inelastic membrane of fibrous tissue that forms a continuous layer throughout the body, covers the surfaces of muscles, or ensheaths them, and often forms an important part of their attachment. It blends with all ligaments with which it comes in contact, and as it passes over the bony surfaces, it fuses with the subjacent periosteum. It may become firmly attached to the body skeleton, and it materially assists muscular action by forming an unyielding membrane against which the muscles contract.

The pelvic fascia consists of a parietal layer and a visceral layer. The parietal layer consists of the aponeuroses and fascial sheaths of the pelvic muscles (the wallpaper of the pelvis). The visceral layer makes up the fascial sheaths of the organs and the fatty tissue filling the space between them (the stuffing of the pelvis).

The connective tissue covering the levator ani is condensed into musculofibrous bands in three areas: (1) the transverse cervical ligament (cardinal ligament) arising from the arcuate line on the side wall of the pelvis; (2) the pubocervical ligaments arising from the fascia of the pubic bone and passing around the bladder neck; and (3) the uterosacral ligaments (posterior part of the cardinal ligaments) arising from the sacral promontory. All three ligaments insert into the upper vagina and supravaginal cervix.

The cellular tissue is continuous above with the extraperitoneal tissue of the abdominal wall, but below it is cut off from the ischiorectal fossa by the pelvic fascia and levator ani muscles. There is a considerable collection of cellular tissue in the wide space of the broad ligament and at the side of the cervix and vagina called the *parametrium.*

The pelvic fascia may be regarded as a specialized part of this connective tissue. It contains parietal and visceral components. The parietal pelvic fascia lines the wall of the pelvic cavity, covering the obturator internis and pyramidalis muscles. There is a thickened white line (the arcus tendineus) on the side wall of the pelvis from which the levator ani muscle arises and where the cardinal ligament gains its lateral attachment. Where the parietal pelvic fascia encounters bone, as in the pubic region, it blends with the periosteum. It also forms the upper layer of the urogenital diaphragm (triangular ligament).

Each viscus has a fascial investment, which is dense in the case of the vagina and cervix and at the base of the bladder but sparse or absent over the body of the uterus and the dome of the bladder. Various processes of the visceral pelvic fascia pass inward from the peripheral layer of the parietal pelvic fascia. From the point of view of the gynecologist, certain parts of the visceral fascia are of particular importance, as will be noted.

The essential support of the uterus and vaginal vault is provided by the cardinal ligaments, the transverse cervical ligaments. These are two strong, fan-shaped, fibromuscular expansions that pass from the cervix and vaginal vault to the side walls of the pelvis on either side.

The uterosacral ligaments run from the cervix and vaginal vault to the sacrum. In the erect position, they are almost vertical and support the cervix.

The bladder is supported laterally by condensation of the visceral pelvic fascia on each side. There is also a sheath of pubocervical fascia that lies beneath it anteriorly.

RELAXATION OF PELVIC SUPPORTS

The possible sequelae of damage to the pelvic floor may cause prolapse of the anterior vaginal wall, which in turn results in prolapse of the bladder (cystocele), or of the urethra (urethrocele), or commonly both. Depending upon the degree of damage to the pelvic floor, a variety of incontinence problems may develop. Prolapse of the anterior vaginal wall is much more common and progresses to a more serious condition than does prolapse of the posterior vaginal wall. Stress incontinence is almost never seen with a large cystocele, but overflow incontinence may be present.

The posterior vaginal wall may prolapse, resulting in herniation of the rectum into the vagina (rectocele). This is often accompanied by a type of constipation in which the patient experiences difficulty in emptying the herniated portion of the bowel. On straining, the feces is directed into the rectocele and pushes up into the vagina. There is lack of stimulation of the sphincter ani, which results in difficulty of defecation. Occasionally the entire vaginal vault prolapses, pulling with it the vagina, bladder, and rectum. This condition is called *third-degree prolapse* or *procidentia.*

It is generally agreed that supportive pelvic structures depend upon the endopelvic fascia, the uterosacral and cardinal ligaments, and the levator muscles. This intact fascial system, with its attachments to the vaginal fornices and upper two-thirds of the lateral vagina, provides a well-supported vaginal tube, which in turn is the most important supporting structure for the uterus and the vaginal vault. Traumatic (obstetric) stretching, wear and tear of living, occupational and unusual athletic endeavors, heredity, and postmenopausal attenuation all contribute in varying degrees to the development of pelvic relaxation. Additional contributing factors that promote uterine descensus are obesity, asthma, and other chronic lung diseases, as well as a variety of metabolic and demyelinating diseases.

URETHROCELE

Descent of a portion of the posterior bladder wall and trigone into the vagina is usually due to the trauma of parturition. Urethrocele (sagging of the urethra) is commonly associated with cystocele and is found in women who have urinary stress incontinence. However, urethrocele is not a cause of urinary incontinence. Occasionally, women with a urethrocele state that after they finish urinating and stand up, they dribble urine for a short period of time. It is interesting that in women with large cystoceles there is seldom any stress incontinence. However, these patients often have repeated bouts of cystitis. Patients with a large cystocele often have difficulty emptying their bladder completely. Some have to put their fingers in the vagina and press up on the cystocele to do so. The patient with a large

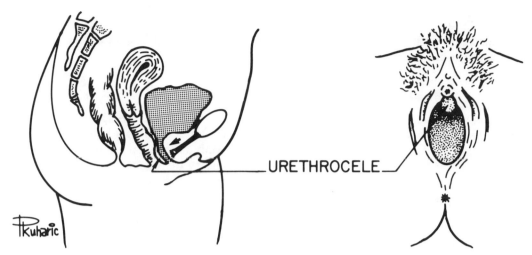

Figure 8-3. Urethrocele.

cystocele often has a constant urge to urinate because of the pull placed on the trigone in the cystocele. Nothing short of surgery will correct this condition (Fig. 8-3).

ENTEROCELE

An enterocele is a herniation of the rectouterine pouch of Douglas into the rectovaginal septum. It presents as a bulge in the upper part of the vagina in the posterior fornix. It is a true hernia in that it is surrounded by peritoneum and contains small bowel. The enterocele was formerly called a *high rectocele.* However, it is now accepted that a rectocele and an enterocele are entirely different entities. Uterine prolapse is almost always accompanied by some degree of enterocele. Prolapse of the vaginal vault after a hysterectomy is also invariably accompanied by an enterocele.

The symptoms associated with an enterocele are usually vague or absent. Since the hernia may drop down as far as the perineum, there is occasionally a drag on the mesentery of the bowel, causing upper abdominal discomfort. Some enteroceles may lead to obstruction and occasionally rupture spontaneously through the vaginal vault. The diagnosis is best made with the patient in a standing position, with the physician placing the index finger in the rectum and the thumb in the vagina and asking the patient to cough. The small intestine will produce a ballottement effect against the fingers. It is also possible to distinguish the enterocele from a rectocele by this method of examination.

Since an enterocele is a true hernia, it must be treated as one. There must be high ligation of the sac and closure of the fascia. To protect against recurrence, the uterosacrals must be brought together or the cul-de-sac obliterated surgically (Fig. 8-4).

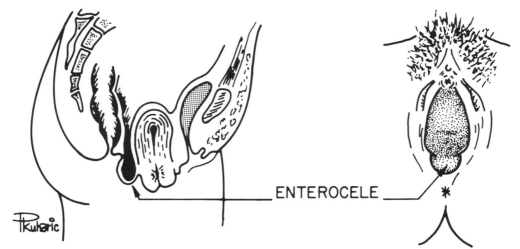

Figure 8-4. Enterocele.

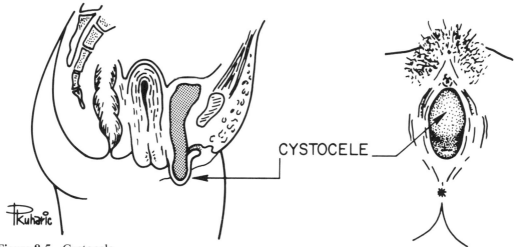

Figure 8-5. Cystocele.

CYSTOCELE

Prolapse of the bladder and the anterior vaginal wall is known as a *cystocele.* A clinical diagnosis of cystocele includes (1) a sensation of vaginal fullness, pressure, or falling out; (2) the feeling that the patient is sitting on a ball; (3) feeling of incomplete emptying of the bladder, urinary frequency, and perhaps a need to push the bladder up in order to empty it completely; (4) the presence of a soft, reducible mass bulging into the anterior vagina and distending the vaginal introitus; and (5) with straining or coughing, increased bulging and descent of the anterior vaginal wall as well as the urethra (Fig. 8-5).

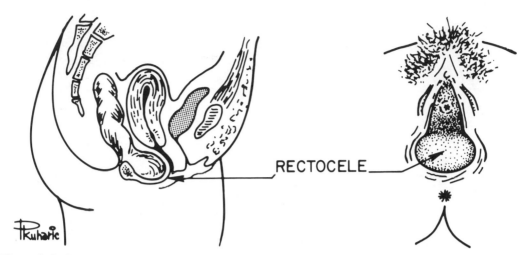

Figure 8-6. Rectocele.

Surgical repair is required if there are repeated bouts of cystitis and trigonitis, or if the cystocele becomes so large that the patient cannot empty her bladder adequately, or if the cystocele protrudes to the vaginal introitus and causes ulceration of the vaginal wall. Some patients have a constant urge to urinate because of the pull on the trigone. Pessaries usually do not help in the management of cystoceles and often create stress incontinence or, in some instances, total incontinence.

RECTOCELE

A rectocele is a bulging of the posterior vaginal wall and the underlying rectum through the rectovaginal fascia. In the presence of a large rectocele, the patient often has constipation and experiences difficulty in emptying the herniated portion of the bowel. There may also be prolapse of the vaginal vault, resulting in a falling of the womb through the inverted vagina. A small rectocele (rarely causing symptoms) is usually present in all multiparous patients. A large rectocele may cause a sensation of pelvic pressure, rectal fullness, or incomplete evacuation of stool. Occasionally, a patient may find it necessary to reduce the posterior vaginal wall manually in a backward direction in order to evacuate the lower rectum effectively. Distinguishing a high rectocele (involving the entire rectovaginal septum) from an enterocele may sometimes be difficult. Generally, with the patient straining, a rectovaginal examination will confirm the presence of abdominal contents sliding into the enterocele sac. An impulse of the small bowel is almost certain to be associated with an enterocele. Since pessaries are not helpful in managing this condition, if the symptoms interfere with the quality of life, surgical repair is indicated (Fig. 8-6).

UTERINE OR UTEROVAGINAL PROLAPSE

These types of prolapse represent a herniation of the genital tract through the pelvic diaphragm. The uterus and vagina are held in the pelvis by the cardinal and uterosacral ligaments and by the pelvic floor muscles, mainly the levator ani. When these ligaments and muscles become ineffective, the uterus and vagina descend (prolapse) through the gap between these muscles.

The term *prolapse* is usually applied to prolapse of the uterus. This condition is always accompanied by prolapse of the vagina. Some investigators think that prolapse of the vagina antedates prolapse of the uterus.

That the vagina may be the principal offender in prolapse of the uterus is demonstrated in patients who have had their uterus removed in anticipation of correcting the problem. However, unless the vagina is well supported, it continues to prolapse and actually turns inside out.

The cause of prolapse in almost every case is childbearing. In less than 1 percent of the cases, a congenital weakness secondary to spina bifida oculta is the primary cause. Contributing factors, but not primary causes, include malnutrition, metabolic disorders, and inanition. The actual cause of the descent in all cases is increased intra-abdominal and pelvic pressure. When this rises above atmospheric pressure, a force is set up within the pelvis that tends to push the viscera and their contents down; thus, constipation, coughing, and lifting of heavy weights are the final factors in the development of prolapse.

The uterus normally lies at right angles to the vagina, with the fundus just above the pelvic brim and the cervix on the level with and adjacent to the ischial spine. The cervix is fixed with the body of the uterus, which lies free in the pelvic cavity and is extremely mobile.

The supports of the uterus can be classified anatomically as direct and indirect. The direct supports include the vagina and the pelvic connective tissue and fascia forming the pubocervical ligaments, transverse ligaments of the cervix, and uterosacral ligaments, as well as the broad and round ligaments. The indirect supports include the levator ani and coccygeus muscles, the urogenital diaphragm, and the central point of the perineum.

Three degrees of prolapse are recognized: (1) the cervix appears at the vaginal introitus (first degree); (2) the cervix and half of the uterus appear at the vaginal orifice (second degree); (3) the entire uterus appears through the orifice, and the vaginal walls are completely everted (third degree or procidentia) (Fig. 8-7).

Symptoms

The symptoms of prolapse are all anatomic: (1) a dragging sensation at the vulva and pain in the back are due to the weight of the protrusion; (2) urination is frequent; (3) stress incontinence is due to the herniation of the bladder wall, though some patients cannot empty the bladder until they put their fingers into the vagina and push the hernia back; (4) a type of constipation follows herniation of the rectum for the same reason; and (5) the patient develops ulceration of the vaginal wall, and chafing and excoriations occur because the organ is exposed.

Surgery is indicated to relieve these symptoms. In young women, the pelvic floor should be restored. The Manchester operation is carried out if conservation of the uterus is important. Otherwise, vaginal hysterectomy with correction of the hernial defects may be elected. Uterine prolapse can

UTERINE PROLAPSE

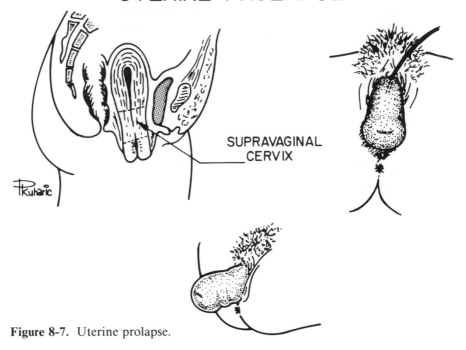

SUPRAVAGINAL CERVIX

Figure 8-7. Uterine prolapse.

be managed by an abdominal approach that includes total abdominal hysterectomy and the obliteration of any associated enterocele. However, this method is more difficult and has greater morbidity than the repair carried out from below.

Palliative Treatment

Treatment of prolapse with a pessary may be considered and should be given a trial for at least 3 months. Occasionally a pessary may be advised when the patient is either unfit for anesthesia or refuses the operation.

A ring pessary made of polyethylene or flexible vinyl is used. The diameters are given in millimeters; the correct size for the patient is the largest size of which she is unaware. If the ring is too small, it may be expelled from the vagina on straining. If it is too large, it will cause discomfort and may cause pressure, necrosis, and ulceration of the vaginal walls.

Before a pessary is inserted, a vaginal examination is done to exclude any other abnormality, to replace the uterus if it is retroverted, and to determine the probable size of the ring required. The pessary is compressed into an ellipse for passage through the vaginal introitus. As the ring passes into the vagina and above the pelvic floor, it returns to its circular form. The forefinger guides the upper part of the ring into the posterior fornix so that the cervix lies within the ring. The patient is then reexamined to make sure that the vaginal walls are not unduly stretched. She is then asked to strain down in order to make sure that the ring is large enough not to be expelled.

Rubber ring pessaries should not be used because they cause vaginitis. The polyethylene pessary causes little irritation, and douching is not required. The ring need only be changed for a new one after 12 months. However, if any purulent discharge or bleeding occurs, the patient should report it at once. The ring should be removed before full investigation for the cause of the staining or bleeding.

SUMMARY

The morphology of the pelvic floor is reviewed. The functions of the pelvic floor are discussed and the anatomy is reviewed. The possible sequelae of damage to the pelvic floor are outlined. The genital prolapses most commonly seen include cystocele, rectocele, uterine prolapse, and enterocele. The causes, anatomy, and suggestions for repair are discussed. Palliative treatment for patients with prolapse who are poor surgical risks is given.

The genital and urinary systems are intimately related both embryologically and anatomically. Therefore, it is difficult to discuss one without discussing the other. As an example, a cystocele or any prolapse may also be complicated by a rectocele and an enterocele.

It is accepted that the support of the pelvic structures depends on the endopelvic fascia, the uterosacral and cardinal ligaments, and the levator muscle. This intact musculofascial system, with its attachment to the vaginal fornices and the upper two-thirds of the lateral vagina, provides a well-supported vaginal tube, which in turn is the most important supporting structure for the uterus and vaginal wall. In uterovaginal prolapse there is damage to or weakness of the structures that support the pelvic organs, so that some of these descend from their normal position and finally herniate through the vaginal opening.

It is important to distinguish the perineum from the pelvic diaphragm. The perineum is the anatomic region at the inferior end of the trunk, below the pelvic floor. The perineal floor is composed of skin and two layers of superficial fascia, the superficial fatty stratum and a deeper membranous one. Superficial fatty fascia is continuous anteriorly with the superficial fatty layer of the abdomen called *Camper's fascia* and posteriorly with the ischiorectal fat. The deeper membranous layer of the superficial perineal fascia (Colles' fascia) is limited to the anterior half of the perineum. Laterally it is attached to ischiopubic rami; posteriorly it blends with the base of the urogenital diaphragm; and anteriorly it is continuous with the deep layer of the superficial abdominal fascia called *Scarpa's fascia*. The urogenital triangle includes a superficial and a deep perineal compartment. The deep perineal compartment is made up of the urogenital diaphragm. It is a strong musculomembranous partition stretched across the anterior half of the pelvic outlet between the ischiopubic rami. It is composed of superficial and inferior fascial layers that enclose the deep perineal muscles, the sphincter of the membranous urethra, and the pudendal vessels and nerves. It is pierced by the urethra and vagina.

The pelvic diaphragm forms the musculotendinous, funnel-shaped partition between the pelvic cavity and the perineum. It is composed of the levator ani and coccygeus muscles sheathed in a superior and inferior layer of fascia. The muscles of the pelvic diaphragm extend from the lateral pelvic wall downward and medially, to fuse with each other, and are inserted into the terminal portions of the urethra, vagina, and anus. Anteriorly they fail to meet in the midline just behind the pubic symphysis, exposing a gap in the pelvic floor that is completed by the urogenital diaphragm. In this area, the inferior fascia of the pelvic diaphragm fuses with the superior fascia of the urogenital diaphragm.

The genital prolapses include cystocele, which is often accompanied by urethrocele. Urethrocele is the prolapse of the bladder and anterior vaginal wall. Rectocele is the prolapse of the rectum and posterior vaginal wall. It is usually accompanied by a deficiency of the perineal body.

Uterine prolapse is often accompanied by descent of the vaginal vault. Cystocele or rectocele or both may occur without uterine descent. The uterine prolapse is accompanied by descent of the bladder because of the close attachment of the bladder to the anterior aspect of the supravaginal cervix.

Prolapse of the uterus may result in the descent of the cervix to the introitus (first degree), protrusion of the cervix through the introitus (second degree), or prolapse of the entire uterus (third degree). Rarely, because of severe medical conditions in an elderly patient, a pessary may be indicated; however, the preferred treatment is operation. There are a number of operations that can be selected to correct a prolapse of the uterus.

Enterocele is a true hernia and must be differentiated from a high rectocele. Enterocele is a hernia of the rectovaginal peritoneal pouch through the posterior vaginal fornix. Small intestine may be found in the peritoneal sac behind the uterus. An enterocele may occasionally occur after the uterus has been removed by abdominal or vaginal hysterectomy. It is usually combined with some degree of prolapse of the vaginal vault.

Nearly all patients suffering from prolapse have borne children, and some cases of prolapse becomes evident soon after a particular delivery. Prolapse is almost invariably the result of damage to the supporting structures during childbirth, yet in many cases the condition does not become evident until after the menopause, when some atrophy of the structures occurs. Prolapse often becomes more marked after the menopause, and most cases of procidentia are seen in elderly women in whom the uterus and its supports are atrophic. Atrophy of the ligaments and fascial structures is associated with diminished estrogen secretion, and there is lowered muscle tone with increasing age. Rare cases of prolapse in nulliparous women are explained by atrophy of the pelvic supports with age. In these cases, descent of the uterus and the vaginal vault occurs with little cystocele or rectocele.

Symptoms consist of local discomfort, backache, urinary symptoms, bowel symptoms, ulceration, and bleeding. If these symptoms interfere with the quality of life, surgical repair is definitely indicated. However, palliative treatment with a pessary may be considered as a temporary measure. Unless the geriatric patient has marked cardiovascular or pulmonary compromise, the surgery required to correct these pelvic floor relaxations can be carried out with relative safety.

REFERENCES

Ardekany, M. S., and R. Rafee. 1978. A new modification of colpocleisis for treatment of total procidentia in old age. *Int. J. Gynaecol Obstet.* 15:358.

Baden, W. F. 1969. Geriatric gynecology. *Postgrad. Med. J.* 46:241.

Comfort, A. 1979. *The Biology of Senescence,* 3rd ed., Elsevier, New York, p. 265.

Curtis, A. H., B. J. Anson, and C. B. McVay. 1939. The anatomy of the pelvic and urogenital diaphragms in relation to urethrocele and cystocle. *Surg. Gynecol. Obstet.* 68:161.

Elkin, M., et al. 1975. Ureteral obstruction in patients with uterine prolapse. *Radiology* 110:289.

Macer, G. A. 1978. Transabdominal repair of cystocele, a 20 year experience compared with the traditional vaginal approach. *Am. J. Obstet. Gynecol.* 131:203.

McCall, M. L. 1957. Posterior culdoplasty: Surgical correction of enterocele during vaginal hysterectomy: A preliminary report. *Obstet. Gynecol.* 10:595.

Milley, P. S., and D. H. Nichols. 1969. A correlative investigation of the human rectovaginal septum. *Anat. Rec.* 163:443.

————.1971. The relationship between the pubourethral ligaments and the urogenital diaphragm in the human female. *Anat. Rec.* 170:281.

Moschcowitz, A. V. 1942. The pathogenesis, anatomy and cure of prolapse of the rectum. *Surg. Gynecol. Obstet.* 15:7.

Nichols, D. H. 1972. Types of enterocele and principles underlying choice of operation for repair. *Obstet. Gynecol.* 40:257.

————. 1978. Effects of pelvic relaxation on gynecologic urologic problems. *Clin. Obstet. Gynecol.* 21:759.

Nichols, D. H., and P. S. Milley. 1970. Surgical significance of the rectovaginal septum. *Am. J. Obstet. Gynecol.* 108:215.

Nichols, D. H., and C. L. Randall. 1977. *Vaginal Surgery,* Williams & Wilkins, Baltimore.

Smout, C. F. V., and F. Jacoby. 1948. *Gynecological and Obstetrical Anatomy,* 2nd ed., Arnold, London.

TeLinde, R. W. 1966. Prolapse of the uterus and allied conditions. *Am. J. Obstet. Gynecol.* 94:444.

Ulfelder, H. 1956. The mechanisms of pelvic support in women: Deductions from a study of the comparative anatomy and physiology of the structures involved. *Am. J. Obstet. Gynecol.* 72:856.

Zacharin, R. F. 1980. Pulsion enterocele: Review of functional anatomy of the pelvic floor. *Obstet. Gynecol.* 55:135.

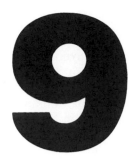

Lower Genital Tract

INTRODUCTION

The lower genital tract consists of the vulva, vagina, and cervix. Epidemiologically, these three organs have many factors in common, and although the vulva is not a mullerian derivative, it is responsive to hormonal stimulation and therefore shares this property with the vagina and the cervix. It is well known that inflammatory processes affecting any one of these organs may also affect the other two. It is also recognized that an in situ lesion in any of these organs may be found in the others. Therefore, it is proper to group them together as the lower genital tract.

VULVA

The vulva tissues of every woman who is several years postmenopausal and who does not take estrogens are more or less atrophic. The word *atrophic* is not synonymous with *senile. Atrophic,* literally translated, means "without nourishment," and in this sense is an accurate term for this condition. During the premenarchal years and again after the menopause, the vulva lacks the stimulation and nourishment of estrogen. Since the vulva is a skin appendage, atrophic changes resemble those seen in the skin of the face and abdomen. In the postmenopausal years, the symmetric shape of the vulva is lost. The skin often hangs in folds. There is shrinkage, loss of elasticity, and dryness due to hormonal withdrawal. Puckering of the vulva tissue with atrophy of the introitus, even in the multiparous woman, may make penile intromission exquisitely painful, and deflection of the penis anteriorly by a rigid perineum may create pressure on the urethra meatus, causing urethritis, local inflammation, and dysuria.

Monkeys, baboons, and chimpanzees have a vulva skin that is referred to as a *sexual skin*. It looks different and undergoes obvious changes. The changes are most marked during sexual heat and at different times of the cycle. Although these changes are not as marked in humans, the skin of the vulva can vary with the cycle and with sexual stimulation.

The vulva, like the skin of the rest of the body, is in contact with the environment. It is a membrane that, as such, allows secretion and perhaps even excretion of substances, as well as absorption. It is recognized that water is lost from all body surfaces. It has been shown that the transdermal water loss of the labia exceeds that of other areas of skin by a large amount. The vulva is "wetter" as part of its normal state than are other areas of skin. However, as the postmenopausal years pass into the geriatric years, these responses are greatly diminished.

Diseases of the Vulva

Many vulva diseases are similar in different age groups. In the postmenopausal and geriatric groups, there is an increase in the incidence of diabetic vulvitis and vulva dystrophies. Persons with these lesions often present with burning, pruritus, or difficulty in coitus.

Intertrigo, is a nonspecific inflammatory condition usually found in the genitourinal folds and beneath the panniculus, and although encountered in patients of all ages, it is frequently seen in older patients, particularly those who are obese and who have difficulty in bathing and cleansing the perineum and vulva. In consequence, the skin covering the perineum, genital crural folds, labia majora, labia minora, and thighs is constantly moistened by perspiration and soiled by urine. Patients with intertrigo usually complain of perineal itching and burning. Inspection shows the area to be superficially denuded, shiny, hyperemic, and moist; a scanty, malodorous discharge may cover the infected area. It is important to teach these women proper hygiene. They should be instructed not to have nylon in contact with the skin and to use only baby soaps or soaps that do not contain detergents. Ivory soap is alkaline and causes marked drying and itching. These patients should be advised to avoid all perfumed toilet papers and perineal sprays. They should be told not to wash too vigorously and to dry the area carefully; cornstarch powder is recommended.

Senile angiomata are small, usually multiple red, elevated papules up to 3 mm in diameter that bleed freely when scrubbed or scratched. They are actually a form of telangiectasia. They are quite benign; bleeding occurs when they are traumatized and frightens the patient. This bleeding often occurs after a hot shower or bath followed by the rough use of a large bath towel. Atrophic angiomata are not excised unless the patient is unduly alarmed or unless they are very large. If they bleed, the patient is instructed to lie down and apply pressure with a handkerchief or a towel; the bleeding will stop promptly. She should be told to have a follow-up examination.

Sebaceous cysts of the vulva form small (barely 1 cm in diameter) yellowish-gray nodules in the skin covering the labia. The foul-smelling, purulent material extruded from the cyst becomes infected and ruptures, or a small lump may develop in the vulva. At the time of the examination, the lump should be drawn to the patient's attention and an explanation given. Thereafter, when the patient finds the lesion, or when it becomes infected or breaks, she will not be frightened. A very large sebaceous cyst that becomes repeatedly infected should be removed. If the cyst is incised and drained in the office, the base should be treated with silver nitrate to destroy the linings so that it will not re-form.

Clitoral phimosis may cause an inspissated smegma to collect beneath the prepuce, producing discomfort. The area is usually very red and resembles balanitis. In women, this is not an uncommon finding. As they grow older, they are less inclined to practice careful vulva hygiene and with the atrophy that occurs, the material becomes inspissated beneath the prepuce. It is easy to evacuate this material in the office. The patient should then be taught the proper care of the area.

Located deeply and toward the perineum are the bilateral Bartholin's glands (vulvovaginal glands). The orifice of each gland's major duct is located at the middle of the lateral margin of the introitus. As one proceeds proximally, the epithelium changes from stratified squamous to transitional to a mixture of columnar to cuboidal, mucus-secretory cells. It is very rare to find a Bartholin cyst in the postmenopausal patient unless it was present during the menopausal years. However, any abscess should be drained and marsupialized. If there is a suggestion of hardness in the cyst, malignancy must be suspected and proper biopsies performed. Since lubricating fluid from Bartholin's glands begins when atrophy occurs, even when sexual stimulation has taken place, the gland secretes less mucus, with resultant frictional irritation during coitus. Therefore, this development in the geriatric patient requires attention and treatment.

The vulva may be affected by *Candida albicans*. The appearance of a fungal infection on the vagina should always arouse a suspicion of diabetes, and the patient should be tested for this condition. *Trichomonas vaginalis* and *Hemophilus vaginalis,* which cause a discharge, may also result in vulvitis. Whenever there is a vulvitis, it is important to inspect the vagina and carry out the proper tests for the major types of vaginitis, including *Candida, Gardnerella, trichomonas,* and, of course, atrophy. Fungal infections should be treated with an antifungal agent, trichomonas with metronidazole, *Gardnerella* with ampicillin or cephradine, and the atrophic condition with an estrogen preparation. A generation ago, a discussion of the sexually transmitted diseases in this age group would have been considered improper. However, with the sexual revolution, older women have been affected by this freedom, and they are much more liberal in their acceptance of having more than one sexual partner. The most important bacteria and viruses infecting the vulva are human papilloma virus, genital herpes simplex virus infection, chlamydia trachomatis, gonorrhea, syphilis, and condylomata. There are certain parasitic skin infections, such as pediculosis pubis and scabies, which must be considered particularly in those who have no response to the usual treatments.

Folliculitis is a common disorder of vulva skin, especially where there is poor hygiene or lowered resistance to infection. It may be caused by a variety of organisms, including pyogenic bacteria such as staphylococcus and streptococcus. Multiple red, tender papules surround hair follicles, resulting eventually in tiny pustules. Folliculitis is treated first by cleansing with a germicidal soap prior to the application of gentamycin or neosporin ointment. Cases that do not respond within 1 week merits systemic antibiotic therapy, and penicillin or erythromycin are the drugs of choice.

Allergic vulvitis is not an uncommon finding. Contact with a wide variety of chemical and physical agents may induce vulva irritation. These agents include synthetic fibers, fabric dyes, hygienic feminine douches, deodorant sprays, and self-medications. Excessive washing with soap and douching can also be irritating. One of the most common causes of vulva irritation at present is tight synthetic garments. Sweating in the perineum can be excessive, and wearing such underclothes for long periods prevents evaporation. The distribution of the lesions reflects their etiology. For example, involvement of the labia majora and the inner part of the thigh points to synthetic garments, whereas involvement of the labia minora and vestibule indicates products employed in relation to intercourse. Allergic vulvitis is characterized by intense erythema and infiltration of the dermis by inflammatory cells, including eosinophils, and vasculitis may be prominent.

Several systemic inflammatory conditions of unknown etiology may also involve the vulva. For example, Crohn's disease may cause vulva ulceration and the formation of fistulae. Chronic relapsing genital and oral ulcers may occur in Behcet's disease in association with ocular, neurologic, gastrointestinal, and other manifestations of the disease.

Vulva Dystrophies

The vulva dystrophies are more common during the postmenopausal years, but there are no good data to implicate estrogen deprivation as a primary etiologic factor. Estrogen therapy does not always improve these patients, and some, in fact, complain of marked burning when estrogen is applied topically. The dystrophies are classified as (1) lichen sclerosus (hypoplastic dystrophy): thin epithelium with loss of rete pegs and dermal elastic tissue; (2) hypertrophic dystrophies: acanthosis, hyperkeratosis, and normal stratification that increase the cell numbers; atypia may be seen at various levels and are graded as mild, moderate, or severe; (3) mixed dystrophies: both appearances can be present in samples from the same vulva.

The vulva dystrophies are characterized by a high incidence of recurrence following treatment. It can be anticipated that at least 50 percent will recur. The malignant potential of these lesions depends upon the degree of cellular atypia. It is estimated that approximately 10 percent of vulva dystrophies with dysplasia will eventually progress to squamous cell carcinoma. This is more common in the hyperplastic and mixed types. Therefore, it is important to take multiple biopsies and attain baseline levels for tissue diagnosis. Lesions with a great deal of cellular atypia are at increased risk for the development of neoplasia. Dystrophies of the vulva are discussed in Chap. 12.

In addition to sebaceous cysts, mucous cysts, and hernias that may occur in the vulva, squamous papillomas, fibroepithelial polyps, hidradenoma, urethral caruncle, nevi, and lentigo may also occur.

Vulvar Intraepithelial Neoplasia (VIN)

There are two varieties of VIN: (1) squamous cell carcinoma in situ and (2) the rare adenocarcinoma (Paget's disease).

VIN is being seen with increasing frequency, especially in younger age groups. Many lesions are asymptomatic and are suspected on routine examination of the vulva. Itching is common. The clinical appearance is highly variable. The lesion may be brown, red, gray, white, or any combination of these colors. The particular shade depends on the histologic construction of the lesion. Most lesions are raised and usually roughened. They may involve small areas or the whole vulva. Seventy-five percent of vulva carcinomas in situ are multicentric. The lesions can extend to the anus, vagina, urethra, and glans clitoris. Twenty-five percent of these patients have a history of premalignant or malignant changes in another organ; half of these conditions are carcinoma-in-situ of the cervix and/or vagina.

Condyloma acuminata are associated with increasing frequency and occur in 7 to 31 percent of the cases. Human papilloma virus has become the prime suspect in vulvar neoplasia. However, women are smoking far more than previously, and it is known that 2000 carcinogens are present in cigarettes, many of which are excreted through the urine. Therefore, vulva contact with these carcinogens may play a role in the production of carcinoma in situ of the vulva. The disease has a higher incidence in patients who have autoimmune disease or are receiving immunosuppressant therapy.

There must be a high degree of suspicion that these lesions are on the increase. Colposcopy may be of value in diagnosing nonkeratotic lesions. The application of 4 percent aqueous acetic acid will present the lesion as pseudowhite epithelium, punctation, and atypical vessels identifying the site for biopsy. The colposcopic appearance is generally less pronounced than that of cervical lesions with similar histology.

Toluidine blue, which is a nuclear stain, is applied as a 1 percent aqueous solution for 1 minute. The skin is then decolorized with dilute acetic acid. In general, carcinoma in situ stains are faint blue; those of invasive cancer are deep blue. The stain identifies a site for biopsy.

The treatment should be individualized. Several options are available: (1) wide local excision, (2) simple vulvectomy, (3) skinning vulvectomy, (4)

CO_2 laser surgery, (5) cryosurgery, and (6) nonsurgical methods. Recently, it has been found that the topical application of a 5-fluorouracil (5-FU) ointment, massaged gently into the lesion twice a day for 6 weeks, will eradicate the lesion. However, ulcerations, sloughing, and pain are fairly marked. 5-FU is now seldom used. Since these lesions are multicentric, CO_2 laser surgery is presently the preferred method of treatment. The major advantages are that it eliminates the disease and produces an excellent cosmetic result. However, more aggressive surgery may be needed.

Paget's disease of the vulva may be either an in situ or an invasive lesion. The mean age at occurrence is approximately 63 years, and the lesion characteristically presents as white islands of hyperkeratosis over a bright red base. The lesions are usually confined to the apocrine (sweat) gland region of the vulva. Histologically, they are characterized by the presence of Paget's cells. One-third have underlying sweat gland carcinoma that can only be diagnosed after excision. Twenty-five percent of these lesions are associated with a prior malignancy elsewhere, usually in the breast. The breast is the most frequent site.

The treatment is by wide excision down through the fat to the fascia. It should extend at least 2 to 3 cm beyond the visible margin, and the lines of excision must be checked histologically for Paget's cells. Only by obtaining this type of specimen is it possible to rule out invasive cancer.

The recurrence rate for squamous cell carcinoma-in-situ and adenocarcinoma-in-situ (Paget's disease) is high.

Microinvasive Carcinoma of the Vulva

Microinvasive vulva carcinoma is defined as a lesion 2 cm or less in diameter, with a 5-mm or less stromal invasion. The presence of vascular confluence, vascular channel permeation, and cellular anaplasia does not exclude the case from this category.

Microinvasive carcinoma constitutes up to 17 percent of all vulva cancers. The mean age at occurrence is the late fifties. However, it is being diagnosed with increasing frequency in younger women. Pruritis is the most frequent presenting symptom. It may be associated with a lump, swelling, soreness, or ulcer, and, more recently, with increasing frequency, condylomata. Ten percent are asymptomatic and are detected on routine vulva inspection.

The appearance of these lesions is extremely diverse. A clinical diagnosis is possible only in lesions between 1 and 2 cm in diameter, where there is obvious cancer. In the remainder, suspicion will be aroused in the clinician with experience in vulva pathology. However, any long-standing dystrophy associated with pruritus, especially if accompanied by ulcerations, bleeding, soreness, pigmentation, or hyperkeratosis, should be biopsied. The most common site is the labia majora, but any part of the vulva, perineal, anal, or perianal epithelium may be affected. The lesions are frequently multifocal and multicentric. Antecedent or coexisting vulva dystrophy is a feature in 80 percent of the cases. The associated lesion may be atrophic or hypertrophic, with or without atypical epithelial hypertrophy or intraepithelial neoplasia.

Vulva condylomata precede or coexist with over 10 percent of microinvasive vulva lesions. The lesion may present as a condyloma. Preclinical or clinical squamous carcinoma precedes or coexists in other sites of the anogenital epithelium in about 12 percent of the cases; the majority of these lesions are found in the cervix.

The true incidence of lymph node metastases remains to be determined. The results from several series indicate that 8 percent have superficial femoral and inguinal and 2 percent deep pelvic node metastases. The positive nodes are more common in tumors more than 1 cm in diameter and in those situated in the clitoral and periclitoral area, the urethra, or the periurethral region. Recurrent or new vulva lesions are a feature of this disease and are noted in up to 20 percent of the cases.

The diagnosis is made by biopsy. Toluidine blue or 4 percent acetic acid help identify the area for biopsy. The biopsy must be adequate and must include at least 1 or 2 cm of normal or apparently normal skin.

Treatment options vary from wide local excision to radical vulvectomy, with or without superficial lymphadenectomy and with or without deep pelvic lymphadenectomy. Sexual function should be preserved whenever possible. The extent of surgery is individualized after assessment of each biopsy specimen and evaluation of the patient. Coexistent cervical, vaginal, and anal lesions may need treatment.

Invasive Carcinoma of the Vulva

Invasive tumors of the vulva comprise 3.5 percent of all gynecologic malignancies. Over 80 percent are squamous cancers. They may be unilateral or bilateral. They may be divided into central (clitoral), lateral (labial, including fourchette), and perineal (in view of different types of lymphatic drainage). Approximately 20 percent of these patients have inguinal node metastases, and 25 percent of those with metastases to the inguinal area have pelvic node metastases. Clinical assessment of the nodes is a poor indicator of the presence of gland metastases.

The standard operation is extended vulvectomy with bilateral inguinal and pelvic lymphadenectomy. More recently, individualization of surgical therapy has been recommended. Pelvic lymphadenectomy is omitted on occasion unless the histology shows metastases to the inguinal glands, and more conservative surgery has been advocated for some stage I lesions. Radiation therapy is being employed with increasing frequency to treat the deep nodes.

The vulva region tolerates irradiation poorly because of the nature of the blood supply, the constant moisture, and the constant friction. Therefore, radiation therapy as a primary treatment is not desirable. Acute painful reactions may occur, and possible late complications include edema and radionecrotic ulcers. The principal use of irradiation in vulva cancer is an adjuvant to surgery in patients with a high risk of failure. The use of chemotherapy is still experimental. Recurrences may be local or distant. The overall survival rate with current methods of management should approach 75 percent in the presence of node involvement and 90 percent in its absence.

THE VAGINA

The vagina is an elastic, fibromuscular, tubal structure located between the cervix and the vulva. In the adult, it measures 8 to 10 cm in length, and is situated just posterior to the urethra and the urinary bladder and anterior to the rectum. It is flat anteriorly and posteriorly, with the anterior wall being shorter than the posterior wall as a result of the invagination of the cervix. There is an inexorable weakening of supportive structures associated with pelvic floor relaxation after the menopause, and this condition directly affects the vagina.

With estrogen deprivation, the rugi of the vagina become less prominent, and the vaginal wall becomes pale because of a decrease in underlying vascularity. The epithelium thins, is easily traumatized, and bleeds readily; as a consequence, intravaginal synechiae may develop. Atrophic vaginitis accounts for about 15 percent of all cases of postmenopausal bleeding.

Diseases of the Vagina

In the postmenopausal years, the pH of the vagina slowly changes from about 4.5 to 6. This alkaline environment predisposes the vagina to a multitude of bacterial pathogens, and the incidence of vaginitis increases in the postmenopausal patient. Vaginitis can be caused by bacteria, viruses, fungi, or parasites or by nonliving agents such as chemical and physical irritants. Although some organisms are associated with specific types of vaginitis, the same organism may be found in completely asymptomatic women.

Candida species rank as the most common cause of vaginitis. All postmenopausal women with *Candida* infections should be tested for diabetes. The fungus infection is seldom confined to the vagina; it also affects the vulva and causes marked itching. The patient may have noticed a curd-like discharge, either white or yellow, but the discharge is not the most prominent feature. Occasionally it will be blood-streaked, particularly if there is an atrophic vagina; this causes great alarm to the postmenopausal patient. Although *Candida albicans* is the most common fungus found in the vagina, *C. glabrata* has also been identified recently. It causes a relatively mild inflammation of the mucosa, without the formation of an appreciable discharge. The imidazole drugs are extremely effective as topical agents against *C. albicans.* Unless the patient has a lactose intolerance, she should be told to eat yogurt every day for about 10 days to restore the normal flora around the anus.

Gardnerella vaginitis is a commonly sexually transmitted disease and therefore is seen less often in the postmenopausal patient than in the premenopausal patient. In smears prepared from the discharge, the organisms cling to the surface of the squamous cells and form a cloudy area over the cells, which are then known as *clue cells.* The treatment is usually ampicillin.

Trichomonas vaginitis infection may occur. The classic strawberry appearance of the vaginal and cervical epithelium is noted in about 5 percent of infected women. The diagnosis can be made with a saline wet smear. The patients usually respond to metronizole treatment.

Human papilloma virus causes condyloma acuminata. Herpes simplex virus type 2 may also cause vaginitis. A thin, watery discharge of normal pH may be present in cases of herpes and vaginal cervicitis. On careful inspection of the vaginal walls, small ulcers may be noticed in the mucous membrane. Although these lesions were uncommon a few years ago in the postmenopausal woman, they are now being diagnosed.

Atrophic vaginitis is the most commonly seen vaginitis in the postmenopausal and geriatric patient. The diagnosis can be made on saline smear that shows a great number of parabasal cells, red blood cells and white cells. It is usually easily corrected with the use of estrogenic cream. The atrophic vaginitis is very often accompanied by an atrophic introitus and it is important to have the patient apply the estrogenic cream to the outside of the vulva as well as inserting it into the vagina. It is best to use a quarter to a half an applicator full of the cream. It is just as effective as a whole tube and does not run out from the vagina. The cream mixed with slough, cells and bacteria are very irritating to the vulva when they do run out. Adhesive vaginitis is a little mentioned disorder that may occur and this fibrosis combined with the adherence of adjacent mucosa may actually close off the upper vagina. This leads to difficulty in doing a good pelvic examination and if there is any neoplasia of the cervix, makes it difficult to place the colpostats accurately at the time of therapy.

Fibroepithelial polyps, leiomyomas, fibromas and other benign tumors may be found in the vagina.

Vaginal Intraepithelial Neoplasia (VAIN)

This condition usually is detected through an abnormal Pap smear. Routine colposcopy during cervical examination will assist detection. It is probable that the incidence of vaginal intraepithelial neoplasia is increasing and this may be coupled with an increased incidence of wartlike virus in the genital field. Thus all condylomata and wart-like lesions of the lower genital tract warrant a thorough vaginal examination. The lesion most often occurs in the 4 percent of transformation zones that extend from the cervix to the vaginal wall. This site may be missed at hysterectomy, so that the lesion persists, with the erroneous diagnosis of recurrence. The lesions can also arise in the original squamous epithelium and are often multiple in the cervix, vagina, and vulva. The problem of diethylstilbestrol (DES) has little relevance to the postmenopausal and geriatric patient.

The vagina can be examined with the colposcope. Four percent acetic acid is used to saturate the vagina, and the full length of the vagina should be surveyed. The lesions are usually pseudowhite, with clear, demarcated borders. Punctate vessels are often seen. The diagnosis is made by punch biopsy. Atrophic vaginitis in the postmenopausal woman can be difficult to diagnose. A 2-week course of intravaginal estrogen cream is helpful in differentiating significant changes in these patients.

The available treatments include biopsy excision, CO_2 laser surgery, cryotherapy, electrocoagulation, local chemotherapy, surgical excision, radiation therapy, and watchful expectancy. Since the lesions are multicentric, CO_2 laser surgery usually gives an excellent result. Although 5-FU produces painful ulcers of the vulva, it can safely be used in the vagina.

However, if it is used, the labia must be coated with petroleum jelly or zinc oxide because if the 5-FU cream runs out onto the vulva, it will produce very painful ulcerations.

Invasive Tumors of the Vagina

The great majority of malignant neoplasms of the vagina are the result of spread from other organs. Primarily malignant vaginal neoplasms are uncommon, and most of them are squamous cell carcinoma. Carcinoma of the vagina is an uncommon malignancy, constituting less than 2 percent of all gynecologic malignancies. It occurs between 50 and 65 years of age. It is important to make an accurate diagnosis and rule out a metastatic lesion to the vagina.

There is no accurate information on the incidence of pelvic lymph node metastases. The upper vagina drains in a manner similar to that of the cervix, while in the lower third it simulates that of the vulva; in the middle third, it may drain either way.

Therapy should be individualized. Most physicians select radiation therapy, which includes a combination of interstitial and external high-voltage pelvic irradiation.

This disease has a poor prognosis. Recurrences can be treated with radical surgery, usually pelvic exenteration. This involves a great deal of morbidity and mortality and is not considered a primary treatment. Chemotherapy is receiving a great deal of attention, but there are no data available on the success of this treatment.

Clear cell adenocarcinoma is generally seen in the young woman who has been exposed to DES in utero.

UTERINE CERVIX

The uterine cervix consists of two parts: the portio vaginalis and the endocervix. The portio, or exocervix, protrudes into the vagina and is covered by nonkeratinizing, stratified squamous epithelium. The endocervix is formed by clefts commonly known as *endocervical glands.* They are lined with one layer of tall, columnar, usually nonciliated, mucin-secreting cells, with a few smaller reserve cells close to the basement membrane.

The histology of the cervix is quite different from that of the corpus with regard to its epithelium, glands, and stroma. The postmenopausal cervix presents an atrophic picture similar to that seen in the postmenopausal vulva and vagina. The cervix shrinks and may become flush with the vaginal vault, presenting as a relatively avascular, fibrous nodule; the cervical canal may become atrophic. The combined upper vagina and cervix often are conical in configuration and very inelastic. Cervical mucus production declines as the estrogen concentration diminishes but may be maintained for several years after the menopause. The transformation zone between squamous and columnar epithelium appears to recede and is often found high in the endocervical canal. Cervical ectropion, in which there is visible columnar epithelium at the exocervix, is found in 20 percent of women in their forties but only 5 percent of women past the age of 50. The endocervical glands atrophy and the endocervical canal gradually narrows, often resulting in frank cervical stenosis in the late postmenopausal period.

Cervical erosion, ulcer, and ectropion are three conditions that become increasingly important with aging. In erosion of the acquired type, there is a loss of superficial layers of the epithelium by a local destructive process that may be unclear etiologically. It may be due to the result of pH change, bacterial toxicity, or a combination of the two. The basal cuboidal cells are exposed. A congenital form of erosion may also be a pathogenetic factor. Cervical ectropion is manifested by an inflamed, edematous endocervical mucosa that protrudes from the endocervical canal and is easily visible. True cervical ulcers, like any ulcer, present gross and histologic findings. There is complete loss of epithelium, revealing a base of more or less active granulation tissue with an increasingly fibrous base over time. Bleeding may recur as a result of senile cervicitis, with or without infections, or benign polyps of the cervix. However, cervical cancer can and does occur in the elderly population, and cervical smears, colposcopic examination, biopsies, and possibly fractional curettage are indicated if a lesion is present in the cervix or cervical smear shows abnormal cytologic changes without any evidence of a gross lesion.

Cervicitis is an inflammation in the cervix and may be part of an inflammatory process that involves primarily the endometrium, vagina, or vulva; alternatively, it may be a primary cervical disease. Cervicitis is probably the most common gynecologic disease. It has been estimated that half of all women suffer from it sometime during their lives. The patient presents with leukorrhea. Acute cervicitis is very rare in the postmenopausal and geriatric patient. However, chronic cervicitis may be seen. Nonspecific cervicitis is extremely common and often afflicts almost every multiparous female. A variety of organisms have been implicated. The nonspecific cervicitis most commonly result from pH change, estrogen depletion, and cervical ectropion. Chlamydia is now being found in the menopausal and postmenopausal patient, but not as commonly as in the younger patient. This is also true of human papilloma virus. The number of flat condylomata that are discovered on biopsy or when surveyed with the colposcope is on the increase. HPV type 6/11 are usually found in these lesions. Occasionally, herpes simplex virus type 2 may cause a lesion on the cervix. The increasing incidence of chlamydia, human papilloma virus, and herpes simplex virus type 2 being found in the vagina and on the cervix of menopausal and postmenopausal women may represent a change in lifestyle.

Cervical Intraepithelial Neoplasia (CIN)

Carcinoma in situ of the cervix is a premenopausal disease, the average age of occurrence being 38 years. The invasive phase of this disease affects white women with peak occurrences in the 45- to 49-year age group, after which the rate remains constant with advancing age. In contrast, the rate in black women continues to rise with increasing age.

The term *cervical intraepithelial neoplasia* denotes all precursors of squamous cervical cancer and embraces a continuous spectrum from CIN 1 to CIN 3. Adenocarcinoma in situ is uncommon. However, it seems to be on the increase. The age distribution is from the mid-teens to the mid-eighties, with the median age in the third decade. HPV 16/18 are usually found in CIN lesions.

The condition is usually revealed on an abnormal Papanicolaou smear. CIN is characteristically symptom and sign free. The symptoms are likely to be associated with a coexisting condition, and visible signs of red or white patches are not necessarily the sites of the lesion of significance. They usually occur within the transformation zone. Unfortunately, in the postmenopausal woman, the transformation zone moves farther up into the endocervical canal, and it is difficult to survey the entire zone. Failure to diagnose CIN on colposcopy may be due to a lesion high in the canal. Alternatively, the disease may occur in an acute cervicitis, often with contact bleeding. Warty atypia due to subclinical human papilloma virus can complicate the colposcopic interpretation. It is important to exclude invasive cancer, and this can only be done by biopsy. In the postmenopausal and geriatric patient, it is also essential to do an endocervical scraping.

With the exclusion of invasive cancer by combined colposcopic–histologic study, the management of in situ cancer becomes a matter of clinical judgment. The lesion can be treated by hot cautery, cryotherapy, or CO_2 laser surgery. There are specific indications for a cone biopsy. These consist mainly of positive cytology, with no visible lesion macroscopically or on colposcopic examination.

Adenocarcinoma in Situ

Adenocarcinoma in situ is an uncommon entity. Recently, it has been recognized more frequently by distinctive changes in the Papanicolaou smear. When it is associated with squamous lesions, it is termed *adenosquamous.* The colposcopic appearance of the lesions, when visible, closely mimics that of the villous outgrowths of normal columnar epithelium. The distinguishing feature of the villi, after application of acetic acid, is their striking white color. The lesions are frequently multifocal. Since invasive carcinoma may coexist deep in the cervical clefts or glands, cone biopsy is necessary to exclude it.

Microinvasive Carcinoma

International Federation of Obstetrics and Gynecology (FIGO) distinguishes stage Ia (microinvasion) from stage Ib (occult). Histologists make this separation by arbitrary definitions that are highly specific for each laboratory. The tendency is to treat occult invasive cancer radically and microinvasion more conservatively. However, when microinvasion is found in the menopausal and postmenopausal patient, it is in their interest to have either a conventional conservative hysterectomy or a modified radical hysterectomy with either node dissection or node sampling. Adenocarcinoma, which meets these criteria, should also be treated in a similar manner.

Invasive Cervical Carcinoma

Over 90 percent of invasive cervical tumors are squamous. The average age of occurrence is 45 years, with a trend toward a younger age. However, among blacks, the incidence increases with age.

It is important to make an accurate histologic diagnosis of invasive cancer. Once this has been done, the patient should be evaluated. Treatment modalities available include radical surgery, radical irradiation, and chemotherapy. In patients aged 65 or less with stage Ib or IIa disease, radical surgery may be chosen, but since these patients often have metabolic and cardiopulmonary problems, external and interstitial radiation therapy is usually selected. Follow-up examinations should be carried out at frequent intervals during the first 2 years because it is during this time that the greatest number of recurrences will be detected.

Stages IIB, III, and IV are treated with radiation therapy. In stages III and IV, chemotherapy is being given with increasing frequency. Three courses of combination therapy are given at 3-week intervals. The drugs used are usually cis-platinum, velban, and bleomycin. This is followed by external therapy. The doses total approximately 5000 rads. The patient is then evaluated to see whether intracavitary and intravaginal radiation should also be given.

In stage IV with bladder involvement, it may be necessary to do a urinary diversion prior to the radiation therapy because of the danger of fistula development. Select central stage IV disease patients below age 65 may be suitable for primary pelvic exenteration. However, it is important to select these patients carefully.

FOLLOW-UP: GENERAL CONSIDERATIONS

Follow-up is best undertaken by the same observer who has been responsible for the initial management. Since 75 percent of deaths occur during the first 2 years, special attention must be given to this time period. The patient should be followed for life whenever possible.

Careful documentation of the following is necessary: symptoms, weight, leg edema, supraclavicular nodes, abdomen including girth and liver, vaginal examination, and rectal examination.

In addition, carcinoembryonic antigen (CEA) is a valuable marker; a rising level is frequently an early sign of recurrent disease, particularly in adenocarcinoma. The blood chemistries and an intravenous pyelogram should be performed at regular intervals, together with pelvic ultrasound, computed tomography (CT) scanning, and x-ray/films as indicated. These patients should be given estrogen supplements as needed, and special attention should be given to the vagina so that synechiae do not form. Ideally, an estrogenic cream is used to help keep the vagina patent.

SUMMARY

The lower genital tract consists of the vulva, vagina, and cervix. These three organs share a great deal in common in terms of their epidemiology and their response to hormone stimulation; therefore, they are discussed together.

The vulva in the geriatric patient is subjected to the same trauma and inflammatory disease, as well as neoplastic disease, as is the premenopausal patient.

Vulvar dystrophies are common during the postmenopausal years, but there are no good data to implicate estrogen deprivation as a primary etiology of this disease. Estrogen therapy does not always improve these patients. Indeed, there are some patients that complain of marked burning when estrogen is applied locally.

Squamous cell carcinoma in situ has been seen with increasing frequency not only among the younger age patients, but in the peri- and postmenopausal years. It is important to rule out neoplastic lesions in other parts of the genital system when the diagnosis of squamous cell carcinoma in situ of the vulva has been made. The diagnosis must be made by biopsy so that a more advanced lesion is not overlooked. Although a great variety of treatments have been given in the past, the CO_2 laser currently gives excellent results, and has a good cosmetic effect as well.

Paget's disease of the vulva is usually listed as an in situ lesion, but must be biopsied carefully so that an invasive lesion is not missed. The biopsy should extend down through the fat to the fascia and should extend at least 2 to 3 cm on the visible margin of the lesion.

Microinvasion of the vulva constitutes up to 17 percent of all vulvar cancers. It is important to get a good biopsy specimen of the area so that the aggressiveness of the lesion can be determined. Therapy is scaled to fit the needs of the patient and the extent of disease. Node dissection is occasionally carried out if the microinvasion involves a wide area.

The standard operation for invasive cancer of the vulva has been an extended vulvectomy with bilateral inguinal and pelvic lymphadenectomy. Recently, there has been a trend toward individualization and a less radical procedure, particularly in the elderly. Many gynecologists working in the field of oncology have abandoned the deep node dissection and are giving external radiation therapy to the area. In some stage I lesions hemivulvectomy and ipsilateral lymphadenectomy has been recommended.

The vagina becomes atrophic in the geriatric patient unless estrogen therapy has been administered. Vaginal intraepithelial neoplasia may occur in these patients. The lesions can be identified by swabbing the vagina with 4 percent acetic acid. With the use of colposcopy, biopsy specimens can then be taken from the suspicious areas. Having ruled out an invasive lesion, the patient can be successfully treated with a variety of treatments, including laser therapy, the use of 5-FU cream, and wide excision of the area.

Invasive tumors of the vagina are uncommon. Once the diagnosis is made by biopsy, however, the patient can be treated by either surgery or radiation. Lesions in the upper vagina can be treated with radical hysterectomy, pelvic lymph node dissection and partial vaginectomy. In this age group, however, most patients are treated with radiation therapy—this includes patients with lesions in the upper, middle, and lower thirds of the vagina.

The term cervical intraepithelial neoplasia (CIN) denotes all precursors of squamous cervical cancer and embraces a continuous spectrum from CIN I through CIN III. Adenocarcinoma in situ of the cervix is uncommon, but it has been seen with increasing frequency during the past few years.

Once the diagnosis is made by performing adequate biopsies, the treatment becomes academic. The chief aim of the therapy is to eradicate the lesion. Cryotherapy, cautery, laser therapy, and cone biopsy are all acceptable treatments. In this age group, there is a more liberal indication for the use of hysterectomy, with particular attention directed toward the upper vagina so that spread to the vagina is not overlooked.

Adenocarcinoma in situ is an uncommon entity that has been recently recognized more frequently by distinctive changes in the Pap smear. It is usually associated with squamous carcinoma in situ—it is then called adenosquamous carcinoma in situ. It is a slightly more aggressive lesion, and when the diagnosis is made, cone biopsy should be carried out to make certain that a more aggressive lesion is not being overlooked.

Invasive cancer of the cervix in the perimenopausal and geriatric age group is usually treated with external x-ray therapy and intravaginal and intrauterine implant of cesium. There are some patients who are 65 years of age or less, however, who have a stage IB lesion who are treated with radical hysterectomy and pelvic lymphadenectomy. Occasionally, a stage IIa will receive the same surgical treatment. Stage IIb, III, and IV, however, are always treated with external x-ray therapy and a radiation implant into the vagina and the cervix.

REFERENCES

Anderson, M. D., and R. B. Hartley. 1980. Cervical crypt involvement by intraepithelial neoplasia. *Obstet. Gynecol.* 55:546.

Averette, H. E., and V. W. Jobson. 1979. The role of exploratory laparotomy in the staging and treatment of invasive cervical cancer. *Int. J. Radiol. Oncol. Biol. Phys.* 5:2137.

Baggish, M. S., and J. H. Dorsey. 1981. CO_2 laser for the treatment of vulvar carcinoma in situ. *Obstet. Gynecol.* 57:371.

Baird, P. J., P. M. Elliott, M. Stening, and A. Korda. 1979. Giant condyloma acuminatum of the vulva and anal canal. *Aust. N. Z. J. Obstet. Gynaecol.* 19:119.

Baird, P. J., P. Russell, and C. R. Laverty. 1978. A pathological study of the relationship between lichen sclerosus et atrophicus and squamous carcinoma of the vulva. *Pathology* 10:196.

Barber, H. R. K. 1978. Cervical cancer, in: *Gynecologic Oncology* (L. McGowan, ed.), Appleton-Century-Crofts, New York, chap. 11.

Benson, W. L., and H. J. Norris. 1977. A critical review of the frequency of lymph node metastasis and death from microinvasive carcinoma of the cervix. *Obstet. Gynecol.* 49:632.

Boronow, R. C. 1973. Therapeutic alternative to primary exenteration for advanced vulvovaginal cancer. *Gynecol. Oncol.* 3:233.

Breen, J. L., C. I. Smith, and C. A. Gregori. 1978. Extramammary Paget's disease. *Clin. Obstet. Gynecol.* 21:1107.

Burghardt, E. 1981. Pathology of preclinical invasive carcinoma of cervix. (microinvasive and occult invasive carcinoma), in: *Gynecologic Oncology* (M. Coppleson, ed.), Churchill Livingstone, Edinburgh, chap. 34.

Burke, L., L. Covell, and D. Antonioli. 1980. CO_2 laser therapy of cervical intraepithelial neoplasia: factors determining success rate. *Lasers Surg. Med.* 1:113.

Buscema, J., J. D. Woodruff, T. H. Parmley, et al. 1980. Carcinoma in situ of the vulva. *Obstet. Gynecol.* 55:225.

Collins, C. G., H. L. Hansen, and E. Thercot. 1966. A clinical stain for use in selecting biopsy sites in patients with vulvar disease. *Obstet. Gynecol.* 28:158.

Corey, L., A. J. Nahmias, M. E. Guinan, et al. 1982. A trial of topical acyclovir in genital herpes simplex virus infection. *N. Engl. J. Med.* 306:1313.

Crum, C. P., Y. S. Fu, R. V. Levine, et al. 1972. Intraepithelial lesions of the vulva: Biologic and histologic criteria for the distinction of condyloma from vulvar intraepithelial neoplasia. *Am. J. Obstet. Gynecol.* 144:77.

Deppe, G., C. J. Cohen, and H. W. Bruckner. 1979. Chemotherapy of squamous cell carcinoma of the vulva. *Gynecol. Oncol.* 7:345.

DiSaia, P. J., W. T. Creasman, and W. M. Rich. 1979. An alternate approach to early cancer of the vulva. *Am. J. Obstet. Gynecol.* 133:825.

Forney, J. P., C. P. Morrow, D. E. Townsend, et. al. 1977. Management of carcinoma in situ of the vulva. *Am. J. Obstet. Gynecol.* 127:801.

Friedrich, E. G. 1981. Intraepithelial carcinoma of vulva, in: *Gynecologic Oncology* (M. Coppleson, ed.), Churchill Livingstone, Edinburgh, chap. 23.

Friedrich, E. G., E. J. Wilkinson, and Y. S. Fu. 1980. Carcinoma in situ of the vulva: A continuing challenge. *Am. J. Obstet. Gynecol.* 136:880.

Hernandez-Linares, W. A. Puthawala, J. F. Nolan, et al. 1980. Carcinoma in situ of the vagina. Past and present management. *Obstet. Gynecol.* 56:356.

Jordan, J. A. 1981. CO_2 laser therapy, in: *Gynecologic Oncology* (M. Coppleson, ed.), Churchill Livingstone, Edinburgh, chap. 62.

Kirkup, W., A. S. Evans, A. K. Brough, et al. 1982. Cervical intraepithelial neoplasia and warty atypia. A study of colposcopic, histologic and cytological characteristics. *Br. J. Obstet. Gynaecol.* 89:25.

Kneale, B. L. G., P. M. Elliott, and I. A. McDonald. 1981. Microinvasive carcinoma of vulva: Clinical features and management, in: *Gynecologic Oncology* (M. Coppleson, ed.), Churchill Livingstone, Edinburgh, chap. 24.

Kolstad, P. 1981. Conservative surgery for carcinoma of vulva, in: *Gynecologic Oncology* (M. Coppleson, ed.), Churchill Livingstone, Edinburgh, chap. 66.

Krupp, P. J. 1981. Invasive tumors of vulva. Clinical features and management, in: *Gynecologic Oncology* (M. Coppleson, ed.), Churchill Livingstone, Edinburgh, chap. 25.

Lee, R. A., and R. E. Symmonds. 1976. Recurrent carcinoma in situ of the vagina in patients previously treated for in situ carcinoma of the cervix. *Obstet. Gynecol.* 48:61.

Mattingly, R. F. 1981. Radical hysterectomy with pelvic lymphadenectomy, in: *Gynecologic Oncology* (M. Coppleson, ed.), Churchill Livingstone, Edinburgh, chap. 68.

Monaghan, J. M., J. A. Davis, and P. T. Edington. 1982. Treatment of cervical intraepithelial neoplasia by colposcopically directed cryosurgery and subsequent pregnancy experience. *Br. J. Obstet. Gynaecol.* 89:387.

Morley, G. W., 1976. Infiltrative carcinoma of the vulva: Results of surgical treatment. *Am. J. Obstet. Gynecol.* 124:874.

Park, R. G., and T. H. Parmley. 1978. Vaginal cancer, in: *Gynecologic Oncology* (L. McGowan, ed.), Appleton-Century-Crofts, New York, chap. 17.

Petrilli, E. S., D. E. Townsend, C. P. Morrow, and C. Y. Nakao. 1980. Vaginal intraepithelial neoplasia: Biologic aspects and treatment with topical 5-fluorouracil and the carbon dioxide laser. *Am. J. Obstet. Gynecol.* 138:321.

Pinkus, H. 1977. Skin biopsy: A field of interaction between clinician and pathologist. *Cutis* 20:609.

Piver, M. S., and J. J. Barlow. 1974. Paraaortic lymphadenectomy in staging patients with advanced local cervical cancer. *Obstet. Gynecol.* 43:544.

Piver, M. S., F. Rutledge, and J. P. Smith. 1974. Five classes of extended hysterectomy for women with cervical cancer. *Obstet. Gynecol.* 44:265.

Reid, R., C. R. Stanhope, B. R. Herschman, et al. 1982. Genital warts and cervical cancer (I). *Cancer,* 50:377.

Reid, R. 1983. Genital warts and cervical cancer (II). Is human papillomaviral infection the trigger to cervical carcinogenesis? *Gynecol. Oncol.* in press.

Stallworthy, Sir John. 1981. Clinical invasive carcinoma of cervix: Combined radiotherapy and radical surgery as primary treatment, in: *Gynecologic Oncology* (M. Coppleson, ed.), Churchill Livingstone, Edinburgh, chap. 40.

Townsend, D. E., R. V. Levine, C. P. Crum, and R. M. Richard. 1982. Treatment of vaginal carcinoma in situ with the carbon dioxide laser. *Am. J. Obstet. Gynecol.* 143:565.

VanNagell, J. R., Jr., E. S. Donaldson, J. C. Parker, et al. 1977. The prognostic significance of cell type and lesion size in patients with cervical cancer treated by radical surgery. *Gynecol. Oncol.* 5:142.

Way, S. 1982. *Malignant Disease of the Vulva.* Churchill-Livingstone, Edinburgh.

Wharton, J. T., G. H. Fletcher, and L. Delclos. 1981. Invasive tumours of vagina: Clinical features and management, in: *Gynecologic Oncology* (M. Coppleson, ed.), Churchill Livingstone, Edinburgh, chap. 17.

10 Upper Genital Tract

INTRODUCTION

The endometrium, uterus, ovaries, fallopian tubes, and breast make up the upper genital tract. They share many epidemiologic factors and have a hormone association relationship. Therefore, it is appropriate that they be grouped together, since they share so many things in common.

UTERUS

The uterine cavity is lined with the endometrium, and the outer surface of the uterus is covered with serosa. The endometrium has two components: the stroma and the glands. Both components are highly sensitive to hormones. During the reproductive years, the endometrium shows active cyclic changes in response to ovarian hormones. It is also highly responsive to pregnancy, as well as to other endogenous hormones and to exogenous hormones. Such reactivity makes the endometrium susceptible to functional changes that may be physiologic or pathologic, such as hyperplasia and atrophy.

In the premenopausal woman, the endometrium is divided into three layers. The layer closest to the myometrium is called the *pars basalis.* Above that is the *zona spongiosa* and then the *zona compacta*. The superficial layer (zona compacta) has glandular portions that are straight and narrow and surrounded by an edematous stroma. Here and there the stroma cells are greatly enlarged, containing glycogen; they are ovoid or slightly polygonal in shape, with a pale spherical nucleus, and are individually surrounded by reticular or even collagenous fibers. These cells, which become abundant if pregnancy ensues, are called *deciduous cells,* and the layer they form is called the *compacta*. The middle layer (compacta spongiosa) occupies most of the mucosa, in which the glands are highly sacculated and often distended with secretion, leading to a reduction in the height of the lining epithelium. The zone is aptly called the *spongiosa*. Here a premenstrual leukocytic infiltration is marked. The superior and middle layers, that is, the compacta and spongiosa, make up the *pars functionalis*. There is a thin, only slightly altered basalis layer just above or within the superficial parts of the myometrium.

At the time of the menopause, the endometrium, like other genital tissues, undergoes atrophic changes. Grossly, the endometrium has a flat, glazed, grayish to gray-red appearance with a hint of translucency and a monotonous pattern. The senile endometrium is thin and atrophic, and contains only scattered, inactive glands in the stroma. Cystic hyperplasia is another form of inactive endometrium in which dilated glands exhibit a single flat layer of mitotically inactive cells. Hyperplasia of the endometrium may be present and resemble that found toward the end of menstrual life. The pattern is indicative of active estrogen support even in the postmenopausal patient. This active hyperplasia may be identified in as many as 20 percent of postmenopausal women. It is due to unopposed estrogen stimulation from endogenous or exogenous sources. When the endometrium is active in the postmenopausal years, there is an increased risk that it is premalignant.

In the endometrium that is not stimulated in the postmenopausal years, there are often flat, cuboidal cells that may be discontinuous with underlying glands. There is a dramatic decline in the mitotic activity of the epithelial glands. Therefore, the presence of mitotic activity in the postmenopausal patient may indicate a premalignant lesion, and the patient must be very carefully monitored. The glands in the postmenopausal endometrium are increased in number, usually dilated, and regularly blanched. Retention cysts may occur, and there may be a cystic hyperplasia with a Swiss cheese pattern. The stroma usually undergoes atrophy. However, it remains responsive to LH stimulation longer than the endometrium.

Under normal conditions, the endometrial cavity is sterile due to the effectiveness of the endocervix as a microbiologic barrier. Regular shedding of the endometrium helps to prevent the establishment of bacteria in the uterine cavity. However, in the postmenopausal years, this situation changes. It is rare to see an acute endometritis in the postmenopausal patient unless there has been an attempt to aspirate cells from the endometrial cavity or even to biopsy the area. The organisms that are usually found include streptococcus species, gram-negative bacilli, *Staphylococcus aureus,*

Escherichia coli. Granulomatous endometritis such as that seen in tuberculosis of the endometrium is almost always secondary to tuberculosis of the fallopian tubes. The lesions are usually asymptomatic. Although these lesions are usually detected in the premenopausal period, they are occasionally found in the postmenopausal endometrium.

Pyometrium indicates the accumulation of purulent exudate within the endometrial cavity, which often results in its distention. This uncommon condition is usually the result of a obstruction of the uterine cervix or the lower segment of the uterine body by carcinoma. It may be secondary to obstruction from an endocervical or endometrial polyp, or stenosis of the cervix, or simply atrophy. Whenever a pyometrium is encountered, carcinoma must be suspected. At the time of treatment of the pyometrium, the pus should be drained and no attempt made to do a dilatation and curettage (D&C) at that time. The patient is then followed and allowed to complete the drainage of the pyometrium. The distended myometrium will contract, so that within a month it will be safe to do a D&C.

Any postmenopausal woman complaining of staining should have a thorough investigation to rule out endometrial and uterine pathology. This requires a fractional curettage with a search of the endometrial cavity with a polyp forceps. If no cause of the bleeding can be found, it is important to investigate the bladder and rectum. Many cases of staining and bleeding in the postmenopausal period are a result of atrophic vaginitis or angiomata on the vulva.

Endometrial polyps may be found in the course of investigating unusual vaginal bleeding and may easily be missed when curettage is done. Therefore, it is important to search every part of the uterus with an endometrial polyp forceps. Endometrial polyps are usually benign, but occasionally in the late postmenopausal or geriatric period they may show some malignant changes. It is sometimes difficult to tell whether it is a true atypical polyp or a carcinoma of the endometrium growing in a polyploid fashion. However, either requires aggressive treatment.

DISEASES OF THE ENDOMETRIUM

Endometrial Hyperplasia

In the perimenopausal age group, endometrial hyperplasia and anovulatory cycles are common causes of uterine bleeding. In the postmenopausal patient, carcinoma of the cervix or endometrium, endometrial hyperplasia, endometrial polyps, hypertension, hormonal manipulation, and atrophic vaginitis are among the common causes of uterine bleeding.

Endometrial hypoplasia and atrophy indicate a generalized atrophic appearance of the endometrium. They are most commonly seen in the menopausal years, but they may also occur during the childbearing age. *Endometrial hyperplasia* is an abnormal proliferation of the endometrial glands and stroma. It is characterized by an increase in the thickness of the endometrium and varying degrees of morphologic abnormality such as stratification of the epithelium and abnormal gland patterns. The excessive proliferation of the endometrium is most probably the result of prolonged exposure to unopposed estrogen. Endometrial curettings produce a large amount of rubbery tissue, often containing microcysts. Such abundant curettings suggest endometrial hyperplasia, endometrial cancer, or marked adenomatous hyperplasia. The endometrium shows evidence of hyperplasia of the glands as well as of the stroma. Three types of endometrial hyperplasia have been identified: simple, cystic, and adenomatous.

Simple hyperplasia occurs frequently around the time of the menarche and menopause, but may also occur sporadically at other times. The glands are crowded, uniform, and small, and may show slight pseudostratification. There may be occasional cystic dilatation, but no cellular atypia is evident. There is evidence of estrogen stimulation. *Cystic hyperplasia* is a more advanced form of the disease and shows cystic dilatation of the endometrial glands. These glands are lined with columnar epithelium showing pseudostratification. The cells have large, crowded nuclei with only rare mitotic figures. Cysts may be present, giving the endometrium the appearance of Swiss cheese. Although this is not a cancer or perhaps even a precancerous lesion, one should be very circumspect when ordering estrogen replacement therapy in the presence of a cystic hyperplasia.

Adenomatous hyperplasia is a more advanced type of hyperplasia in which the glands are crowded and arranged back to back. They are lined with tall columnar cells with marked pseudostratification and intraglandular papillary folding. Mitotic figures are usually present in both the glands and the stroma. The glands are abnormal in shape and show evidence of irregular budding into the stroma. This may be considered a precancerous lesion and precludes the use of estrogen replacement therapy. Atypical adenomatous hyperplasia is sometimes referred to as *adenocarcinoma in situ.* In this type of disease, focal cytologic atypia is seen in the form of large vesicular nuclei, prominent nucleoli, eosinophilia of the cytoplasm, and loss of polarity. The cells become stratified. These changes may occur on a background of adenomatous hyperplasia. Since this type of change occurs in the menopausal and postmenopausal years, watchful waiting with frequent endometrial biopsies can be carried out. However, most clinicians feel that hysterectomy with bilateral salpingo-oophorectomy is the method of choice. Since most of these patients present with spotting or vaginal bleeding, this reinforces the statement that after the menopause it is important to screen the endometrium at least every year and a half.

The incidence of endometrial carcinoma is increasing. The majority of patients are postmenopausal, but approximately 20 percent are peri- or premenopausal.

Endometrial Metaplasias

The differential diagnosis of endometrial carcinoma includes not only the well-known hyperplasias but also a group of epithelial metaplasias, some appearing after known etiologic stimuli and others occurring without known antecedents. They have been classified into seven categories: (1) morules and squamous metaplasia; (2) papillary metaplasia; (3) ciliated cell or tubule metaplasia; (4) eosinophilic metaplasia; (5) mucinous metaplasia;

(6) hobnail metaplasia; and (7) clear cell metaplasia. None of these metaplasias have any clinical significance unless they are mistaken for carcinoma. The first four are the most common and thus most likely to be confused with cancer.

Squamous metaplasia and morules are most likely to be confused with adenoacanthoma, in which benign-appearing squamous or morular nests are seen within an adenocarcinoma. Papillary metaplasia has also been called *syncytial surface metaplasia,* because it tends to occur at or near the endometrial surface and is characterized by cells that form papillary projections and syncytia. The appearance is often reminiscence of microglandular hyperplasia of the endocervix. In tubule, ciliated cell, mucinous, or eosinophilic metaplasia, occasional glands are lined with cells with bland nuclei and bright eosinophilic cytoplasm.

Carcinoma of the Endometrium

The high-risk group includes women with obesity, nulliparity or low parity, late menopause, hypertension, diabetes, hormone-secreting tumors of the ovary, a history of polycystic ovary syndrome, exposure to ionizing radiation, exogenous estrogen use, and sequential oral contraceptive use. The most common presenting symptom is abnormal bleeding. A watery vaginal discharge is an uncommon presentation.

Adenocarcinoma makes up 65 percent of endometrial cancers and is followed by adenoacanthoma (20 percent) and adenosquamous carcinoma (12 percent). Rare tumors are clear cell adenocarcinoma, argyrophil cell carcinoma, and squamous carcinoma. The endometrium is involved in 15 to 25 percent of women with ovarian endometrioid cancer, although this may represent a simultaneous neoplastic transformation rather than a metastasis. Grade 3 adenocarcinoma, adenosquamous carcinoma, papillary serous carcinoma, and clear cell adenocarcinoma are aggressive tumors and have a worse prognosis than does adenocarcinoma of the endometrium.

Papillary Serous Carcinoma of the Endometrium

Papillary serous carcinoma is occurring with increasing frequency. Although this form of adenocarcinoma of the endometrium, often containing concentric microcalcifications or psammoma bodies, has been recognized for years, its clinical and pathologic features have only recently been fully characterized. These tumors are best called *papillary serous carcinomas* to indicate their identity, at the light microscopic level, with the similarly named tumor encountered far more frequently as an ovarian primary tumor.

Histologically, these tumors are characterized by papillary structures with broad fibrovascular connective tissue cores. These cores are lined with irregularly stratified cells that form secondary papillary structures and interconnecting arches. Exfoliation of small clusters of cells is quite common. Foci of necrosis are frequently seen. Since the tumors tend to be moderately to poorly differentiated, solid sheets of large, undifferentiated cells are almost invariably present. Psammoma bodies are detectable in approximately 30 percent of these tumors. A very characteristic feature of this cancer is its tendency to infiltrate the myometrium within the lymphatic or blood vessel channels. This is often an unexpected microscopic finding, occurring in a small, atrophic-appearing uterus. Grossly normal-appearing uterine adnexa also frequently show extensive tumor emboli. As would be expected from this pattern of dissemination, the prognosis is extremely poor, and this tumor should be considered one in which adjuvant therapy will almost always be necessary.

Papillary serous carcinoma must be differentiated from papillary endometrioid carcinoma. Papillary endometrioid carcinoma is generally well differentiated and prognostically favorable; thus, its histologic distinction is clinically important. Unlike papillary serous carcinoma, its papillae are narrow and tend to be lined with uniform, stratified cells with their axes uniformly perpendicular to the basement membrane.

Prognostic Factors

Three out of four patients will be found in stage I. Prognostic factors other than clinical stage are important if treatment is to be individualized. These factors, permitting surgical-pathologic classification, are (1) histologic differentiation, (2) myometrial penetration, (3) lymph node metastases, both pelvic and paraaortic, (4) occult involvement of the cervix, (5) unexpected adnexal metastases, and (6) positive peritoneal cytology.

Fractional uterine curettage is necessary for definitive diagnosis. The canal is first curetted (to detect stage II lesions) with a special sharp curette prior to cervical dilatation. Routine D&C follows.

The patient should have a careful preoperative evalution. The standard treatment is total hysterectomy with bilateral salpingo-oophorectomy. Pelvic and paraaortic nodes are sampled if the patient's condition permits it. All patients receive intravaginal radiation therapy 1 month after the hysterectomy. In grade 2 and 3 carcinomas or those in which the uterus is more than 8 cm, patients receive pelvic external x-ray therapy. Intracavitary irradiation is effective in decreasing the incidence of vaginal metastases. Chemotherapy with progesterones and tamoxifen is being used to treat recurrent endometrial cancer.

Follow-Up

Sixty percent of the recurrences occur within 2 years and 90 percent within 5 years. Undifferentiated tumors seem to recur earlier. Recurrences may be found in the vagina, pelvis, or distal organs. Recurrence in the vagina is uncommon if radiotherapy has been given. Plasma carcinoembryonic antigen (CEA) values may be of use in predicting recurrences. Pretreatment CEA values have been raised in 22 percent of well-differentiated, 29 percent of moderately differentiated, and 67 percent of undifferentiated tumors.

After treatment of endometrial carcinoma, follow-up should occur every 3 to 4 months for the first year; at 6-month intervals until the third year; and after that, at 6-month to 1-year intervals, depending upon the stage and the condition of the patient. A Pap smear should be carried out at each visit, as well as plasma CEA. A chest x-ray should be done at least once a year, and ultrasound and scans (either CT or sonography) as indicated.

OVARY

The decline of estrogen production by the ovary is the most clinically significant endocrine alteration of the menopause and the postmenopausal period. In the premenopausal years, 17-beta-estradiol is the principal circulating estrogen. In the postmenopausal period, the estrogens of note are estrone and its precursor, probably androstenedione. When the follicles disappear or become unresponsive to pituitary stimulation, there is a marked decrease in estrogen. The primary steroidogenic element remaining in the postmenopausal ovary is the stroma, which still responds after the menopause to pituitary LH by producing androgens. Androgen production also occurs in the adrenal gland and by peripheral conversion of less potent sex steroids. The relative contribution of each source is difficult to assess.

It has been repeatedly observed that the menopausal ovary exhibits direct secretion of only minimal amounts of estrogen due to a reduced number of functioning follicles. Gonadotropin levels rise due to reduced negative feedback of estrogen. With high LH levels, the ovarian stroma continues to produce androgen. Estrone, a relatively weak estrogen, is formed by peripheral conversion of androgen precursors. It is apparent, therefore, that the endogenous hormonal milieu of the postmenopausal ovary is primary androgenic, and that estrogen production and its effect are dramatically reduced.

The contrast between the premenopausal and postmenopausal ovary is striking. Whereas the premenopausal ovary measures $3.5 \times 2 \times 1.5$ cm, the menopausal ovary tends to atrophy and shrink when the graafian follicles and ova disappear. The tunica albuginea becomes very dense and causes the surface of the ovary to become scarred and shrunken. The cortex is marked by increased thinning, as well as the presence of numerous corpora fibrosa and corpora albuginea, with areas of dense fibrosis and hyalinization. The ovary shows varying degrees of avascularity. Eventually the ovary becomes an inert residue that consists of connective tissue, and clings to the posterior leaf of the broad ligament. Its pink color becomes pure white. It shrinks to $2 \times 1.5 \times 0.5$ cm, and in some women it may be as small as $1.5 \times 0.75 \times 0.5$ cm. Its wrinkled surface resembles the gyri and sulci of the cerebrum. At this point, it cannot be palpated. The postmenopausal palpable ovary (PMPO) is not a normal ovary at this stage of life.

Pure oophoritis is a rare disorder. The most acute and chronic inflammation lesions of the ovary occur in association with similar inflammatory lesions of the fallopian tube, resulting in salpingo-oophoritis or tuboovarian abscess. This rarely occurs in the postmenopausal patient. However, the ovary may become involved in an inflammatory process secondary to an acute diverticulitis or perforation of the bowel secondary to diverticulitis. Occasionally the ovary will be involved in an inflammatory process when there is carcinoma of the bowel, particularly if there is a small perforation that may involve the ovary. Chronic oophoritis is practically unknown in the postmenopausal patient. Tuberculosis and actinomycosis of the ovary may cause oophoritis, but these tumors are usually seen in the premenopausal years.

DISEASES OF THE OVARY

Carcinoma of the Ovary

The ovary may become too old to function, but it never becomes too old to form a tumor. In the postmenopausal years, the ovary should be removed with the uterus. The reason is that if it is late in the postmenopausal period, the ovary is not functioning, either a cancer or a retained ovary syndrome may develop. If the woman insists on keeping her ovaries—and it is difficult to believe that she would not listen to the advice of her physician—she should be made to sign a form stating that she has been thoroughly informed of these problems.

Ovarian cancer is the leading cause of death from gynecologic cancer. It is the most frustrating problem that the physician faces in gynecology. It is not possible to make an early diagnosis, as evidenced by the fact that 60 to 70 percent of these patients are already in stage III or IV when they present for initial treatment. The overall 5-year survival for the patient with invasive common epithelial cancer is seldom better than 25 percent. It is now accepted that over the age of 65, the survival rate is less than it is in patients below this age.

The greatest number of cases appear between ages 45 and 60, but the peak incidence is at about age 77. This pattern tends to reinforce the statement that the ovary becomes too old to function but never becomes too old to form a cancer. Although it has been stated that there are no early symptoms of ovarian cancer, reports in the literature contradict this statement. Many women with ovarian cancer have vague abdominal complaints for a long time before the diagnosis is made. Many of these women have had a complete workup, including barium enema and a GI series, but a thorough pelvic examination was not carried out. It is therefore important to rule out ovarian cancer in any women over age 40, particularly one who is nulliparous or has had a history of involuntary sterility or multiple spontaneous abortions and who presents with vague abdominal symptoms that are not identified by careful workup. These patients must be watched very carefully, and if the suspicion is great enough, surgical exploration is warranted. It is important to examine patients over age 40 every 6 months. They should be instructed to take an enema before coming in for a pelvic examination.

Postmenopausal Palpable Ovary Syndrome

Any women who is 2 years postmenopausal and presents with a palpable ovary that is normal in size for a premenopausal patient should have a careful workup. If on repeat examination the finding is confirmed, surgical exploration should be carried out. This finding has been designated the *postmenopausal palpable ovary syndrome (PMPO).*

Classification

Primary ovarian neoplasms have been divided into gonadal stromal tumors, germ cell cancers, common epithelial ovarian cancers, and metastatic lesions.

The gonadal stromal tumors are very rare in the postmenopausal period. However, a thecoma is occasionally diagnosed. Most often it is a functioning tumor, and when it functions, if there is a uterus present, it is often accompanied by vaginal staining or bleeding. The thecomas are almost uniformly benign tumors. Occasionally there are granulosa cell tumors, about 25 percent of which function and, again, provide endometrial stimulation with vaginal bleeding. Approximately 25 percent of these tumors are malignant and approximately 5 percent are bilateral.

Germ cell tumors are very rare in the postmenopausal period. However, the common epithelial ovarian cancer of the clear cell variety may be confused with the endodermal sinus tumor. However, the histologic pictures, when carefully reviewed, are found to be fairly dissimilar. A clear cell neoplasia consists of epithelial cells, with clear or pale eosinophilic cytoplasm, which are frequently arranged in a hobnail pattern. Since some of these tumors do not consist of clear cells, the term *mesonephroid tumors* is preferred by some authors. These tumors usually occur between the ages of 40 and 70 and are almost always malignant. Very few cases of borderline or benign tumors have been reported. Adenofibromatosis and cytoadenofibromatosis variants also occur. This tumor must be distinguished from the endodermal sinus tumor, which is an extraembryonal germ cell tumor. There are distinctive paravascular structures resembling the endodermal sinuses of the rat placenta, and both intracellular and extracellular hyaline globules give a periodic acid-Schiff reaction. The hyaline bodies resemble Russell's bodies. These tumors are thus extraembryonal derivations of the yolk sac endoderm from embryonal carcinoma. They are highly malignant tumors and usually are not seen in the postmenopausal period except occassionally in orientals. The diagnosis is suspected after pelvic examination, but is confirmed at exploratory surgery. The alpha fetoprotein assay then helps monitor the patient's response to therapy. The therapy is the same as for the epithelial and fallopian tube cancer, which is removal of the uterine tubes, ovaries, omentum, and appendix, followed by combination chemotherapy.

Epithelial tumors arise from the mesothelial surface of the ovary. The International Federation of Gynecology and Obstetrics (FIGO) has classified common primary epithelial tumors of the ovary as serous cystomas, mucinous cystomas, endometrioid tumors, clear cell tumors, undifferentiated carcinoma, mixed epithelial tumors, and tumors with no histology or unclassifiable.

Invasive epithelial tumors comprise about 90 percent of malignant ovarian tumors. The average age of diagnosis is 50 years. The tumors are uncommon below the age of 40. Ovarian carcinoma is rarely diagnosed in the symptom-free patient. The most common presentation is abdominal swelling (mass and/or ascites). Abdominal discomfort, gastrointestinal or urinary symptoms, abnormal bleeding, and weight loss are frequent symptoms. Rarely does the disease present as a surgical emergency.

Physical signs suggestive of a malignant change in an ovarian tumor include bilaterality, fixation in the pelvis, nodularity of the surface or in the pouch of Douglas, solid or semisolid consistency, and ascites. None of these findings are diagnostic.

Diagnosis. Diagnosis is made at laparotomy. The possibility that the disease is metastatic to the ovary must be borne in mind. Reports indicate that 10 to 30 percent of malignant ovarian tumors are metastatic. The most common primary sites are the breast, gastrointestinal tract, uterus, and the opposite ovary.

Staging laparotomy is essential for more accurate staging of the disease. Such procedures will upstage stage I disease by 10 to 20 percent and stage II disease by over 50 to 80 percent. The procedure consists of making an adequate vertical incision so that the entire abdomen and pelvis can be very carefully explored. Any patient who is understaged will be undertreated.

Treatment. The treatment of carcinoma of the ovary is surgical removal of the uterus, tubes, ovaries, omentum, and appendix. The surgery should be aggressive without creating inordinate morbidity and mortality. This can usually be accomplished in stages I and II and, whenever possible, in stages III and IV. Occasionally in advanced stages, subtotal hysterectomy is preferred. Tumor reductive surgery (debulking procedures) has improved chemotherapy response rates, as well as increasing survival when the tumor masses can be reduced to lesions 2 cm in diameter or less.

Superradical surgery in the form of pelvic exenteration has a very limited place and should not be attempted in the geriatric patient. If the ovarian cancer violates its natural history, recurs late, and is confined to the pelvis, pelvic exenteration may be indicated.

Chemotherapy is generally recommended as adjuvant therapy in malignant epithelial tumors of all stages. Adriamycin, which is associated with cardiac toxicity, should be used with great caution in the elderly. Excellent response rates have been reported with cis-platinum and cyclophosphamide. The place of radiation as an adjuvant to surgery is still ill-defined. Most authors have shown no advantage in stages I through IV, although there is some support for its use in stage II cases.

Intraperitoneal use of radionuclide therapy in stage I and II disease is advocated by some authorities, especially with intraoperative rupture of the tumor. ^{32}P is now preferred to radioactive gold. These nuclides give a high dose of radiation to the peritoneal surface that can produce bowel injury, especially if its distribution within the peritoneal cavity is not uniform.

Second-look laparotomy or reexploration to assess the success of chemotherapy and then to indicate the desirability of continuing or ceasing treatment is commonly practiced. Since there are no hard data to support this procedure, it is important to discuss the options, risk, complications, and indications for second-look laparotomy with the patient. At this point in time it should be recommended that the patient have a second-look procedure unless her physiologic age matches her chronologic age.

FALLOPIAN TUBE

Primary carcinoma of the fallopian tube is rare and constitutes 0.3 percent of all gynecologic malignancies. The mean age of occurrence is 55 years, with a range from 18 to 88 years. The disease is seldom diagnosed before laparotomy. Twenty percent of these tumors are bilateral. If they are confined to the tube, a clinical diagnosis of hydrosalpinx or pyosalpinx may be made.

Only half of these cases show the classic triad of bleeding, abdominal pain, and pelvic or abdominal mass. An occasional patient presents with a watery discharge. The most common presentation is abnormal bleeding or discharge; the Pap smear is rarely abnormal. The diagnosis of an unknown pelvic mass is usually made by ultrasound, CT scan, or laparoscopy.

The spread is similar to that of ovarian cancer. The treatment consists of staging laparotomy with peritoneal washings, biopsy, total hysterectomy, bilateral salpingo-oophorectomy, omentectomy, appendectomy, postoperative chemotherapy, and possible pelvic radiotherapy in stage III cases with bulky residual tumor. Cis-platinum, cyclophosphamide and possibly adriamycin is the usual adjunctive treatment given.

BREAST

The breast may be conveniently thought of as three systems: the skin, the ducts, and the paraductal or glandular system. It is helpful to think of these divisions when considering breast changes in the menopause, appreciating the fact that the menopause is characterized by diminution of the hormones that for so many years had so much to do with the physiology of the breast. In the postmenopausal years, the breasts undergo several alterations. These include atrophy of the acini and lobules, with involution progressing from the periphery toward the nipple. The stroma decreases in bulk and the paraductal tissue becomes progressively hyalinized. Although the atrophy of the breast in the postmenopausal years may be related somewhat to the loss of estrogen, there are no satisfactory, reversible changes with estrogen replacement. Histologic changes include flattening of the duct epithelium, with thinning of the ducts and a decrease in alveolar size. The reduction in the proportion of glandular tissues is accompanied by an increase in the proportion of subcutaneous fat. The breast usually becomes flaccid and smaller after the menopause, although some women maintain fairly normal-appearing breasts and often complain of cyclical changes occurring in their breast tissue.

In considering breast changes in the menopause, the physician and surgeon must determine what medication and hormones have been and are continuing to be administered. The normal events in breast physiology are a gradual decline in the size and function of the glandular mass throughout the menopause. The question is raised of whether these regressive changes in the presence of many factors—genetics, environment, pituitary hormones, and other hormones—permit the appearance of abnormal growths or neoplasia.

Breast Cancer

Cancer of the breast is increasing at a rate of about 1 percent a year; most of this increase occurs in patients under age 40. It is generally agreed that up to 20 percent of cancers may not be apparent to the palpating finger of even the most expert examiner. In fact, it has been stated that 30 population doublings are required to develop a 1-cm cancer. This may take 30 to 200 days. However, it has been shown that certain tumors have a phenotypic tendency to metastasize, and will do so within the first 10 to 20 doublings. It is totally impossible to detect this metastasis by any means available today. In addition, some studies show a disturbingly high percentage (about 30 percent) of cancers found within 1 year of a supposedly negative examination.

Detection

Over 90 percent of breast cancers are detected initially by the woman herself. However, the vast majority of women have not learned self-examination of the breast. The discovery of the tumor is accidental and, apparently, too late. Most breast cancers seen by the physician are late cancers with definite nodal involvement.

The three important methods used in screening for breast cancer are clinical examination, including palpation and inspection, mammography, and thermography. CEA and cystic disease protein blood tests can play a role in monitoring the patient with cancer. Mammography can help the clinician detect breast cancer at an earlier, more curable stage than is possible with clinical examination alone. There are certain indications for screening patients with a mammography. These include the following: (1) All women with signs and symptoms of breast disease should have mammography, as well as clinical examination, as often and whenever needed, regardless of age. (2) All women should have a baseline mammogram between ages 35 and 40, whether symptomatic or not. (3) All women over 40 should have a physical examination annually and mammography every 1 or, at most, every 2 or 3 years. (4) All women over 50 should have a physical examination and mammography every year.

Epidemiology

It is estimated that 123,000 new cases of cancer of the breast will occur in the United States during 1987. About 1 out of every 10 women will develop breast cancer sometime during their life. Risk factors include (1) an age of over 50, (2) a personal or family history of breast cancer, and (3) never having had children or having had the first child after age 30. The warning signals are *breast changes including cysts,* a lump, thickening, swelling, dimpling, skin irritation, discoloration, retraction or scaliness of the nipple, nipple discharge, pain, or tenderness.

The mean survival time for women of all ages with breast cancer is 6.6 years; between ages 55 and 64 it is 7.4 years; between 65 and 74 it is 5.9 years; and over 75, the median survival time is only 3.3 years.

Types of Breast Cancer

There are six histologic types of infiltrating breast cancer. The most common is infiltrating duct cancer, which makes up 78 percent of all breast cancers; it has a 60 percent rate of node involvement and a 5-year survival of 54 percent. Infiltrating lobular duct cancer is the next most common form. It constitutes about 8.7 percent of breast cancers, with a 60 percent rate of node involvement and a survival rate of approximately 50 percent. Medullary infiltrating cancer makes up 4.3 percent of these cancers, with a node involvement rate of 44 percent and a 69 percent survival rate. Colloid infiltrating cancer makes up 2.6 percent of all cancers, with a 32 percent node involvement rate and approximately 73 percent 5-year survival. Comedo infiltrating carcinoma makes up about 4.6 percent of all cancers of the breast. It has a node involvement rate of 32 percent and a survival rate of 73 percent. Papillary infiltrating cancer makes up 1.2 percent of breast cancers, with a node involvement rate of about 70 percent and a crude survival of 83 percent.

The estrogen and progesterone receptors have added a new dimension to the management of breast cancers. The estrogen receptor concentration is slightly higher in postmenopausal than in premenopausal women. However, in estrogen receptor-negative tumors, the receptor concentration may not be zero. The tissue simply contains an insufficient amount of receptor to elicit a hormone response, usually less than 3 to 10 femtomoles per milligram of protein. The patient in the postmenopausal period also seems to have a more well-differentiated tumor. Patients with estrogen receptor-negative tumors have a significant earlier recurrence rate than those with estrogen receptor-positive tumors, irrespective of age, menopausal status, size and location of the primary tumor, number of involved axillary lymph nodes, and adjuvant therapy. This has very important therapeutic implications. Patients with estrogen receptor-negative tumors and positive nodes at the time of mastectomy should be treated aggressively with adjuvant chemotherapy because of their poor prognosis. More importantly, these patients have a significantly shorter survival than those with estrogen receptor-positive tumors.

SUMMARY

The endometrium, ovary and fallopian tube, and breast constitute the upper genital tract, and they share a great number of epidemiologic factors and hormonal relationships.

Next to the breast, the endometrium is the site with the greatest number of cancers in the genital tract.

Endometrial hyperplasia in the postmenopausal period indicates that the endometrium is being stimulated either endogenously or exogenously. Any postmenopausal bleeding should be investigated by a fractional curettage. Most patients with cystic hyperplasia and adenomatous hyperplasia without atypical changes can be cured by a simple curettage. These patients should not receive any estrogen therapy after this diagnosis is made. Hysterectomy is reserved for those with any atypical adenomatous hyperplasia.

Grade 3 adenocarcinoma, adenosquamous carcinoma, papillary serous carcinoma, and clear cell adenocarcinoma are aggressive tumors and have a worse prognosis than does adenocarcinoma of the endometrium.

Both pre- and postoperative x-ray therapy give the same survival rate. The value of vaginal vault radiation has been proved. The incidence of recurrence in the vault has been cut from approximately 18 percent down to 1 to 3 percent in those that have been given radiation to the vault.

The postmenopausal ovary loses all its follicles; if there are follicles remaining, they do not function and the ovary does not secrete estrogen. For a period of time in the postmenopausal period, however, the ovary does produce some androgen.

One diagnostic sign of early neoplastic change (not necessarily malignant) in the ovary of the postmenopausal woman has proved to be both valuable and consistent in the hands of the gynecologist—the palpation of what is interpreted as a normal sized ovary in the premenopausal woman represents an ovarian tumor in the postmenopausal woman.

Ovarian cancer is the leading cause of death from gynecologic cancer. It is the most frustrating problem that the physician faces in gynecology. The greatest number of cases appear between ages 45 and 60, but the peak incidence is about age 77. The ovary is always at risk to develop a cancer.

The epithelial tumors arise from the mesothelial surface of the ovary and they are the most common tumors seen in the postmenopausal and geriatric patient. All postmenopausal and geriatric patients complaining of vague abdominal discomfort or any swelling should be carefully investigated to rule out ovarian cancer.

Surgery is the backbone of treatment for common epithelial ovarian cancer and this is usually followed by triple chemotherapy. The geriatric patient may have compromise of the kidney and cardiac systems, and it is therefore very important to evaluate the heart and kidney before giving adriamycin or cis-platinum.

The postmenopausal and geriatric patient definitely have a worse prognosis than the premenopausal patient with common epithelial ovarian cancer.

The breast is at risk for life to form cancer. Any change in the breast of these patients should be biopsied even if the mammography is negative.

The observed mean survival for all ages in woman with breast cancer is 6.6 years, whereas in patients 75 and older, it is only 3.3 years.

The postmenopausal patient with positive nodes and positive hormone receptors should be treated with tamoxifen. Chemotherapy may be considered for postmenopausal women with positive nodes and negative hormone receptor levels, but it cannot be recommended as standard practice. Patients in the geriatric age group who have negative nodes regardless of the hormone receptor levels should not be given routine adjuvant treatment.

REFERENCES

Aalders, J., V. Abeler, P. Kolstad, and M. Onsrud, M. 1980. Postoperative external irradiation and prognostic parameters in Stage I endometrial carcinoma. Clinical and histopathologic study of 540 patients. *Obstet. Gynecol.* 56:419.

Bannatyne, P. M., and P. Russell. 1981.: Early adenocarcinoma of the fallopian tubes. A case for multifocal tumorigenesis. *Diagn. Gynecol. Obstet.* 3:233.

Barber, H. R. K., 1980. Cancer of the breast, in: *Manual of Gynecologic Oncology,* Lippincott Co., Philadelphia, chap. 23, P. 241.

———. 1982. *Ovarian Carcinoma. Etiology, Diagnosis and Treatment,* 2nd ed. Masson Publishing, USA, New York.

———. 1982. Cancer of the breast, in: *Modern Concepts of Gynecologic Oncology* (J. P. VanNagell, Jr., and H. R. K. Barber, eds.). John Wright PSG, Inc., London, chap. 16, p. 443.

———. 1986. Ovarian cancer. *Ca-A Cancer Journal for Clinicians* 36(3):149.

Barber, H. R. K., and S. C. Sommers. 1981. *Carcinoma of the Endometrium. Etiology, Diagnosis and Treatment* (H. R. K. Barber and S. C. Sommers, eds.). Masson Publishing, USA, New York.

Benedet, J. L., and G. W. White. 1981. Malignant tumors of fallopian tube, in: *Gynecologic Oncology* (M. Coppleson, ed.). Churchill Livingstone, Edinburgh, chap. 48.

Boronow, R. C. 1976. Endometrial cancer: Not a benign disease. *Obstet. Gynecol.* 47:630.

Cohen, C. J. 1981. Advanced and recurrent carcinoma of endometrium, in: *Gynecologic Oncology* (M. Coppleson, ed.). Churchill Livingstone, Edinburgh, chap. 45.

Crile, G., Jr. 1984. Breast cancer. A personal perspective. *Surg. Clin. North Am.,* 64(6):1145.

Deppe, G. 1982. Chemotherapeutic treatment of endometrial carcinoma. *Clin. Obstet. Gynecol.* 25:93.

Fisher, E. R. 1984. The impact of pathology on the biologic, diagnostic, prognostic and therapeutic considerations in breast cancer. *Surg. Clin. North Am.* 64(6):1073.

Fox, H., and F. A. Langley. 1981. Malignant gonadal stromal tumors of ovary, in: *Gynecologic Oncology* (M. Coppleson, ed.). Churchill Livingstone, Edinburgh, chap. 52.

Gee, D. C., and P. Russell. 1981. The pathological assessment of ovarian neoplasms. IV. The sex cord stromal tumors. *Pathology* 12:235.

Gordon, A., D. Lipton, and J. D. Woodruff. 1981. Dysgerminoma: A review of 158 cases from the Emil Novak Ovarian Tumor Registry. *Obstet. Gynecol.* 58:497.

Hendrickson, M. R., and R. L. Kempson. 1980. *Surgical Pathology of the Uterine Corpus.* W. B. Saunders Co., Philadelphia.

Jones, H. W. 1975. Treatment of adenocarcinoma of the endometrium. *Obstet. Gynecol. Surv.* 30:147.

Leis, H. P., Jr. 1977. *The Diagnosis of Breast Cancer.* Professional Education Publication. American Cancer Society, New York.

Lippman, M. E., and B. A. Chabner, B.A. 1986. Editorial overview. *NCI Monogr.* no. 1:5.

Morrow, C. P. 1981. Malignant and borderline tumors of the ovary: Clinical features, staging, diagnosis, intraoperative assessment and review of management, in: *Gynecologic Oncology* (M. Coppleson, ed.). Churchill Livingstone, Edinburgh, chap. 50.

Morrow, C. P., and J. B. Chlaerth. 1982. Surgical management of endometrial carcinoma. *Clin. Obstet. Gynecol.* 25:81.

National Institutes of Health Consensus Development Panel on Adjuvant Chemotherapy and Endocrine Therapy for Breast Cancer. 1986. *NCI Monogr.* no. 1:1.

Ng, A. B. P., J. W. Reagan, J. P. Storaasli, and W. B. Wentz. 1973. Mixed adenosquamous carcinoma of the endometrium. *Am. J. Clin. Pathol.* 59:765.

Norris, H. J., and A. E. Adam. 1981. Malignant germ cell tumors of ovary, in: *Gynecologic Oncology* (M. Coppleson, ed.). Churchill Livingstone, Edinburgh, chap. 51.

Parker, R. T., and J. L. Currie. 1981. Metastatic tumors of the ovary, in: *Gynecologic Oncology* (M. Coppleson, ed.). Churchill Livingstone, Edinburgh, chap. 55.

Piver, S. M. 1983. Ovarian malignancies, in: *The Clinical Care of Adults and Adolescents.* Churchill Livingstone, Edinburgh, chap. 1 through 17.

Raju, K. S., G. H. Barker, and E. Wiltshaw. 1981. Primary carcinoma of the fallopian tube. Report of 22 cases. *Br. J. Obstet. Gynaecol.* 88:1124.

Serov, S. F., R. E. Scully, and L. H. Sobin. 1981. International histologic classification of tumors. *No. 9 Histological Typing of Ovarian Tumors.* World Health Organization, Geneva.

Shingleton, H. M., J. W. Orr, Jr. 1983. *Cancer of the Cervix.* Churchill Livingstone, Edinburgh.

Silverberg, S. G. 1984. New aspects of endometrial carcinoma. *Clin. Obstet. Gynecol.* 2(1):189.

Smith, J. P., G. Delgado, and F. Rutledge. 1976. Second-look operation in ovarian carcinoma. *Cancer* 32:1438.

Strax, P. 1984. Imaging of the breast. *Surg. Clin. North Am.* 64(6):1061.

VanNagell, J. R., E. S. Donaldson, E. G. Wood, et al. 1978. The prognostic significance of carcinoembryonic antigen in the plasma and tumors of patients with endometrial adenocarcinoma. *Am. J. Obstet. Gynecol.* 128:308.

Welander, C., K. E. Kjorstad, and P. Kolstad. 1978. Postoperative irradiation and chemotherapy in patients with advanced ovarian cancer. *Acta Obstet. Gynecol. Scand.* 57:161.

Yancik, R., L. G. Ries, and J. W. Yates. 1986. Ovarian cancer in the elderly: An analysis of surveillance, epidemiology and end results program data. *Am. J. Obstet. Gynecol.* 154:639.

11 Breast Tumors in the Aged

INTRODUCTION

The breast may be the site of contusions and lacerations secondary to trauma. Elderly women often fall against objects, and it is not uncommon to see a contusion of the breast, with or without a hematoma.

Fat necrosis may resemble a neoplastic process in the elderly female patient. It may be defined as an isolated, localized, inflammatory process with subsequent scarring that results in a focus of increased consistency grossly resembling a carcinoma. The entity is also termed traumatic fat necrosis, which arises out of the common history of prior trauma to the site of the lesion and is followed by the appearance of a mass. It may not be as sharply circumscribed as cancer, but the fibrosis in and around the area fixes the mass to the adjacent breast as well as to the overlying skin. A mass may be present for a period of time. A fresh specimen may look exactly like a scirrhous carcinoma with radiating hard white bands extending from a central focus. Histologically, a lesion that has been present for a short period of time may show intense neutrophilic or chronic infiltration, necrotic fat cells, lipid-filled macrophages, fibroblastic proliferation, and dense scarring with crystalline lipids and foreign body giant cells, calcium salts, and hemosiderin.

Inflammatory lesions do occur in the geriatric patients; most are secondary to scratching or insect bites. Sebaceous cysts occasionally become infected and cause great concern to the patient.

Fibrocystic changes, especially in the form of nodules, are occasionally seen in the postmenopausal patient. Nodular fibrosis, a distinct entity from fibrocystic changes, occurs in the patient over 65 years of age. Intraductal papilloma and ductic ectasia, which usually occur in the patient under age 55, may occur postmenopausally. The relationship of fibrocystic changes to the subsequent development of carcinoma has been extensively studied, and the general consensus is that a patient with fibrocystic changes is approximately four times more likely to have or to develop a cancer in one breast than a woman who has not had these changes. There is fairly good agreement that cancer of the breast relates principally to certain patterns of more or less diffuse ductal hyperplasia with prominent epithelial overgrowth and increasing atypism.

A nipple discharge, especially if there is any discoloration or blood, must be suspect for a neoplastic process. Papilloma, papillomatosis, and papillary carcinoma are entities in a spectrum of growth that develop within ducts or cysts; these occur most often in women just prior to or during the climacteric. There may be painless nipple discharge—the closer to the nipple, the greater the chance of the appearance of the discharge. On clinical examination, the lesions are small and, therefore, difficult to locate. However, by examining the breast carefully, by starting at the 12 o'clock axis and proceeding around the breast, it is often possible to identify the exact area that is producing the discharge.

Paget's disease of the nipple does not conform to the usual clinical picture of a carcinoma. It usually presents with eczema of the nipple, and the patient complains of itching and scaling. The lesions require adequate biopsy to ensure that there is no underlying invasive neoplasm. Approximately 25 percent of the patients presenting with Paget's disease of the nipple have had or will have Paget's disease of the vulva.

BREAST CANCER

An estimated 135,000 new cases of cancer of the breast will occur in the United States during 1988. About one out of 10 women will develop breast cancer sometime during her life. In several areas in the United States, this incidence drops to one in nine or one in eight women that will develop breast cancer.

An estimated 41,000 deaths, caused by breast cancer, occurred in 1987. Breast cancer is second only to lung cancer as the foremost site of cancer deaths in women.

The risk of breast cancer increases as a woman grows older. Genetic and lifestyle variances—a history of breast cancer and a close family relative, giving first birth after age 30, never giving birth, high fat diet, obesity (body weight 40 percent above normal)—may increase the risk further.

The warning signals include breast changes that persist, such as a lump, thickening, swelling, dimpling, skin irritation, distortion, retraction or scaliness of the nipple, nipple discharge, pain, or tenderness.

The median age of cancer of the breast is 40 to 71 years.

Histology

The common histologic types include infiltrating duct carcinoma, infiltrating lobular carcinoma, infiltrating medullary carcinoma, infiltrating colloid carcinoma, infiltrating comedo carcinoma, and infiltrating papillary carcinoma.

Among all histologic types, white women with mucinous producing adenocarcinoma and black women with medullary carcinoma experience the poorest survival rate. The highest proportion of women in both races was diagnosed with distant metastases when the tumor was classified as inflammatory carcinoma—one third of the white patients and more than two thirds of the black patients were diagnosed in this advanced stage. Also in both races, mucin-producing adenocarcinoma was diagnosed more often in older patients, while medullary carcinoma occurred more frequently in younger women.

Survival Trends

The observed median survival time by age among all white patients of all ages was 6.6 years; under 45, it was more than 10 years; from 45 to 54 years, it was more than 10 years; from 55 to 64 years, it was 7.3 years; from 65 to 74 years, it was 5.9 years; and 75 years and above it was 3.3 years.

This shows that age definitely plays a role in the overall prognosis and survival rate.

The observed median survival time by age among all black patients of all ages was 3.7 years; under age 45, it was 4.1 years; from 44 to 54 years, it was 4.4 years; from 55 to 64 years, it was 3.8 years; from 65 to 74 years, it was 3.5 years; and for those 75 years and above, it was 2.3 years.

This demonstrates poor survival among black patients with breast cancer. This may be a reflection of earlier detection and diagnosis for white women, with a higher proportion of them diagnosed as having localized disease. Furthermore, the proportion of black patients diagnosed with distant metastases was almost twice that of white patients during all time periods.

Early Detection of Breast Cancer

The modalities of early detection include breast self examination (BSE)—physical examination is the means by which breast cancer can be detected. Retrospective studies of BSE in a prospective randomized trial of screening mammography have shown a reduction in breast cancer mortality. The recommendations of the American Cancer Society and National Cancer Institute are that all women over the age of 50 have a routine annual mammography.

Since definitions of menopausal status vary widely among clinical trials, age (below 50 versus 50 or over) can be substituted as a prognostic variable.

The pathologic status of the axillary lymph nodes remains the single most important diagnostic variable. Four lymph node categories have been defined: negative; 1 to 3 positive nodes; 4 to 9 positive nodes; and 10 and over positive nodes.

Early Versus Small Breast Cancer

The biology of breast cancer is all too often considered by the physician as a relatively stereotyped time-related progression of events. This concept follows a pattern where once the tumor has reached a certain size, it spreads to the lymph nodes, and then, throughout the system. Current work contradicts this concept.

Breast cancer represents a heterogeneous group of neoplasms. Recent evidence suggests biologic heterogeneity of cells comprising individual breast cancers.

It is accepted that breast cancers cannot generally be palpated until they are at least 1 cm in size or 1 billion cells. Kinetic studies indicate that such a size requires 30 population doublings. When it is recognized that a doubling time might encompass anywhere from 30 to 200 or more days, it becomes apparent that a tumor that is regarded as clinically early is in truth biologically late, requiring only 10 to 20 more doublings before causing death of the host. A small 0.5-cm breast cancer detected by mammography, although regarded as early clinically, has already traversed through 27 doublings and is a biologically late tumor. The most important consideration is when a tumor, when it does contain metastasizing phenotypes, exhibits such a phenomenon. Current research indicates that when metastasis occur, they may do so within the first 10 to 20 doubling times, or at a stage undetectable by prevailing methodologies. It has been estimated that 50 percent of women with a breast cancer measuring 1 cm already have systemic disease. There is no evidence at the present time to indicate whether the elderly are more inclined to have systemic spread early or not. The poor survival rate in the elderly, however, may support the concept.

Familial occurrence is operationally defined as two or more first degree relatives with verified breast cancer. If the patient's mother had breast cancer before the menopause or bilateral breast cancer, however, she is at risk regardless of whether other blood relatives have had breast cancer.

One percent of women presenting with breast cancer have frank clinical disease on both sides. Approximately 15 percent of those who have survived the treatment of initial breast cancer for 3 or more years will develop a cancer in the opposite breast. Contralateral occult cancer is seen in about 25 percent of the patients with breast cancer recently proved on one side. This latter statement has been subject to some controversy.

Breast cancer is more common in white women; but black women are rapidly gaining parity. In the past 10 years, there has been a 2 percent increase in the death rate from breast cancer in white women, but an increase of 5 percent in nonwhites.

Thirty-five percent of women with untreated breast cancer have been known to survive for 5 years. Sixty-eight percent who have presented with localized disease and were untreated survived at least this long. Unfortunately, some cancers still elude present methods of detection. Some 10 percent of cancers will become apparent within 1 year of a negative examination. Reliance must be placed on self examination of the breast to detect these tumors.

It must be emphasized that neither palpation nor mammography used singly or in combination can detect 100 percent of the cancers present. Ninety percent of all breast lumps are found by women themselves, and the incidence of malignancy increases as patients get older.

Estrogen Receptor (ER) Assay

The discovery of estrogen-binding receptors in mammary carcinomas has lead to the development of sensitive quantitative assays. These assays can be performed on tumor tissue excised by biopsy. The results of these assays have been evaluated as a possible prognostic index of clinical response to antiestrogen or estrogen-ablative therapy. Tumors that have a strong affinity for estrogen are more likely to regress when estrogen levels are significantly increased.

Estrogens are carried down to plasma transport protein. The ability of the tissue to bind to hormones is secondary to specific hormone receptors located within or on the surface of the cells. These receptors apparently interact with a given hormone by combining with it, thereby initiating the biochemical events characteristic of the function of that particular hormone (Figs. 11-1 and 11-2).

It is believed that estrogens may be able to enter the cytoplasm of all cells, whether they are target tissue or not. The steroid hormone enters the cell, presumably by passive diffusion, and combines with specific receptor proteins that are termed *receptors* (estrogen receptors, ER). The reaction is labeled *uptake.* Following this initial binding step, the steroid receptor complex undergoes a temperature-dependent activation. This activation allows the steroid receptor complex to enter the nucleus of the cell and bind to the chromatin, which is the genetic information of the cell. This is labeled *translocation.* Once inside the nucleus, the steroid hormone receptor complex associates with the nuclear chromatin. This is labeled *retention.* Once bound to the chromatin by a little understood process, the interaction of the steroid receptor complex with the genetic information of the cells leads to an elaboration of a new species of messenger RNA. These messenger RNA molecules can be translated on polysomes into new proteins. It is this new protein that leads to the induced effects of the steroid hormone.

From current knowledge of hormone receptor interactions, it is obvious that a cell will not respond to a specific hormone unless the cell contains specific receptors. In the absence of specific receptors, the cell will not respond to the hormone. This is true of neoplastic as well as normal cells.

Antiestrogens have been introduced as a therapeutic modality in the treatment of breast cancer. The mechanism of action simply indicates that antiestrogens, in part, competitively prevent the binding of estrogen to the receptor protein. However, the action is slightly more complicated than described by this simplistic statement.

Antiestrogens, when administered pharmacologically, are also transported in the plasma and readily enter all cells, whether they be target tissue

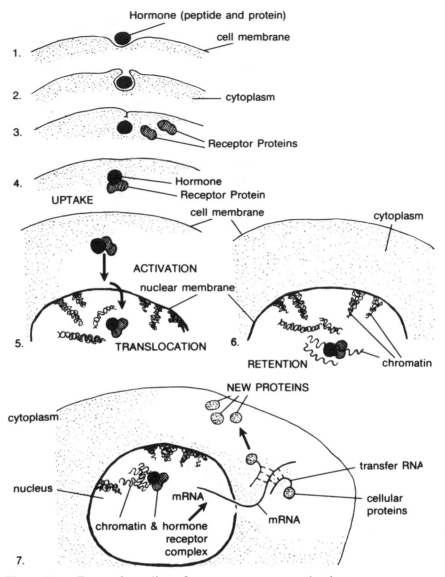

Figure 11-1. Dramatic outline of estrogen receptor mechanism.

or not. Once again, as with estrogens, these molecules combine to the estrogen receptor. Their action, however, is greater than simply preventing a binding of radioactive estrogens to the receptor. Recent experiments have shown that antiestrogen can bind to the receptor and activate, and that the antiestrogens bound to the estrogen receptor can translocate to the nucleus and also bind to chromatin sites. At this time, there is no absolute clear cut documentation of what is happening. In terms of two criteria—nuclear occupancy time and salt extractability—these complexes are very different in their biologic behavior from that of the normal estrogen receptor complex. Additional activity of these antiestrogen compounds involves this nuclear interaction.

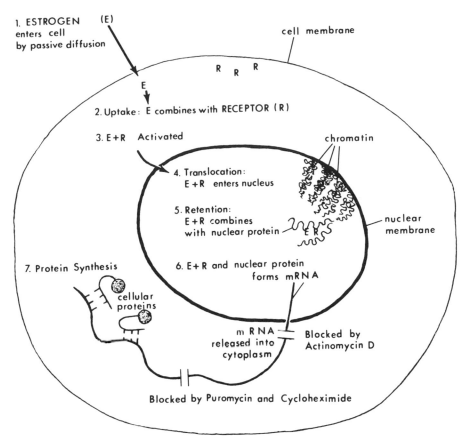

Figure 11-2. Response of cells to steroid hormones.

In summary, antiestrogens can exert their effect by two mechanisms. They can compete with biologically active estrogens for the receptor protein, and thus prevent their binding, or the antiestrogen compounds can bind to the receptors themselves. These antiestrogens, vertical line estrogen receptor complexes, can translocate the nucleus, where they can alter the transcriptive process of the cell in a manner that leads to tumor regression.

Progesterone receptor assays have been added to the estrogen receptor assays; combined, they give a more accurate predictive value for the response of the tumor to antiestrogen therapy.

The estrogen receptor mechanism is very useful in clinical practice. The following are generally accepted guidelines for therapy from the estrogen receptor assay: (1) if a tumor is positive for estrogen receptors, there is a 50- to 60-percent chance that the tumor will respond favorably to antiestrogen or estrogen ablative therapy; (2) if a tumor is negative for estrogen receptors, there is a less than 10-percent chance that the tumor will respond to similar therapy; (3) postmenopausal women tend to have higher positive estrogen receptor results (60 percent) than premenopausal women (45 percent). Invasive lobular carcinoma has a high incidence of positive results (90 percent), whereas tumors with a high lymphocyte count, notably medullary carcinoma, have a low incidence of positive results (25 percent).

Other morphologic features, such as histologic grade and involvement of axillary nodes, show no correlation with the presence or absence of estrogen receptors.

Diagnosis

A thorough history and clinical examination is required whenever there is a suggestion of breast disease. It is also important to do a very thorough breast examination on any patient who is having a physical examination. More than 90 percent of breast cancers are discovered by the patient herself. A well informed public that is taught self-examination of the breast will identify lumps or thickening at an earlier period than they have previously, and they will seek help earlier.

The typical presentation is a lump or thickening of the breast that is isolated, freely movable, and painless in the early stages. Later, the more dramatic findings that are identified with breast cancer will appear. About 50 percent of breast cancer patients will present with a cancer in the upper outer quadrant, 20 percent will present centrally, 10 percent will present in the lower outer quadrant, and 20 percent, will present in the medial half. If the patient reports that the lump has been present for at least 1 month, axillary nodes will be found to be positive in 50 percent of the cases. If the lump has been present for 6 months or more, axillary nodes are positive in about 70 percent of the cases.

In addition to careful examination of the breast, mammography, and xerography are available as modalities for making a diagnosis. The combination of a carcinoembryonic antigen assay and a cystic disease protein assay may be useful in monitoring the patient and should be obtained as a baseline.

The final decision as to whether it is cancer or not depends upon excisional biopsy. Recommendations have been advanced for doing contralateral biopsies in women found to have a cancer of the breast because there is a rate of 10 to 15 percent of simultaneous bilateral breast cancer. Although aspiration biopsy of the breast or nodal mass is advocated by several medical centers in the United States, it is important to obtain a biopsy specimen for a definitive diagnosis in this age group.

Cancer of the breast usually presents as a solitary, unilateral, solid, hard, irregular, poorly delineated, nonmovable, painless, and nontender lump. It is usually in the upper outer quadrant of the breast; and as it advances the signs become more pronounced. Certain cancers of the breast, however, do not conform to this clinical picture. Paget's disease, for example, presents with eczema of the nipple. Medullary colloid papillary cancers can be present with a well delineated mass that is not hard and gives the impression of mobility. Sarcoma also presents with a well-delineated mass and closely resembles a fibroadenoma.

Biopsy is mandatory in patients in this age group with any suspicious area present, including eczema or marked scaling of the nipple.

The indications for mammography in the perimenopausal and geriatric age group have been presented by the American Cancer Society. All women over the age of 50 should have an annual mammography.

There are numerous benefits of mammography. Most cancer experts believe that early detection offers the best cure rate. In the American Cancer Society and National Cancer Institutes Screening Centers, the earliest breast cancers, which are called minimal tumors, cannot be felt and are only detectable through mammography, a 5-year cure rate of up to 95 percent has been reported, compared to only 45 percent after the disease has spread to nearby lymph nodes. The risk from a mammography producing a cancer is infinitesimal, particularly when equated against the chance for a cure.

Schematic Anatomic Staging Outline (Clinical Observations)

The term *clinical staging* refers to a method of staging that applies only to clinical examination prior to histologic assessment of regional lymph node areas.

Clinical diagnostic staging systems have been devised by the American Joint Committee for Cancer Staging and End Results Reporting—the *TNM classification.* For the gynecologist, this a fairly elaborate type of staging. The following is proposed as a simplified method:

Stage I—Breast mass localized, all nodes negative
Stage II—Breast mass localized, axilla positive
Stage III—Breast mass locally extensive; axilla, supraclavicular, and internal mammory nodes positive
Stage IV—Distant metastases

In addition to the preceding classifications, there is the postsurgical treatment, pathologic staging system of the American Joint Committee for Cancer Staging and End Results Reporting: the TNM classification. These elaborate stagings have value when a detailed study of cancer of the breast is being conducted. The simpler classification, however, meets the needs for the practicing gynecologist (Table 11-1).

Type of Surgery

The operation is tailored to the type of lesion and extent of disease. If a patient has localized breast cancer without grave signs suggesting or establishing curability by regional means of therapy, many treatment alternatives are available and a choice must be made. There are data suggesting there is no particular advantage to any approach, but there are few reliable data for establishing truly optimal treatment.

Treatment alternatives vary from lumpectomy to extended radical mastectomy or supraradical mastectomy. Data at this time appear to have reliably answered some of the questions raised by consideration of these treatment alternatives. There is general agreement that: (1) no benefit from surgical removal of the internal mammary lymph nodes (as a routine operative approach) has been demonstrated, (2) no benefit has been demonstrated in the administration of postoperative radiation therapy, and (3) radiation therapy can control breast cancer effectively, but its relative effectiveness, in comparison to that of surgical methods, has not been clarified completely.

Table 11-1. Clinical-Diagnostic Staging System of the American Joint Committee for Cancer Staging and End-Results Reporting: TNM classification

Primary tumor (T)

TX   Tumor cannot be assessed

TO   No evidence of primary tumor

TIS   Paget disease of the nipple with no demonstrable tumor

     NOTE: Paget disease with a demonstrable tumer is classified according to the size of the tumor.

T1*   Tumor 2 cm or less in greatest dimension

     T1a   No fixation to pectoral fascia or muscle

     T1b   Fixation to pectoral fascia, muscle, or both

T2*   Tumor more than 2 cm but not more than 5 cm is greatest dimension

     T2a   No fixation to pectoral fascia or muscle

     T2b   Fixation to pectoral fascia, muscle, or both

T3*   Tumor more than 5 cm in greatest dimension

     T3a   No fixation to pectoral fascia or muscle

     T3b   Fixation to pectoral fascia, muscle, or both

T4   Tumor of any size with direct extension to chest wall or skin

     NOTE: Chest wall includes ribs, intercostal muscles, and serratus anterior muscle but not pectoral muscle.

     T4a   Fixation to chest wall

     T4b   Edema (including peau d'orange), ulceration of the skin of the breast, or satellite skin nodules confined to the same breast

     T4c   Both of above

     T4b   Inflammatory carcinoma

Nodal involvement (N)

NX   Regional lymph nodes cannot be assessed clinically

NO   No palpable homolateral axillary nodes

N1   Movable homolateral axillary nodes only

     N1a   Nodes not considered to contain growth

     T1b   Nodes considered to contain growth

N2   Homolateral axillary nodes considered to contain growth and fixed to one another or to other structures

N3   Homolateral supraclavicular or infraclavicular nodes considered to contain growth, or edema of arm

     NOTE: Edema of the arm may be caused by lymphatic obstruction and lymph nodes may not then be palpable.

Distant metastases (M)

MX   Not assessed

MO   No (known) distant metastasis

M1   Distant metastasis present

*Dimpling of the skin, nipple retraction, or any other skin changes except those in T4 may occur in T1, T2, or T3 without affecting the classification

Lumpectomy has two disadvantages. One is that cancer of the breast is often diffuse and there may be more cancer present than appreciated. Between one third and one half of breast tumors are found outside the original site. The other disadvantage is that nodes are not removed and examined; thus, there is no way of knowing if the nodes are involved.

With a reasonably early lesion, a modified radical mastectomy, leaving the pectoralis major muscle intact, is being selected with increasing frequency. This avoids the major defect in the axilla and affords a rather good cosmetic result. The nodes are taken out and are available for pathologic examination.

The nature and description of the various methods of treatment of breast cancer that apply to the tumor itself are:

1. Extended radical mastectomy or supraradical mastectomy—surgical removal of the internal mammary chain of lymph nodes, the entire involved breast, the underlying chest muscles, and the lymph nodes in the axilla.

2. Halsted radical mastectomy—surgical, en bloc removal of the entire involved breast, the underlying chest muscles, and the lymph nodes in the axilla.

3. Modified radical mastectomy—surgical removal of the entire involved breast and the lymph nodes in the axilla. The underlying chest muscles are removed in part or left in place after removal of the axillary nodes.

4. Simple mastectomy (more recently called total mastectomy)—surgical removal of the entire involved breast. The underlying chest muscles and the lymph nodes in the axilla are not removed.

5. Limited procedures have a variety of names, including lumpectomy, local excision, partial mastectomy, and tylectomy (comparable to lumpectomy). In each instance, the tumor is surgically removed with a varying amount of surrounding tissue.

In the perimenopausal patient modified radical mastectomy, simple mastectomy, and limited procedures can be carried out. There is practically no place for the extended radical mastectomy or supraradical mastectomy, or for the Halsted radical mastectomy;

In the geriatric patient particularly those in their late eighties and nineties a simple mastectomy is usually the procedure chosen. Nodes are only removed if they are palpated and enlarged.

It is interesting that in the postmenopausal patient, even up to 65 years of age, some are inquiring about reconstruction. Reconstruction has now become a very important part of treatment and rehabilitation.

Radiation Therapy

The use of radiation therapy as an adjuvant to surgery has been debated from the beginning of clinical x-ray therapy. A higher survival rate has been reported for patients with a large primary tumor and extensive axillary involvement when they receive postoperative radiation therapy, not only to the regional nodes, but also to the chest wall. Radiation therapy is usually given postoperatively to patients with inner-quadrant, infiltrating cancer, regardless of axillary nodal status. It is also given to those with outerquadrant lesions with multiple, positive axillary nodes.

Other indications for considering postoperative x-ray therapy are large primary tumors (more than 5 cm in size), cancer cell permeation of intramammary lymphatic vessels, skin involvement or ulceration, chest wall invasion, or massive axillary involvement.

As tests such as the estrogen receptor become better understood and more readily available in predicting accurately biologic behavior of an individual's breast cancer, a rational approach to therapy can be established. At that time, the role of chemotherapy, immunotherapy, castration, and radiation therapy can be presented accurately.

Radiation versus Mastectomy

Bloomer (1976) has reported encouraging preliminary results with radiotherapy as primary care for women with Stage I, II, and III disease. He has shown that an adequate dose of radiation is essential for success. The breast usually retains a good cosmetic appearance. The addition of chemotherapy may, in the future, further improve survival.

The treatment consisted of external beam irradiation using a 4-MEV linear accelerator, supplemented in many cases with interstitial implantation of iridium-192 ribbons or radium needles. Two opposed, tangential portals included the breast, chest wall, adjacent pleura, and ipsilateral internal mammary lymph node chains. Wedge filters were used as compensators to achieve homogeneity of dose within the tangential breast portal. A third portal encompassed the axillary and supraclavicular nodes.

Bloomer reported that there is only minimal breast retraction and no significant discoloration with the use of supervoltage irradiation. Despite radiographic changes of fibrosis in the skin, subcutaneous tissue, and supporting stroma, definitive radiation therapy often produces a breast that is cosmetically acceptable in appearance. This is especially true with Stage I and II tumors.

This investigator also reported that no local failures developed in 64 patients with Stage I and II disease. Of the 86 patients with locally advanced and unresectable Stage III tumors, 70 percent had local control. These results have been obtained after a minimum follow-up period of 1 year in 100 patients followed for at least 2.5 years. This was a preliminary study, but it is encouraging in that as shown by the experience of many centers most local recurrences occur within the first 2 years of treatment. Based on this, Bloomer believed that local control is likely to be excellent in patients with operable breast cancer.

Calle and Pilleron (1979) have reported that exclusive radiation is a difficult procedure, and is more complex than lumpectomy followed by irradiation. First of all, the irradiation technique requires a great deal of supervision. Tumor doses must be adequate for local control, but must not jeopardize the chances for performing salvage surgery if radiotherapy fails to control the tumor. Because of the high doses delivered to the breast and nodes, radiation sequelae are more severe and cosmetic results are not as good as those obtained by lumpectomy followed by irradiation. Second, surgery after irradiation is more difficult to perform than primary surgery and, at 10 years, 50 percent of patients required such secondary surgery. In contrast, only 16 percent of the cases treated by lumpectomy required secondary surgery. Of the two regimens, lumpectomy followed by irradiation appears to be an excellent therapeutic modality and has a definite place in the treatment of breast carcinoma. On the other hand, exclusive irradiation is more complex than the combination of surgery and irradiation, and the author does not encourage its general use. It requires a meticulous technique, and cosmetic results are not as satisfactory. When utilizing radiation therapy, it is advisable not to promise the patient conservation of her breasts, but rather to propose an attempt to do this.

Palliation

X-ray therapy has been employed as a palliative measure in the treatment of local recurrence in soft tissue metastases, as well as for osseous and visceral metastases. The majority of patients with widespread metastatic breast cancer often have painful and disabling bone lesions. Although disseminated osseous metastases must be treated by systemic therapy, irradiation to localized symptomatic areas offers the greatest chance for relief. Subjective improvement, as evidenced by a decrease in pain, is achieved in the majority of patients.

Radiation should also be given to relatively asymptomatic, weightbearing bone lesions that appear likely to cause a pathologic fracture. At times, prophylactic nailing of a long bone should be carried out prior to irradiation.

Since the ovary is not producing hormone in this age group, there is no indication for oophorectomy.

A certain number of elderly, postmenopausal women have better results from adrenalectomy than do younger women. One predictive test is to give high doses of cortisone over a short period of time. If the bone pain eases, the patient can be considered a candidate for adrenalectomy.

Hypophysectomy suppresses prolactin and growth hormone. For practical purposes, adrenalectomy and hypophysectomy seem to provide the same effects in so far as tumor stimulation is concerned. If one treatment is not effective, the other will also offer little, if anything.

Currently there is practically no indication for these surgical procedures and reliance is made totally on medical suppression of estrogen through the use of antiestrogen agents.

Adjuvant Chemotherapy and Hormonal Therapy

These are effective treatments for breast cancer patients. While significant advances have been made in the past 5 years, optimal therapy has not been defined for any subset of patients.

Outside the context of a clinical trial, and based on the research data presented at the 1985 Consensus Development Conference, the following statements can be made:

1. For the postmenopausal patient with positive nodes and positive hormone receptors, Tamoxifen is the treatment of choice.
2. For postmenopausal women with positive nodes and negative hormonal receptor levels, chemotherapy may be considered, but cannot be recommended as standard practice.
3. For postmenopausal women with negative nodes, regardless of hormone receptor levels, there is no indication for routine adjuvant treatment. For certain high risk patients in this group, adjuvant therapy may be considered.

SUMMARY

An estimated 135,000 cases of cancer of the breast are anticipated in the United States during 1988. About one out of 10 women will develop breast cancer at some time during her life. An estimated 41,000 females will die of cancer of the breast, which is second only to lung cancer as the foremost site of cancer deaths in women.

Breast changes, such as a lump, thickening, swelling, dimpling, skin irritation, distortion, retraction, scaling of the nipple, nipple discharge, pain, or tenderness must be carefully evaluated in this age group. Liberal indications for biopsy should be the rule in this age group.

There are certain risk factors that include patients over 50 years of age; personal or family history of breast cancer; never had children; first child after age 30, and those that have been on a high fat diet.

The American Cancer Society recommends the practice of breast self examination (BSE), particularly in women over the age of 40 (Figs. 11-3–11-10). Although most breast lumps are not malignant, this is not so in the perimenopausal and geriatric age group, and most represent a neoplastic change.

Mammography should be done in all women over the age of 50. A low dose x-ray examination is able to find cancers too small to be palpated by the most experienced examiner.

Once a lump is found, mammography is carried out to determine if there are other lesions in the same or opposite breast that are too small to be palpated.

All suspicious lumps or thickening should be biopsied for definitive diagnosis even though the mammography is described as normal.

Several methods of treatment may be used, depending upon the individual's preferences and medical situation. Surgery ranges from local removal of the tumor to mastectomy, radiation therapy, chemotherapy, or hormonal manipulation. A combination of methods is often used. It is important to explain the options to the patient very carefully, and it is wise to make a recommendation as the responsible physician.

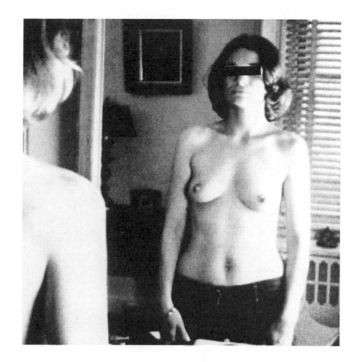

Figure 11-3. Breast self-examination (BSE): 1. Observe the breast in front of a mirror.

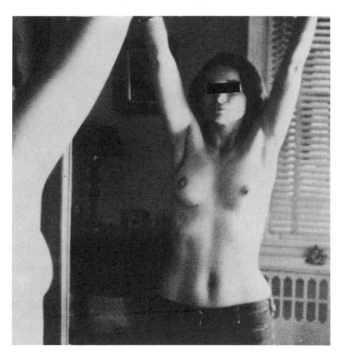

Figure 11-4. BSE: 2. Arms elevated.

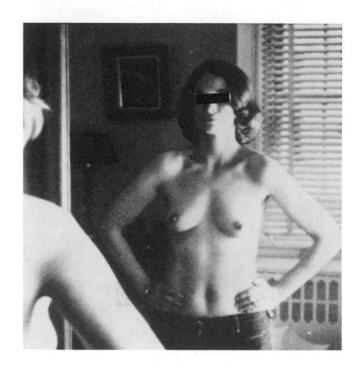

Figure 11-5. BSE: 3. Hands pressed against hip.

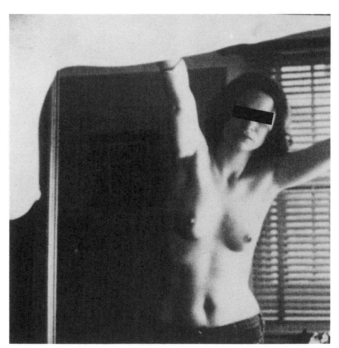

Figure 11-6. BSE: 4. Bending forward.

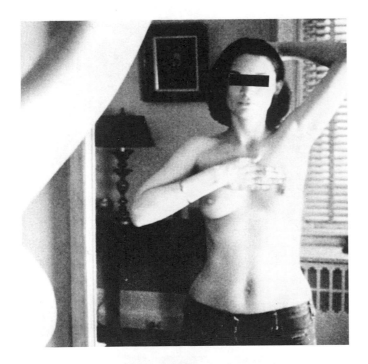

Figure 11-7. BSE: 5. Palpate the breast while starting in the upper quadrant.

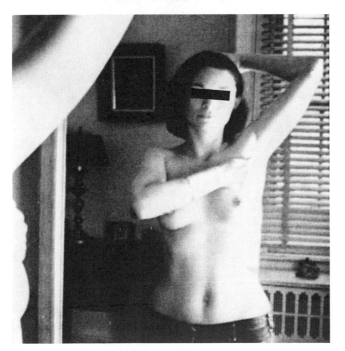

Figure 11-8. BSE: 6. Palpate the breast while standing, progressing medially downward.

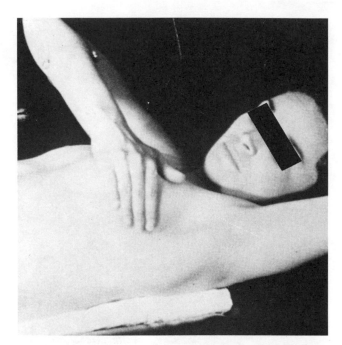

Figure 11-9. BSE: 7. Examine the breast while supine.

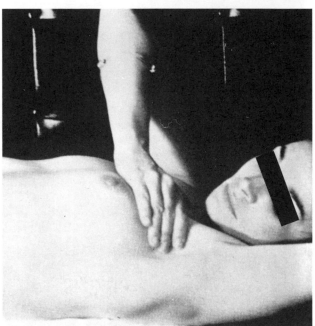

Figure 11-10. BSE: 8. Examine the breast while supine, progressing medially downward.

The observed median survival among white patients 55- to 64-years old is 7.3 years; from 65 to 74 years, it is 5.9 years, and for those over 75, it is 3.3 years. Among black patients, the observed median survival time is 3.8 years in patients 55- to 64-years old; in patients 65- to 74-years old, it is 3.5 years, and for those 75 and over, it is 2.3 years.

In postmenopausal women with positive nodes and positive hormonal receptor level, Tamoxifen is the treatment of choice and should be recommended. The problem is a little bit different for the postmenopausal women with positive nodes and negative hormone receptor levels —chemotherapy may be considered, but cannot be recommended as standard practice in these patients. In the postmenopausal patient with negative nodes, regardless of hormone receptor levels, there is no indication for routine adjuvant treatment. For certain high risk patients in this group, adjuvant therapy may be considered. If the patient is an octogenarian or older, however, it is probably wise to withhold aggressive chemotherapy.

REFERENCES

Barber, H. R. K. 1982. Cancer of the breast, in: *Modern Concepts of Gynecologic Oncology* (J. R. Van Nagell, Jr., and H. R. K. Barber, eds.) John Wright PSG, Inc., Boston, p. 443.

Beatson, G. T. 1896. On the treatment of inoperable cases of carcinoma of the mamma: Suggestions for a new method of treatment, with illustrative cases. *Lancet* 2:104.

Bloomer, W. D. 1976. Radiotherapy vs. mastectomy. *The Female Patient* 1:35–38.

Bonadonna, G., E. Brusamolino, P. Valagussa, et al. 1976. Combination chemotherapy as an adjuvant treatment in operable breast cancer. *N. Engl. J. Med.* 294:405.

Burnet, F. M. 1970. The concept of immunological surveillance. *Prog. Exp. Tumor Res.* 13:1.

Calle, R., and J. P. Pilleron, 1979. Radiation therapy, with and without lumpectomy of operable breast cancer: Ten-year results. *Dis. Breast* 5:2.

Cooperman, A. M., and R. Hermann, 1984. Breast cancer: An overview. *Surg. Clin. N. A.* 64(6):1031.

Crile, G., Jr. 1984. Breast cancer. A personal perspective. *Surg. Clin. North Am.* 64(6):1145.

Fisher, E. B. 1984. The impact of pathology on the biologic, diagnostic, prognostic and therapeutic considerations in breast cancer. *Surg. Clin. North Am.* 64(6):1073.

Jensen, E. V., and E. R. DeSombre, 1973. Estrogen-receptor interaction. *Science* 182:126.

Lippman, M. E., and B. A. Chabner, 1986. Editorial Overview. NCI Monographs, Number 1:5.

McGuire, W. L., P. P. Carbone, and E. P. Volimer, eds. 1975. Estrogen receptors, in: *Human Breast Cancer,* Raven Press, New York.

McGuire, N. I., and G. M. Clark, 1983. Progesterone receptors and human breast cancer. *Eur. J. Cancer Clin. Oncol.* 12:1689.

National Institutes of Health Consensus Development Panel on Adjuvant Chemotherapy and Endocrine Therapy for Breast Cancer: Introduction and Conclusions. 1986. NCI Monographs Number 1:1.

Peters, M. V. "Local" treatment of early breast cancer. Surg. Clin. North Am. 64(6):1151–1154.

Russell, K. P. 1976. The gynecologist and the asymptomatic patient. *Doctor* 4:48.

Strax, P.: 1984. Imaging of the breast. A perspective. *Surg. Clin. North Am.* 64(6):1061.

Strax, P. 1976. Results of mass screening for breast cancer in 50,000 examinations. *Cancer* 37:30.

Urban, J. A. 1978. Management of operable breast cancer. *Cancer* 42:2066.

Young, J. O., et al. 1986. Mammography of women with suspicious breast lumps. *Arch. Surg.* 121:807.

12 Vulvar Dystrophy

INTRODUCTION

The vulva is sensitive to physiologic and pathologic changes and to sex hormones, similar to the sex skin of monkeys. Estradiol is the main estrogen produced by the ovary, although small amounts of estrone are also produced. These ovarian hormones are derived from androgenic precursors. They influence the sexual organs by being selectively attached to specific hormone receptors. Membrane permeability is increased, and the synthesis of RNA and probably that of DNA is influenced. The hormone remains unaltered for some time within the cell. Progesterone also acts on specific receptor sites and tissues that have been previously processed by estradiol, but it is destroyed rather quickly.

The vulva may exhibit cyclic changes with the menstrual cycle. The inner aspects of the labia minora are similar to those seen in the vagina. The skin of the labia majora and of the outer surface of the labia minora is more responsive to androgens that induce thickening. At the menopause, atrophic changes occur in the vulva and the epithelium is reduced to a few layers of uniform cells, mostly of the intermediate and parabasal cell types. The labia majora and minora, as well as the clitoris, gradually become less prominent. The pigmentation decreases and eventually the pubic hair becomes gray and very often scant.

The hormonal sensitivity of the vulva predisposes it to various maturational and degenerative changes in response to variations in the levels of hormones and hormone receptors during life. *Dystrophic diseases* are defined as disorders of epithelial growth and nutrition that may result in a white surface change. Therefore, the term *vulvar dystrophy* indicates a clinical and nonpathologic entity and is used to standardize the terminology of a clinically confusing group of vulvar disorders. Microscopic examination of adequate biopsy specimens remains the only way to make an accurate diagnosis.

Pruritus is common and is often difficult to treat in older women. If it is associated with an obvious skin lesion and is accurately diagnosed, treatment is usually prompt and effective. However, pruritus associated with ill-defined, variable changes in vulval skin, for which no specific cause is apparent, is much more difficult to manage.

White lesions of the vulva have been traditionally treated as a group, with the misguided perception that they are premalignant. Three factors, operating independently or in concert, account for their white appearance: keratin, deep pigmentation, and relative avascularity. When a patient presents with a vulvar lesion that is white, gray, or simply pale, in which there is a change in skin surface and architecture, and to which a specific cause cannot be ascribed, the clinician should biopsy the lesion for diagnosis. Based upon the findings of a microscopic report, the changes can be assigned to one of the various dystrophies and then given the proper treatment.

With the growing realization of the organ status of the vulva, the International Society for the Study of Vulvar Disease was founded and, after careful study, suggested that the term *dystrophy* should be used to encompass the several lesions that, by growth and by chemical changes, result in a white appearance of the skin of the lesion.

ETIOLOGY

The etiology of vulvar dystrophy is unknown. Achlorhydria has been noted in a significant number of these cases. There is general agreement that achlorhydria is often an autoimmune phenomenon, so evidence of other autoimmune conditions—pernicious anemia, hypothyroidism, and hyperthyroidism—has been sought in association with vulvar dystrophy. It was found more often in this group of patients than in age-related controls. An association has been demonstrated between primary biliary cirrhosis and lichen sclerosus.

It has been shown that G cells in the lower end of the stomach give rise to gastrin, which, in turn, acts on the parietal cells in the stomach to produce hydrochloric acid. Urogastrone has been shown by Lavery to be related to vulvar changes. If the action of urogastrone on the vulvar skin were unopposed, achlorhydria would be associated with only hypertrophic dystrophy. However, the local homeostatic mechanism in the vulva responds to the hypertrophy caused by urogastrone stimulation by releasing somatostatin locally, which, in turn, cause atrophy. Thus, while the skin fluctuates between hypertrophy and atrophy, gastric hydrochloric acid secretion under the opposed influence of urogastrone remains constantly depressed, there being no rise in the level of somatostatin in the plasma. It is interesting that the urogastrone stimulation causing hypertrophy results in extremely high rebound levels of somatostatin, which remain elevated in the skin even after atrophy has occurred. As found in serial biopsies, high somatostatin levels persist for a time even in the atrophic skin, but eventually fall.

The constant and opposing actions of urogastrone and somatostatin lead to hypertrophy and atrophy, respectively, continually stimulating the skin cells; even atrophic skin has been shown to be metabolically active. It has been proposed that elevated urogastrone levels occur in patients with chronic vulvar disease.

The exact mechanism of development of vulvar dystrophy is not known. However, local factors may play an important role. These factors include chronic irritation, hormonal deficiency, alteration of hormonal receptivity, and disturbances of connective tissue factors. *Chalones* are recently discovered reversible, tissue-specific proteins with hormone-like receptivity. They are elaborated in and act upon that tissue, and, like hormones, act upon other tissues. Also, they develop mainly in the epithelium. Epidermis extracts (chalones) inhibit cell flux at various transitions in animal epidermis, but they are not the only substances that may be involved: the chain of mitotic change and control is probably also associated with other water-soluble compounds (e.g., glucosaminoglycans) in the regulatory system of epidermal development. Chalones may play a part in the interplay of deep and superficial tissues, perhaps inhibiting mitotic growth and differentiation. Various hormones or other agents may modify the effect of these compounds, either by stimulating or by blocking chalone receptor sites.

WHITE LESIONS

The vulvar dystrophies are a group of conditions characterized by disordered growth, and sometimes disordered maturation, of the vulval squamous epithelium. Their etiology is unknown, though recently an association between vulval dystrophy and achlorhydria has been demonstrated and papilloma virus has been identified in a few cases. A rationalized and simplified classification and nomenclature of vulvar dystrophies has been established. It includes lichen sclerosus, hypertrophic dystrophy, and mixed dystrophy.

Dystrophic lesions appear as white patches in the epithelium known as *leukoplakia.* In addition, the mucocutaneous tissue becomes dry, shriveled, and brittle, a condition clinically known as *kraurosis vulvae.* These are clinical terms, similar to *dystrophy,* used to describe the gross appearance of the lesion. They do not indicate specific pathologic disease entities. Leukoplakia can be caused by a wide variety of abnormalities other than dystrophy. The diagnosis of specific conditions depends entirely on careful histologic evaluation.

White lesions of the vulva were once treated as a group. They were considered premalignant. The white appearance of the lesion is due to keratin, deep pigmentation, and relative avascularity. All three of these mechanisms are present in the vulvar dystrophies. It is now recognized that white lesions of the vulva are not premalignant or malignant. Much of the confusion in the past resulted from the fact that there was no uniform terminology.

The skin of the vulva consists of two parts: dermis and epidermis, which interact and therefore modify each other. Each part does not necessarily respond to the same nutritional or other conditioning patterns. Estrogen lack has little effect on vulvar epidermis. However, it has a considerable effect on the dermis, causing fibrosis and shrinking of the introitus and loss of fat from the labia majora. The vulva is not part of the integument. Embryologically, from the mons pubis to the anus, it is an organ. Its lymphatic drainage and blood supply are its own, and not merged with those of the surrounding skin, although they are related in varying degrees to the connecting vaginal mucosa.

DYSTROPHY

Based on clinical and histologic characteristics, the vulvar dystrophies may be subdivided into three groups: lichen sclerosus, hyperplastic, and mixed. In the latter two groups, it may occur with or without atypia.

Lichen Sclerosus

Lichen sclerosus is the most common of the three groups of white lesions. It usually occurs in postmenopausal patients, but it can affect persons of all ages, including children. Clinical examination reveals the skin of the vulva to be thin, atrophic, parchment-like, dry, white or yellow.

Vulvar itching is a common symptom among postmenopausal patients. The scratching that usually takes place results in ulcerations and the formation of ecchymosis. The architecture of the vulva is slowly destroyed, and the small labia undergoes adhesions to the adjacent large labia. The edema and scarring that occur around the clitoris result in its disappearance behind this white tissue. The change continues progressively, with marked loss of subcutaneous fat. The lesions involve the vulva in a symmetrical fashion, resulting in a butterfly shape or a figure-of-eight. The lichen sclerosus involves the small and large labia, the clitoris, and occasionally the skin of the thigh, anal region, and trunk.

Histologically there is marked thinning and atrophy of the epidermis, with hyperkeratosis. Focal areas of cellular nuclear atypia are extremely rare. The epidermis is edematous in the early stages, but later it becomes fibrous, with loss of dermal appendages. Chronic inflammatory cells are seen in the deeper part of the dermis. Senile atrophy, which also occurs in postmenopausal patients, reveals no epithelial dysplasia on histologic examination.

An increased incidence of pernicious anemia, achlorhydria, and auto-immune disorders has been reported in patients with lichen sclerosus.

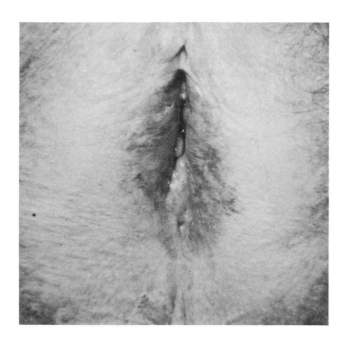

Figure 12-1. Lichen sclerosus.

Although these observations are of interest, there is no known etiology of lichen sclerosus. (Fig. 12-1).

Management. Lichen sclerosus is, by interpretation of the involutional changes and by the histologic appearance, an epithelium that requires thickening and activation; the natural hormone that does this is testosterone. This form of dystrophy appears to be permanent in the sense that it does not, as far as is known, revert to normal because the collagen deposition cannot be replaced by elastic tissue. Testosterone applications result in some epithelial activation, perhaps by blocking chalone receptor sites or by simply activating their growth potential and increasing the blood supply to the epithelium. Current reports indicate that testosterone is metabolized in much larger quantities in skin from lichen sclerotic patients than in normal vulvar skin. Although not always successful, testosterone ointment can be applied freely for 2 to 3 weeks, then once or twice a week or more frequently if the pruritus returns, and finally as needed to promote patient comfort. Testosterone propionate ointment has its greatest benefit when there is burning rather than itching. Judicious use of corticosteroid ointment may help to reduce the disturbing edema of the prepuce and clitoris, but if it is continued for long it may be dangerous, because the thin skin is then easily ulcerated.

Hyperplastic Dystrophy

Hyperplastic dystrophy is also called *hyperplastic vulvitis, neurodermatitis,* and *leukokeratosis.* It usually occurs in patients who are less than 50 years of age but is also found in the postmenopausal and geriatric patient. The resulting clinical picture is one of thickening and lightening of the vulva and adjacent skin. In contrast to lichen sclerosus, the perineal and

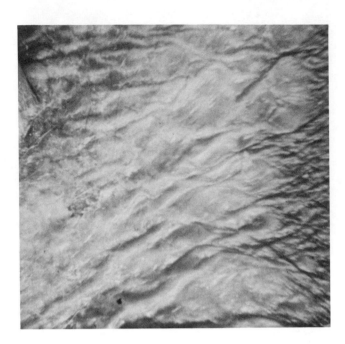

Figure 12-2. Characteristic wrinkling of superficial layers.

perianal areas are seldom affected. The vulva is often affected in a patchy manner. The vulvar folds are preserved and show generalized thickening of the epithelium. There are often patches of white, sometimes raised, skin. The vulvar folds may be exaggerated, but narrowing of the introitus is usually not a prominent feature unless the patient is sexually inactive.

Isolated areas of involvement are seen more frequently than with lichen sclerosus, and dystrophic remodeling of the labia minora and clitoris is usually absent. In black women, the appearance of hyperplastic dystrophy may be dramatic and is often confused with vitiligo.

Pruritus is always present, and due to the uncontrollable urge to scratch, changes occur in the primary lesion. The gross appearance of the lesion cannot accurately determine the histology. The epidermis shows marked acanthosis due to the thickening of the prickle cell layer and elongation of the rete pegs. Acanthosis, hyperkeratosis, and normal stratification with increased numbers of cells may be seen. Atypia may be present at various levels and are graded as mild, moderate, and severe. Cellular atypia or carcinoma in situ can be seen in approximately 10 percent of cases. The atypia is marked by hypercellularity, disordered polarity of epidermal cells, variation in nuclear size, hyperchromasia, and premature individual cell keratinization. Mitosis can be seen high in the epidermis. A dense, chronic inflammatory cellular infiltrate is usually seen in the dermis. Since the potency of the lesion depends upon the severity of the atypical change, it is important to do biopsies (Fig. 12-2).

In making a differential diagnosis, it is important to consider carcinoma in situ, Paget's disease, lichen sclerosus, and mixed dystrophies. They may all present a similar clinical picture. It is therefore important to have biopsy proof of the histology. Multiple biopsies should be carried out.

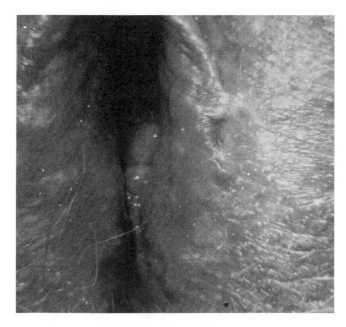

Figure 12-3. Early adhesions of labia minor.

Management. Since these patients present with marked itching, therapy must be directed to controlling this symptom. It is important to teach the patient proper hygiene. Any soap with detergent should be excluded. For example, Ivory soap is very alkaline; it dries the area and often aggravates the itching. The patient should be told to use baby soap or Neutrogena when bathing. The tense, nervous patient, particularly one who is focused on the vulvar itching, should be treated with a mild tranquilizer for a period of time. Atarax is used widely among dermatologists as an adjuvant treatment for itching. Topical corticosteroids provide the backbone for treatment. They should be applied twice a day. Although the itching is controlled rather rapidly, it takes about 6 to 8 weeks before any visible change is seen in the gross lesion. Patients who do not respond to corticosteroids should have a cream made up of Urax and corticosteroids, consisting of 30 percent Urax (3 parts) and 70 percent corticosteroid (7 parts), in 45-g lots. It should be applied twice daily until the itching is controlled. The patient can then resume using the topical corticosteroids, switching to the Urax–corticosteroid combination only when the itching is bad. Burning is best treated with testosterone propionate 2 percent in white petrolatum. Progesterone in oil 400 mg in 4 oz. Aquaphor has been successfully used in those cases of dystrophy that were unresponsive or unsuited to testosterone.

Mixed Dystrophy

Approximately 15 percent of all cases of vulvar dystrophy show a mixed pattern. Both lichen sclerosus and hyperplastic dystrophy may be found on the same vulva and constitute the condition then known as *mixed dystrophy.* In studying these lesions, some areas show the gross and microscopic features of lichen sclerosus, while others show the features of

175

hyperplastic dystrophy. A wrinkled, parchment-like appearance usually signifies an area of lichen sclerosus, and heaped-up white plaque is usually associated with a hyperplasia. It is important to take multiple biopsy specimens from this lesion (Fig. 12-3).

In the differential diagnosis, lichen sclerosus with hyperkeratotic plaques, superimposed fungal infections, and carcinoma in situ must be considered.

Management. The treatment is similar to that for the other dystrophies. Attention should be given to soap, underclothing, and personal hygiene. The vulva should be treated with corticosteroids, and when the hyperplastic areas disappear, it may be necessary to treat the lichen sclerosus with 2 percent testosterone propionate in a petrolatum base. The corticosteroid and testosterone preparations may have to be alternated. In order to control the itching in some resistant cases, it is necessary to give alcohol injections.

OTHER WHITE LESIONS

Vitiligo may occur in the vulva. It is usually associated with a generalized condition of the skin. It usually occurs early in life and is seen more often in the female than in the male. Hyperkeratosis presents clinically as elevated, thickened patches of white skin or mucosa. Chronic inflammatory lesions may become hypertrophic because of the irritation from scratching. Senile atrophy occurs in elderly women. It is usually accompanied by shrinkage and by very dry, thin tissue, often with multiple telangiectasias present.

SUMMARY

The etiology of vulvar dystrophy is unknown. Theories include lack of hydrocloric acid, imbalance of somatostatin, lack of chalones, and poor hygiene.

The International Society for the Study of Vulvar Diseases has divided the category of dystrophy into three groups: lichen sclerosus, hyperplastic dystrophy, and mixed dystrophy. *Dystrophy* denotes a disturbance of nutrition. There may be dystrophy with or without atypia.

In studying the lichen sclerosus lesions, it was found that the epithelium is very active, with uptake of tritiated thymidine and radioactive phosphorus. Therefore, the name *lichen sclerous et atrophicus* was changed to *lichen sclerosus* when it was found that these lesions had an active epithelium. It is important to make a diagnosis by means of multiple biopsies. The presenting symptom is usually marked pruritis. After biopsies have been done, this should be treated by the use of corticosteroids and testosterone. The usual hygienic measures should be carried out. The use of Urax combined with corticosteroid is effective in controlling some of the resistant cases of pruritis. Alcohol injection is rarely needed but occasionally is employed and gives relief. Vulvectomy has not been particularly effective, and often the dysplasia recurs right at the edge of the excision line. Laser therapy has been employed in some of these patients, but there are not enough data to determine its value accurately. In making up the testosterone preparation, it must be remembered that testosterone separates from petrolatum rather easily. A good mixture is made with testosterone propionate in sesame oil. This holds the mix well. Testosterone propionate ointment is most effective if burning of the vulva is the chief complaint. The overuse of testosterone may result in priapism. The overuse of hydrocortisone may result in ulceration of the vulvae.

REFERENCES

August, P. J., and T. M. Milward. 1980. Cryosurgery in the treatment of lichen sclerosus et atrophicus of the vulva. *Br. J. Dermatol.* 103(6):667. 1981.

Elgio, K., O. P. E. Clausen, and E. Thorud. 1981. Epidermis extracts (chalone) inhibit cell flux at the G1–S2, S–G2, and G2–M transitions of Mouse epidermis. *Cell Tissue Kinetics* 14:21.

Friedrich, E. G. 1971. Topical testosterone for benign vulva dystrophy. *Obstet. Gynecol.* 37:677.

———. 1976. Lichen sclerosus. *J. Reprod. Med.* 17:147.

———. 1976. White lesions, in: *Vulvar Disease* W.B. Saunders Co., Philadelphia, chap. 6.

Gregory, H. 1980. Urogastrone, in: *Gastrointestinal Hormones* (G.B.G. Grass, ed.). Raven Press, New York, p. 317.

Harrington, C. J. 1979. An investigation into the incidence of autoimmune disorders in patients with lichen sclerosus et atrophicus. *Br. J. Dermatol.* 100(suppl. 17):12.

Harrington, C. J., and I. R. Dusmore. 1981. An investigation into the incidence of auto-immune disorders in patients with lichen sclerosus and atrophicus. *Br. J. Dermatol.* 104:563.

International Society for the Study of Vulvar Disease. New nomenclature for vulvar disease. 1976. *Obstet. Gynecol.* 47:122.

Jeffcoate, T. N. A. 1966. Chronic vulvar dystrophies. *Am. J. Obstet. Gynecol.* 95:61.

———. 1962. The dermatology of the vulva. *Obstet. Gynecol. Br. Commonw.* 69:889.

Jeffcoate, T. N. A., and A. S. Woodcock. 1961. Premalignant conditions of the vulva with particular reference to chronic epithelial dystrophies. *Br. Med. J.* 2:127.

Kaufman, R. H., and H. L. Gardner. 1978. Vulvar dystrophies. *Clin. Obstet. Gynecol.* 21:1081.

Lavery, H. A. 1984. Vulval dystrophies: New approaches. *Clin. Obstet. Gynecol.* 11(1):155.

Sutherst, J. R. 1979. Treatment of pruritus vulvae by multiple intradermal injections of alcohol—a double blind study. *Br. J. Obstet. Gynaecol.* 86:371.

Woodruff, J. D., M. I. Barmouf, E. A. Carnold, and J. Knaack. 1965. Metabolic activity in normal and abnormal vulvar epithelia. *Am. J. Obstet. Gynecol.* 91:312.

Zelle, K. 1971. Treatment of vulvar dystrophies with topical testosterone. *Am. J. Obstet. Gynecol.* 109:530.

13 The Postmenopausal Palpable Ovary Syndrome (PMPO)

INTRODUCTION

The postmenopausal palpable ovary syndrome (PMPO) is a clearly established entity. However, even after 16 years of investigation, there is still confusion about its meaning. This confusion is caused by the fact that what is interpreted as "a normal sized ovary in the premenopausal woman represents an ovarian tumor in the postmenopausal woman." This statement by Barber and Graber may appear to be insignificant in terms of the total problem of ovarian neoplasms, but it has been the experience of the author that all such palpable findings prove to be new growths; they are not all necessarily malignant, but none have been functional or dysfunctional. The PMPO syndrome does not mean that anything that can be felt is abnormal. Occasionally in a thin, relaxed woman with poor musculature, it is possible to feel a 2 × 2 cm ovary that clearly would not qualify for the PMPO syndrome. The next important point is that the PMPO syndrome represents a new growth but not necessarily a malignant growth. It is the author's opinion that the postmenopausal palpable ovary is a most significant finding because it does not represent a functional change, but rather a neoplastic change.

Normal ovary
Premenopausal
3.5 x 2 x 1.5 cm

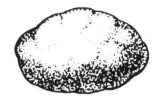

Early menopause
(1 - 2 years)
2 x 1.5 x 0.5 cm

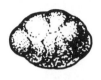

Late menopause
(2 - 5 years)
1.5 x 0.75 x 0.5 cm

Figure 13-1. Relative sizes of premenopausal, menopausal, and late menopausal ovaries.

The menopause is peculiar to the human race, and with it comes the cessation of cyclic hormone activity within the ovary. At about the fifth month of fetal life there are 9 million oocytes present, and by birth this number has decreased to about 700,000 to 2 million. Because of the continuing process of atresia, the human ovary in the pubertal female contains an average of 380,000 primordial follicles, and in the 40- to 44-year old woman this number decreases to about 8,000. The efficiency of the atretic process and the total number of oocytes at puberty apparently determine, to a large extent, the age of menopause. The large variation in these factors may explain the differences among individuals and the number of primordial follicles at any given age, as well as the age of menopause. The ultimate exhaustion of primordial follicles has been blamed for the phenomenon of menopause. Almost invariably, however, at least some primordial follicles can be found in the ovaries of postmenopausal women. Some developing follicles may also be identified, but they will usually appear to be in varying stages of atresia. These data suggest that the remaining primordial follicles are functionally abnormal, either in their sensitivity to gonadotropin stimulation or in their inability to withstand atresia. Therefore, even though an occasional primordial follicle is found in the postmenopausal and geriatric patient, it does not function and no estrogen is produced.

ANATOMY OF THE OVARY

In the normal course of events, the postmenopausal ovary shrinks and becomes densely fibrous, the external convolutions increase, and its appearance can be likened to that of a very small walnut (Fig. 13-1).

After menopause the ovaries are smaller and more fibrotic, and usually exhibit pits on their surface. Besides the diminution of primary and differentiating follicles, ultrastructural studies indicate a great increase in fibroblasts and connective tissues throughout, especially in the cortex, where germinal structures are largely absent. The advanced follicles identified in postmenopausal ovaries are usually undergoing atretic changes. Although there is a great increase of atretic follicles in the postmenopausal ovaries, normal-appearing follicles are occasionally found; the granulosa cells, however, are smaller. Any observed corpus luteum is usually undergoing atresia. The luteal cells appear vacuolated, with an increase in the dense bodies and lipofuscin droplets. An infiltration of connective tissue can be observed in the atrophying corpus luteum. Although the ovarian cortex is becoming atrophic, the medullary region, with stromal and interstitial cells, is more abundant and usually active. Groups of functional stromal cells may be found throughout the postmenopausal ovary, especially around the hilar region. On occasion, single cells or smaller clusters of very active cells are apparent near the atretic follicle or corpus luteum. It is difficult to define these cells as either follicle cells, follicle cells differentiating into stromal cells, or a type of stromal cell. Stromal cells show similarity to Leydig's cells of the testes. When the stromal cells atrophy, they revert back to fibroblastic cell types. Active stromal cells have the ability to synthesize androgen.

A postmenopausal ovary exhibits an increase of connective tissue and a decrease of germinal elements. Although follicles, when present, appear to be undergoing atresia and the cells lining these follicles are in regression, activity in some cells may be present. Thick internal cells from atretic follicles differentiate into stromal or interstitial cells. An abundance of stromal cells are seen in postmenopausal ovaries, and in vitro experiments indicate that these cells are the source of androgens.

An occasional follicle that was developing in the early postmenopausal period may stay as a 1-cm follicular cyst and remain during the postmenopausal period. This often causes confusion for the physician reading the sonogram. It has no significance, and within a 2-month period a second sonogram will confirm the fact that it has remained unchanged.

The size of the ovary varies with age. During the reproductive period, the ovaries are approximately 3.5 to 4 cm in length, 2 cm in breadth and 1.5 cm in thickness. Postmenopausally, the ovaries decrease in size to approximately 0.5 cm in each dimension in the geriatric patient. The postmenopausal ovary measures approximately 3.5 to 4 × 2 × 1.5 cm. It has its own mesentery, the mesovarium from the posterior leaf of the broad ligament, and is attached to the cornua of the uterus by the ovarian ligament, which is continuous with the round ligament, the vestigial gubernaculum. The ovary is developmentally an abdominal organ, and its blood supply is from the abdominal aorta. The ovarian vessels lie in the infundibulopelvic ligament. The left ovarian vein empties into the left renal vein. The free surface of the ovary has no peritoneal covering, only a surface epithelium. The part attached to the mesovarium, through which all vessels and nerves pass, is the hilum. In the postmenopausal period, the ovary eventually becomes an inert residue that consists of connective tissue, and it clings to the posterior leaf of the broad ligament. Its normal pinkish color becomes pure white. It shrinks from 2 × 1.5 × 0.5 cm, and in some cases it may be as small as 1.5 × 0.75 × 0.5 cm. Its wrinkled surface resembles the gyri and sulci of the cerebrum. At this point, it cannot be palpated. At the time of laparotomy the ovary is often found on the lateral pelvic wall in the geriatric patient, presenting as a small, white, wrinkled, cord-like structure.

In the menopause, the geriatric ovary tends to atrophy and shrink when the graafian follicles and ova disappear. The tunica albuginea becomes very dense and causes the surface of the ovary to become scarred and shrunken. The cortex is marked by increasing thinning, as well as numerous corpora fibrosa and corpora albuginea, with areas of dense fibrosis and hyalinization. The ovary shows varying degrees of avascularity. The ultrastructure indicates a great increase in fibroblasts and connective tissue throughout, especially in the cortex, where germinal structures are largely absent. The advanced follicles identified in postmenopausal ovaries are usually undergoing atretic changes. These changes in the follicle granulosa and stroma continues until the ovary is practically replaced by connective tissue.

Additionally, a woman in this age group who is amenorrheic is clinically considered menopausal. However, chemically and anatomically, the changes described previously do not occur precipitously, but rather over a period of time. Although they appear to occur quite rapidly, it takes approximately 3 to 5 years for the final histologic changes to take place. It must then be concluded that if an ovary is palpated as premenopausal in size 3 to 5 years after clinical menopause, it is pathologic until proved otherwise. The author recommends that the patient have the benefit of an expedited examination under anesthesia, and if the previous impression is verified, the patient should undergo laparotomy. On opening the abdomen, washings should be taken from the pelvis and upper abdomen immediately, followed by careful abdominal exploration. A total hysterectomy with bilateral oophorectomy should be the treatment chosen. The ovaries should be removed without biopsy in the postmenopausal group when they are the size of premenopausal ovaries.

INTERVAL FOR PELVIC EXAMINATION

The literature suggests that a pelvic examination should be done every 6 months. This routine helps to detect early changes in the ovary. Despite the protocol for regular examinations, however, the chance of detecting an ovarian neoplasm during routine pelvic examination in an asymptomatic woman is only 1 in 10,000. It is obvious that the detection rate is very low. In most instances, physicians judge any ovarian cyst under 5 cm to be of little significance. This concept must be challenged, especially in the postmenopausal and surely in the geriatric woman.

POTENTIAL TO FORM A CANCER: PRESENT THROUGHOUT LIFE

Although physicians may accept the axiom that an ovary may be too old to function but never too old to form a tumor, they are still often lulled into a sense of false security if the mass has not reached a size of 5 cm. Until recently, it was felt that the common epithelial ovarian cancer rarely occurs before age 40 and peaks by age 60. However, recent figures show that at age 25 there is an annual incidence rate of 3 per 100,000 women; at age 60, 40 per 100,000 women; the rate continues to climb, and the peak incidence is at age 77. If physicians accept the premise that a cancer starts as a derangement within the cell and progresses from atypia to dysplasia to in situ and then to invasive cancer, there is a greater possibility of making an early diagnosis when any change is detected in the ovary in the postmenopausal patient.

SMALL CANCER VERSUS EARLY CANCER

An early cancer is not a tumor in the sense that a mass is necessarily present. A volume of tumor must be present before a mass can be detected. In fact, the earliest the tumor can be detected by any means is when it reaches 1 cm^3. By that time, the cancer contains 10^9 or 1 billion cells with the potential to metastasize and to kill. Therefore, even though it is small in size, this tumor is not truly an early cancer but rather a small cancer. This distinction will keep the physician alert to the danger of ignoring a change in the size of the ovary in the postmenopausal or geriatic patient. It usually takes 30 population doublings to reach the size of 1 cm. Therefore, a tumor that is regarded as clinically early is in truth biologically late, requiring only 10 to 20 more doublings before causing the death of the host. A 0.5-cm cancer, although regarded as early clinically, has already gone through 27 doublings and is biologically a late tumor. An important consideration is that some cancers have metastasizing phenotypes. These are the cancers that metastasize early. Most evidence suggests that when metastases occur, they may do so within the first 10 to 20 doubling times or at a stage undetectable by prevailing methodologies. Using the breast as a model, it has been estimated that 50 percent of women with a breast cancer measuring 1 cm already have systemic disease. However, by better education of the public and the profession, earlier diagnoses are definitely being made. Hopefully an early diagnosis will eventually be achieved through a serologic assay.

DIAGNOSTIC SIGNS

One diagnostic sign of early cancer in the ovary of a postmenopausal patient has proved both valuable and consistent. Stated simply, it is that the palpation of an ovary that is interpreted as a normal-sized ovary in a premenopausal woman represents an ovarian tumor in the postmenopausal woman. This is the keystone of the PMPO syndrome. This suggestion may appear to be insignificant in terms of the total problem, but it has been the experience of the author that all such palpable findings have proved to be a new growth; they were not necessarily malignant, but none were functional or dysfunctional. It is unfortunate that a registry has not been established to collate the material on the postmenopausal palpable ovary.

The PMPO syndrome is a misnomer, and it is unfortunate that a more descriptive term had not been chosen when this observation was published.

It must be emphasized that it does not mean that anything that is palpated in the adnexa is abnormal in the postmenopausal or geriatric patient. Expediency in carrying out the exploration is the choice of management when the PMPO syndrome is diagnosed. Exploratory surgery should be carried out in 2 to 4 weeks and not longer than 6 weeks.

There is no such thing as physiologic enlargement of the postmenopausal ovary. A physiologic cyst can arise only from the nonrupture of a graafian follicle or from cystic degeneration of a corpus luteum (lutein cyst). There are no functioning follicles or lutein cysts in the postmenopausal ovary simply because there are no follicles; or, if they are present, they are totally unresponsive, and there are no corpora lutea.

The only cause of the growth must be a neoplasm that is not necessarily malignant. It is neither functional nor dysfunctional and requires expedient management.

By strict definition, *menopause* means the cessation of menses. It has a definite endpoint, unlike the climacteric, which includes physiologic, psychologic, and anatomic changes and has no clear conclusion. Traditionally, a woman in this age group who is amenorrheic for 1 year is considered menopausal. However, chemically and anatomically, these changes occur over a period of time.

INCIDENCE OF CANCER OF THE OVARY

Cancer of the ovary is the most frustrating problem that a gynecologist faces. It is on the increase and has a high death rate. It is badly neglected by both patient and physician. Ovarian cancer is now the leading cause of death from gynecologic cancer in the United States. The figure that is most impressive is that ovarian cancer makes up about one-quarter of all gynecologic cancers but accounts for one-half of all gynecologic deaths. Of newborn girls, 1.4 percent, or 1 in 70, will develop ovarian cancer during their lifetime. The tragic feature of ovarian cancer is that at least 70 percent have advanced to stages III or IV by the time they are diagnosed. Therefore, the treatment of ovarian cancer is usually directed to the far advanced patient or to the terminal care of the patient with advanced or recurrent disease. The challenge presented by ovarian cancer is that more than 11,000 patients will die from it each year in the United States and that the results in 1988 are no better than they were in the previous two decades. By an aggressive approach directed to diagnosis and therapy, patients with ovarian cancer are living longer and, hopefully, more comfortably, but there has still been no significant improvement in the overall 5-year survival.

Ovarian cancer reaches a peak incidence at age 77, and then drops slightly and remains steady for the remainder of life. It is essential that these figures and the distribution of this curve be kept in mind when making a decision on whether to retain the ovaries at the time of hysterectomy in women over age 40. Since the incidence of ovarian cancer is on the increase in the highly industrialized nations, an effort must be made to achieve earlier diagnosis or to practice prophylaxis by removing the ovaries at the time of surgery in women over age 40. Currently in the United States, almost 700,000 hysterectomies are being performed annually, mostly in women over age 40. It is obvious that some cancers of the ovary could be prevented in these women if oophorectomy was done at the time of hysterectomy. It is important for the physician to explain that with the retained ovary the patient is always at risk of developing a tumor, as well as a retained ovary syndrome. If the patient wishes to retain her ovaries, she should sign after these warnings have been written into the infomed consent form.

If more women are to be saved and mortality from ovarian cancer is to diminish, a more liberal approach and an indication for surgery must be employed. Palpation of what appears to be a normal-sized premenopausal ovary in the postmenopausal period is indicative of ovarian pathology and should be investigated immediately. To wait until one feels a solid mass of up to 5 cm and expect a cure is an exercise in fancy and futility.

It is difficult to make a decision on the management of a menopausal patient who has fibroids. All too often, an ovarian neoplasm is followed under the false impression that it is a fibroid. Ovarian tumors may enlarge and grow against the uterus, and both the uterus and the ovary can rise from the pelvis as a midline mass. Therefore, if the ovaries cannot be palpated as separate entities from the fibroids, the patient should have a sonogram. If this is inconclusive, it is in the patient's best interest to be examined under anesthesia. The decision on whether to perform surgical exploration must be based on the findings at that time.

EVALUATION OF THE GERIATRIC OVARY BY SONOGRAPHY

Sonography can often give useful information about the nature of a pelvic mass. For instance, a cystic ovarian tumor can be homogeneous to ultrasound, whereas a malignant tumor can produce diffuse reflection, demonstrating its irregular internal pattern.

Loculations in a multicystic ovarian tumor may be seen. It is rarely possible to differentiate between irregular types of gynecologic tumors such as tuboovarian abscesses and cystadenomas of the ovary. Since it is extremely rare to have a tuboovarian abscess in the geriatric patient except occasionally when a diverticulitis abscess is present, the finding of a multicystic ovarian tumor would indicate a new growth.

A 1- or 2-cm cyst in the geriatric patient identified on sonography requires careful follow-up. However, this in itself is not an indication for immediate surgery. After an enema, the patient should be given a careful pelvic examination. If nothing is detected clinically, the patient should be reevaluated in approximately 6 weeks. The sonography and pelvic examination should be repeated. CT scans and nuclear magnetic resonance tests often add another dimension to the diagnosis. The patient should also have a ^{125}Ca and a CEA test. Any ovarian tumor that measures more than 3.5 cm is an indication for examination under anesthesia and possible exploratory laparotomy.

SUMMARY

The PMPO syndrome is a clearly established entity. It indicates that the palpation of what is interpreted to be a normal-sized ovary in a premenopausal woman represents an ovarian tumor in a postmenopausal woman. The ovary becomes too old to function but never becomes too old to form a cancer. Therefore, women who will be receiving a pelvic examination should be advised to take an enema so that it will be easier to detect changes that occur in the ovary.

The finding of what appears to be a normal premenopausal-sized ovary in a geriatric patient is an abnormal finding. The patient should have a workup and an examination under anesthesia.

The finding of a 1- to 2-cm cyst by sonography or CT scan in the postmenopausal woman requires careful evaluation. The patient should be reevaluated in about 6 to 8 weeks; if the findings are unchanged, the workup can be repeated in 2 more months. If there is no growth, the patient can then be followed carefully at stated intervals.

REFERENCES

Barber, H. R. K. 1979. The postmenopausal palpable ovary syndrome. *Comp. Ther.* 5(9):58.

————,ed. 1982. The postmenopausal palpable ovary syndrome (PMPO), in: *Ovarian Carcinoma. Etiology, Diagnosis and Treatment,* 2nd ed. Masson Publishing USA, New York, p. 173.

————. 1986. Ovarian cancer. *Ca-A Cancer Journal for Clinicians* 36(3):149.

Barber, H. R. K., and E. A. Graber. 1971. The PMPO syndrome (postmenopausal palpable ovary syndrome). *Obstet. Gynecol.* 38:921.

Creasman, W. T., and J. T. Soper. 1986. The undiagnosed adnexal mass after the menopause. *Clin. Obstet. Gynecol.* 29(2):446.

Osteoporosis

14

INTRODUCTION

The aging population in the United States is steadily increasing in number, and the majority are women who may be predisposed to an osteoporotic fracture syndrome. Osteoporosis is called the *silent disease*. Technically this is because it produces absolutely no symptoms until a fracture occurs. Osteoporosis is not a specific disease. Osteopenia, the state of having less than a normal amount of bone, results from normal bone loss associated with aging. Osteoporosis is the pathologic state of osteopenia, in which bone mass is so reduced that the skeleton becomes unable to perform its supportive function. Bone loss is normal. Bone loss great enough to prohibit proper functioning is not normal, although it occurs frequently.

The term *osteoporosis* is used to describe a reduced amount of bone. It is the end result of severe or prolonged bone loss. By *bone loss* is meant the gradual thinning and increased porosity of bone (hence the name *osteoporosis*) that occurs naturally with aging but that can be dangerously accelerated or beneficially slowed down by a multitude of factors. The chemical composition of the bone is unchanged in osteoporosis; there is simply less

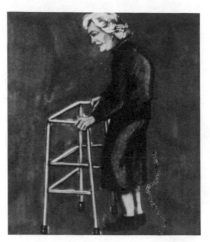

Figure 14-1. Typical picture of patient with advanced postmenopausal osteoporosis.

bone mass. In the trabecular bone, the trabeculae are abnormally thin and sparse; in cortical bone, the cortical width is reduced and the Haversian canals are enlarged. Osteoporosis must be distinguished from osteomalacia. Osteoporosis is due to an increased breakdown or reduced formation of whole bone. In *osteomalacia,* the amount of bone is normal but its mineral content is reduced. Osteomalacia is due to delayed mineralization of new bone.

As previously noted, osteoporosis has been called a silent disease because it frequently produces no symptoms until a fracture occurs. There is, however, another sense in which this disorder is silent, perhaps even invisible. Despite the fact that osteoporosis is extremely common, it is largely unknown among the general population and is not always appreciated by physicians. It is important for the public and the physician to understand what osteoporosis is, and to recognize that it can be accelerated or reduced by many factors. Osteoporosis is a painful, disfiguring, and debilitating process. It has been referred to as a "woman's issue" because the loss of bone begins sooner and proceeds twice as rapidly in women as it does in men. Osteoporosis affects 25 percent of women after natural menopause. Of those who have undergone surgical menopause without hormone replacement, up to 50 percent will develop osteoporosis. It has been stated that osteoporosis cannot be cured but it can be prevented. Although prevention is easier to achieve than cure, progress has been made in reversing or slowing down the osteoporotic process (Fig. 14-1).

BONE FORMATION

Bone contains 99 percent of the body's calcium, 88 percent of the phosphorus, 50 percent of the magnesium, 35 percent of the sodium, and 9 percent of the water. Bone is composed largely of protein, particularly collagen. About 12 percent of bone is calcium; however, it is the calcium and phosphorus that comprise the supporting structures of bone. These minerals are of equal importance in bone nutrition. Both are involved in bone formation, so that when bone loses calcium, it also loses phosphorus.

Bone is constantly being broken down and reformed in a process called *bone remodeling.* The process occurs when a small quantity of bone is lost through breakdown (resorption) on the inner surface lining the bone marrow cavity, while at the same time new bone tissue is formed on the outer surface. The same remodeling process occurs on the microscopic surfaces throughout the bone. The result is that bones grow bigger and denser. *Bone mass,* which is the total amount of bone in the skeleton, is maintained by a delicate balance between these two processes. The balance is dynamic and is constantly changing in response to the needs of the body.

Bone is a living tissue and is constantly being broken down and reformed, like all tissues of the body. Bone formation is needed for growth, for repair of microscopic fractures that result from everyday stress, and for the replacement of worn-out bone.

FORMATION OF NEW BONE

Bone remodeling begins with bone breakdown. The *osteoclasts,* the bone-resorbing cells, dig microscopic cavities along the inner surface of the bone. Next, bone-building cells, called *osteoblasts,* begin filling in these cavities with new bone cells. Many osteoblasts are required to replace the bone removed by one osteoclast. The osteoblasts begin the bone rebuilding process by first producing the collagen matrix. This is followed by the laying down of calcium and phosphorus crystals within the matrix, a process called *bone mineralization.* The entire cycle lasts for approximately 3 to 4 months. It is estimated that every year 10 to 30 percent of the entire skeleton is remodeled in this way (Figs. 14-2 to 14-5).

BONE STRUCTURE

There are 206 bones in the body, and although all of them undergo age-related changes, not all are affected in the same way. The differences are due to the structural makeup of the two basic kinds of bone tissue.

Cortical bone, the first type, is solid and dense. Trabecular bone, which is more porous and looks like a honeycomb, is the second type. Every bone in the body is composed of both types, with the trabecular inside, surrounded by the cortical. The relative proportions of each differ from one bone to another, moving within parts of an individual bone. The vertebrae of the spine consist mostly of porous trabecular bone surrounded by a thin cortical shell. The long bones of the arms and legs are mostly cortical, with areas of trabecular bone concentrated at both ends. Trabecular bone has a delicate, lacy appearance that is actually very strong. The lattice work gives a porous appearance to the bone and decreases its weight. Otherwise, if trabecular bone had the same structure as cortical bone, it would be very difficult for the human to walk around. Therefore, bones that have the greatest amount of trabecular tissue are most vulnerable to disturbances in the bone remodeling process. Spinal vertebrae, for example, consist mostly of porous, trabecular bone with a thin cortical shell. Since osteoporosis affects trabecular bone more than cortical bone, the spine is one of the first areas to be affected by the disease.

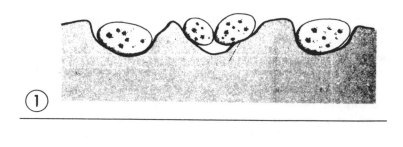

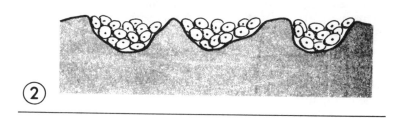

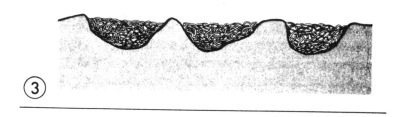

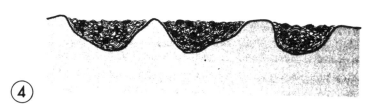

Figure 14-2. Four-step sequence of new bone formation: 1) osteoclasts, bone-resorbing cells, 2) osteoblasts, bone-forming cells, 3) collagen matrix of the new bone, and 4) bone mineralization.

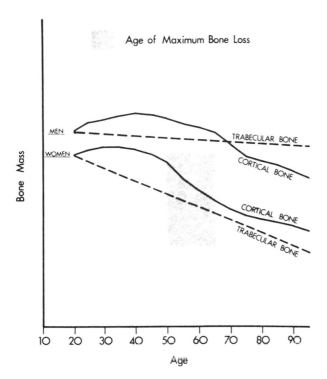

Figure 14-3. Bone loss with age: a comparison of men and women.

Bone is composed of a variety of tissues and minerals. It consists of tiny crystals of calcium and phosphorus embedded in a framework of interlocking protein fibers. These protein fibers are made primarily of collagen. It is the calcium crystals that give bones their strength, hardness, and rigidity, and it is the collagen fibers that give them their relative capacity for flexibility. A number of other minerals are also present in bone, including fluoride, sodium, potassium, magnesium, and citrate, as well as a variety of trace elements. These minerals act as the mortar holding the "bricks" of calcium and phosphorus crystals together.

The Three Surfaces of Bone

The cross section of a bone presents three surfaces called *envelopes.* Each envelope has different anatomic features, even though the cell makeup is identical throughout. The surface facing the marrow cavity is known as the *endosteal envelope;* the outer surface is called the *periosteal envelope;* and the material in between is called the *intracortical envelope.* The rate of bone formation in these three surfaces occurs at different rates in different age groups. During childhood, new bone formation occurs in the outer or periosteal envelope, and a smaller amount of breakdown occurs on the inner endosteal envelope. During adolescence, bone formation occurs on both surfaces, leading to large overall gains in bone mass. During early adulthood, the aging process starts. Bone breakdown begins on the endosteal or inner envelope; this is the start of the age-related decline in bone mass. Bone loss in the aged occurs on the osteal surface, while bone loss associated with immobilization or prolonged bed rest takes place in the intracortical envelope.

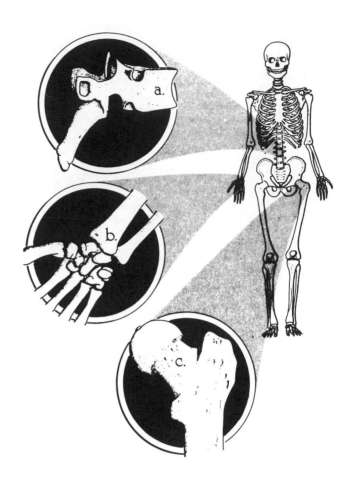

Figure 14-4. Three principal sites of osteoporotic fractures: a) vertebra, b) wrist, and c) hip bone.

OSTEOPOROSIS

Epidemiology

Women are more susceptible to develop osteoporosis than men. It occurs more often after the menopause, and the likelihood of its development increases with advancing age. The vertebrae and long bones are in greatest danger. The bones at the wrist (the radius), the upper arm (humerus), and the hip (femur) are common fracture sites. In many women, the weakness also affects the back, producing collapsed or flattened vertebrae and curvature of the spine *(kyphosis)*.

Generally, a woman's bones, even at the peak of her bone strength in her twenties, are not as strong as the bones of a man. After the menopause, the ovaries stop producing the hormone estrogen. The estrogen deficiency that results leads to an accelerated loss of bone content in all parts of the skeleton. As women grow older, they tend to reduce their calcium intake, which is the chief component of bone. Predisposing causes can be divided generally into three factors: genetic, insufficient dietary calcium, and estrogen deficiency.

Genetic factors play a role in osteoporosis. The osteoporotic syndrome is less common among black women, who tend to have denser bone structure. White women have more delicate bone structure and may be at greater risk than those with originally heavy bone structure and thick cortices. It has definitely been shown that heredity plays an important role in determining the amount of bone that will be present at maturity and the rate of bone loss with age. Many women with osteoporosis have a family history of the disorder. An accurate recording of the family tree would be helpful in predicting whether or not osteoporosis will occur. This is based on the assumption that no metabolic problems occur and that the person's lifestyle follows a moderate pattern. However, if more than two first-degree relatives have osteoporosis, the patient is at high risk.

Risk Factors

The risk factors in osteoporosis include (1) a thin body with a light frame, (2) a mother, grandmother, or sisters with osteoporosis, (3) early menopause, either surgical or due to natural causes, (4) a light-skinned Caucasian or Oriental background (5) a low intake of dietary calcium (milk, cheese, ice cream), (6) a long period of immobilization from disease or injury, (7) poor nutrition, (8) long-term treatment with high doses of steroid drugs (cortisone, prednisone), (9) heavy smoking and drinking, and (10) excessive intake of coffee or other caffeine containing beverages.

Detection of Bone Loss

Tests for calcium and other products of bone breakdown produce no specific biochemical signal, but the process that leads to the osteoporotic state produces various biochemical abnormalities. The bone-losing state may be recognized by (1) a fasting urine calcium value. A high fasting urinary calcium/creatinine ratio (upper normal limit, about 0.4 mmol/mmol) generally indicates a negative calcium balance, whether due to a high rate of bone resorption or a low rate of bone formation. The converse does not hold, however. In severe calcium malabsorption, a negative calcium balance may be present when the fasting urinary calcium level is in the normal range. It is important to emphasize that since meals result in sporadic elevations of calcium and other compounds in the blood, tests should be performed in the morning after a 12-hour overnight fast. (2) A fasting urine hydroxyproline test may be of help. A raised fasting urinary hydroxyproline/creatinine ratio (upper normal limit, about 0.017 mmol/mmol) indicates an increased rate of bone resorption and generally indicates a negative bone balance. However, if the bone formation rate is also high, as in Paget's disease and hyperthyroidism, the bone balance may be zero. (3) Plasma alkaline phosphatase is in the high normal range in patients who are losing bone and developing osteoporosis. High values suggest osteomalacia, Paget's disease, or some other bone condition, unless, of course, they are due to liver disease. The plasma alkaline phosphatase level is, therefore, most useful in the sense that a value in the low normal range makes rapid bone loss very unlikely. There is no satisfactory routine procedure for separating bone and nonbone phosphatase; the former is more heatlabile than the latter, and the "heat stability" value is sometimes of assistance.

It has been stated that the most important tests are the calcium/creatinine ratio (reflects loss of calcium from bones) and the hydroxyproline/creatinine ratio (reflects loss of collagen from bone).

There are a number of methods available for screening women for osteoporosis, as well as several noninvasive methods for quantitating appendicular bone mass. *Routine x-ray examinations* have been of little value, since at least 30 percent of bone must be lost before obvious changes are radiographically demonstrable. In the past, bone biopsy provided the best technique to evaluate osteoporosis. However, the method is painful and expensive, tissue samples are difficult to process, and most patients are unwilling to be subjected to the series of biopsies required for evaluation. Hand x-rays assess cortical bone only and are the least accurate of all the testing procedures. However, they are the most readily available; virtually every community is capable of taking hand x-rays.

Radiogrammetry is the measurement, on a simple x-ray plate, of cortical bone volume and total bone volume. The bone of the middle finger between the wrist and the metatarsal is typically used. The identified width of the bone marrow cavity is subtracted from the total width of the bone to yield an estimate of cortical bone thickness. This test is easy to perform and requires no special or expensive equipment. Only a small dose of radiation exposure is required, and the test can be safely and easily repeated at specific intervals to estimate the rate of bone loss. The disadvantage is that it is not sensitive enough to measure bone mass and, therefore, loses value as a screening tool for osteoporosis. It gives a rough estimate of cortical bone loss but cannot measure changes in trabecular bone and, therefore, is of little or no value in predicting spinal bone loss.

Norland-Cameron single-photon absorptiometry is most commonly used to measure the mineral content in the long bones. A monoenergetic photon source of ^{125}I is coupled with a sodium iodide scintillation counter. The difference in photon absorption in bone and in soft tissue allows measurement of the mineral content in the extremities, especially in the radius, in which normally the diaphysis is 95 percent cortical bone and 5 percent trabecular bone, and the distal metaphysis is 75 percent cortical bone and 25 percent trabecular bone. The densitometer measures the mineral content in the bones of the forearm (the radius and ulna) by calculating how many gamma rays are absorbed. The greater the absorption, the greater the bone mineral content and the greater the bone density. The densitometer is sensitive enough to detect a 1 to 3 percent loss of bone, whereas, as previously noted, with x-rays there has to be at least a 30 percent loss of bone. Single-photon absorptiometry offers a simple and noninvasive measure of skeletal status with high precision and accuracy. However, it has the drawback of correlating only moderately with the actual amount of bone in the spine. This is because the midpoint of the radius is mostly cortical bone.

X-rays of the jaw as carried out by the dentist may make a significant contribution to the diagnosis of osteoporosis. Bone loss in the jaw may precede and, therefore, warn of bone loss elsewhere in the body. X-rays of the jaw that reveal reduced bone density identify the patient as being at increased risk for osteoporosis.

The rate of turnover in trabecular bone is nearly eight times that in cortical bone, and is, therefore, a sensitive indicator of early metabolic changes. Currently, the two most useful techniques for assessing the bone mineral content in axial skeleton are the dual-photon absorption technique and the *dual-energy quantitative CT scan.*

The specially modified CT scanner can measure the exact amount of trabecular bone in an individual vertebrae. The procedure can be completed in about 30 minutes. The measurement is usually taken at the midportion of the first and second lumbar vertebrae. It is a very accurate method of determining early bone loss in the spine. The CT scan does have the disadvantage of exposing the patient to relatively high amounts of radiation. The test is expensive, and CT scan units are usually not available for screening asymptomatic patients.

In *dual-photon absorptiometry,* which is a modification of the Norland-Cameron technique, a radioisotope is used that emits photons at different energy levels and allows differentiation of fat and soft tissue components of bone. Thus it is more accurate than Norland-Cameron single-photon absorptiometry and quite applicable for quantitative imaging of the axial skeleton, in which more marrow-laden trabecular bone predominates. Therefore, it is a practical method of measuring the trabecular bone content in the spine. Since it uses an isotope with two different energies to measure the density of bone situated in deeper tissue, it gives a more accurate picture than single-photon absorptiometry. Both single- and dual-photon absorptiometry involve very little radiation.

The noninvasive methods for quantitating bone mass have been reviewed. The radiogrammetry and single-energy photon absorptiometry measure primarily cortical bone. In some sites, such as the distal radius and the calcaneus, trabecular bone is measured but changes in these areas may not always reflect what is occurring in the spine, and precision of repeated measurements is decreased because of the problem of repositioning. Measurements of cortical bone in themselves are of clinical importance. Eighty percent of the skeleton is cortical bone, and its loss is important in the pathogenesis of fracture. Hip fractures may be primarily caused by loss of cortical bone, and it has been suggested that even in the spine, the small amount of cortex present provides much of the strength of the vertebrae.

Single-photon absorptiometry offers a sensitive measurement of cortical bone, and is very practical and safe for large-scale screening and monitoring of treatment. Its main limitations are that it is less accurate in measuring trabecular as opposed to cortical bone. Dual-photon absorptiometry provides a method for identifying women at risk of losing bone in their spines. It is becoming increasingly available. CT scans may be the most accurate means of assessing bone loss in the spine, but the enormous cost of CT scan units and the relatively large radiation dose to the patient dampen the enthusiasm for using them on a large scale.

Total bone neutron activation analysis is a procedure that is used only in clinical research. A source of high-energy neutrons activates all the calcium in the body from ^{48}Ca to ^{49}Ca. The radioactive decay back to ^{48}Ca is measured with a gamma radiation counter. Ninety-nine percent of total body calcium is sequestered in the skeleton; therefore, the technique provides an extremely accurate assessment of bone mass. Major limitations include the total bone marrow radiation dose and the lack of differentiation between axial and appendicular calcium.

Histomorphometry refers to techniques and methods that allow preparation and processing of ultrathin (5- to 10-um), undecalcified sections of bone. With these sections, the relationship between fully mineralized, hypomineralized, and nonmineralized portions of bone can be studied. Currently this does not have wide application in clinical medicine.

Fracture Epidemiology

Osteoporosis is the main health hazard associated with the menopause. It consists of the increased porosity (rarefaction) of bone. It is a disease of the axial skeleton, with most of the loss occurring in trabecular bone or thinning of the cortex. Osteoporosis has been associated with decreased estrone and androstenedione levels. Bone loss is most rapid after oophorectomy resulting in castration or in women with gonadal dysgenesis. The consequences of osteoporosis include fractures of the vertebral body (often compression fractures), humerus, upper femur, and distal forearms and ribs. Osteoporosis, as noted earlier, is more common in white women than in black women. Approximately 25 percent of white women over age 60 have spinal compression fractures. In addition, approximately 32 percent of white women can expect to have one or more hip fractures at some time in their lives if current inadequate methods of prevention and treatment are maintained. On average, 16 percent of women with hip fractures die within 4 months of the fracture. Exercise and proper diet have a beneficial effect on bone integrity, and estrogen therapy can retard the process of osteoporosis.

Recently, it has been established that five main fractures are indicative of osteoporosis. These are fractures of the distal radius (Colles'), vertebrae, humerus, pelvis, and femoral neck. In general, Colles' fractures occur within the first 10 to 15 years after the menopause; spine fractures occur within 15 to 20 years after the menopause; and hip, humerus, and pelvic fractures occur within 20 to 40 years after the menopause.

Osteoporosis develops slowly and silently after the menopause, and the first sign is the occurrence of a fracture. Thus, when one sees the first major fracture, with the exception of Colles' fracture, one is really looking at the beginning of end-stage disease. Although it is important to consider fracture epidemiology in terms of its impact on health care systems, it is equally important to examine the pattern of bone loss with age, since knowledge of these factors holds the most promise in terms of preventive therapy (Fig. 14-6).

It is accepted that clinical manifestations of osteoporosis include fractures and their complications. Characteristically, fractures occur in the thoracic and lumbar vertebral bodies, the neck and intertrochanteric regions of the femur, and the distal radius. Osteoporotic individuals may fracture any bone more easily than their nonosteoporotic counterparts (Fig. 14-7).

Vertebral compression fractures occur more frequently in women than in men and typically affect T8–L3. These fractures may develop during routine activities such as bending, lifting, or rising from a chair or bed. Immediate, severe local back pain often results. The pain usually subsides within several months. Some individuals experience persistent pain due to altered spinal mechanics. In contrast, some vertebral fractures do not cause pain. Gradual, asymptomatic vertebral compression may be detected only upon radiographic examination. Loss of body height and/or the development of kyphosis may be the only signs of multiple vertebral fractures. Discomfort, disability, and, rarely, pulmonary dysfunction may accompany thoracic shortening. Abdominal symptoms may include early satiety, bloating, and constipation.

Hip fractures are another important manifestation of osteoporosis. The affected population tends to be older and the sex distribution more even than is the case in vertebral fracture. Acute complications including hospitalization, depression, and mechanical failure of the surgical procedure are common. Most patients fail to recover normal activity, and mortality within 1 year approaches 20 percent. Distal radial fractures limit the use of the extremity for 4 to 8 weeks, although long-term disability is uncommon. These fractures promote fear of loss of independent living, fear of additional falls, and fractures and depression.

In a study of the natural history of fractures, there are two terms that are often used: *incidence rate* and *prevalence rate.* The incidence rate is the number of fractures that occur in an age group in 1 year divided by the total number of individuals in that same age group, ascertained from census studies. The prevalence rate is concerned with the cumulative number of people who have had a fracture during a certain period of time divided by the total number of individuals in that same age group. In other words, the prevalence rate of a fracture at age 70 represents the cumulative incidence rate for each year up to age 70. This is a useful measurement to have because it gives some idea of the size of the health problem for that age group; however, the characteristics of that group may not be truly representative because these people are also survivors. When one compares the incidence rate of fractures among various populations, one finds that it may vary because one particular community may have a higher proportion of younger or older people in the population.

Detection of low skeletal mass and/or a fracture after minor trauma should alert the physician to the presence of metabolic bone disease. The physician should evaluate further to exclude osteomalacia, hyperparathyroidism, multiple myeloma, metastatic disease, syndromes of glucocorticoid excess, and other causes of secondary osteoporosis. No blood or urinary tests can establish specifically the diagnosis of primary osteoporosis, but they may exclude secondary causes.

Pathogenesis

Primary Osteoporosis. The term *osteoporosis* implies that the condition is not associated with any of the disorders or conditions that are known to produce an osteoporotic state, notably hyperthyroidism, Cushing's syndrome, and corticosteroid therapy. Primary osteoporosis cannot be traced to one single cause; it is usually the result of interaction among genetic, nutritional, and environmental factors. Primary osteoporosis may be either simple or accelerated.

Simple primary osteoporosis in women is the result of increased bone resorption associated with the menopause. Estrogenic hormones tend to protect bones against the resorbing action of PTH. It is felt that the estrogen effect is mediated through calcitonin, since calcitonin levels are low in menopausal females and blood calcitonin rises during estrogen therapy. It is difficult to say whether the action of estrogen on bone is direct or indirect. The menopausal increase in bone resorption is associated with small but significant rises in the fasting plasma calcium, phosphate, and alkaline phosphatase levels, as well as in urinary calcium and hydroxyproline excretion. Currently, the primary mechanism of action of estrogen in the bones of mammals is known to be the suppression of osteoclastic bone resorption. Whether the effect is direct or indirect is unclear. Estrogen therapy in the osteoporotic woman has been shown to decrease urinary hydroxyproline excretion, decrease serum calcium and phosphate concentrations, and increase serum parathyroid hormone and 1-alpha, 25-dehydroxy vitamin D [1,25(OH)2D] concentrations; calcium absorption is increased and urinary calcium excretion is generally decreased.

Decelerated osteoporosis has been seen in a variety of patients. The principal metabolic abnormality that has been defined in men and women with vertebral depression fractures (accelerated osteoporosis) is malabsorption of calcium, which is present in a high proportion of cases. The cause of this malabsorption is uncertain. It has been suggested that it is due to a deficiency of 1,25(OH)2D caused by the functional depression of 1 alpha-hydroxylase, but there is no agreement on this point. An alternative explanation might be that these patients (or some of them) are suffering from end organ failure in the gastrointestinal tract.

There are several other risk factors that probably contribute to accelerated osteoporosis in various ways. The best documented of these is alcohol. There is strong evidence that alcoholics are more liable to develop osteoporosis than the population at large, and a history of high alcohol intake has been obtained from a number of male osteoporotics. The mechanism is obscure. Gastrointestinal surgery probably constitutes another factor because of the effect of certain bypass surgeries on calcium operation. Diabetes is probably another risk factor, possibly due to the adverse effect of insulin deficiency on protein synthesis. However, diabetes is not a common finding in osteoporotic men or women. Another risk factor is alactasia (malabsorption of lactose due to a deficiency of lactose), which has been reported in 30 percent of osteoporotic subjects in several series. It is not clear whether the connection with osteoporosis is malabsorption of the calcium secondary to the bowel defect or the low calcium intake of alactasic subjects. Low calcium intake is a risk factor for osteoporosis in both males and females, but it has not often been identified as the only causal factor. It is recognized that a high protein intake increases urinary calcium and produces a negative calcium balance. Calcium requirement is a function of protein intake, and the low fracture rate in developing countries despite the low calcium intake reflects the low calcium requirements in the presence of low protein intake. Liver disease may constitute another risk factor, but the evidence on this point is weak.

Secondary Osteoporosis. Secondary osteoporosis is usually the result of a drug or disease that causes bone loss.

Hyperadrenocorticism. Reports indicate that vertebral crush fractures are a well-recognized feature of Cushing's disease and are also associated with corticosteroid therapy. The cause of the increase in bone breakdown is not entirely clear, but it may be secondary to inhibition of calcium absorption in the presence of corticosteroids, for which there is a great deal of clinical and experimental evidence.

Hyperthyroidism. Hyperthyroidism has long been associated with spinal osteoporosis. The changes reported probably reflect a direct effect of thyroid hormone on bone. Reports indicate that there is a rise in urinary calcium and hydroxyproline excretion and a significant elevation in plasma alkaline phosphatase. In addition, plasma calcium and phosphate levels tend to be slightly elevated.

Disuse. The third major cause of secondary osteoporosis is disuse or weightlessness. Once again, it has been classically attributed to reduced new bone formation, since it is well established that mechanical stresses on bone stimulate new bone formation. Why bone resorption should increase in response to weightlessness is unknown. The effect of exercise on bone loss became an issue when the first astronauts came back from space. NASA physicians found evidence of measurable bone loss even after a short time in space. The medical consultants decided that although physical activity is necessary to preserve bone mass, ordinary calisthenics are ineffective. Therefore, it was recommended that upright exercise, such as walking or jogging, which involves gravity, movement, and muscle pull on the bones, is an important factor. It is also important to exercise and spend time outdoors whenever possible. Sunlight helps the body create the active form of vitamin D, which helps metabolize calcium.

Hyperparathyroidism. Hyperparathyroidism has also been associated with osteoporosis. Trabecular osteoporosis is relatively uncommon, but cortical osteoporosis occurs. Cortical bone loss is accelerated in primary hyperparathyroidism, and cross-sectional measurements demonstrate reduced cortical width in these cases, particularly in the postmenopausal woman. Hyperparathyroidism affects cortical bone rather than trabecular bone. Vertebral osteoporosis does occur occasionally in primary hyperparathyroidism, but probably no more often than would be expected by chance.

Economics of Osteoporosis

By age 80, 33 percent of all women will have sustained a hip fracture and 24 percent of all women will have had a Colles' fracture. Although a number of patients will have had one or more hip fractures, it is clear that the number of women who have age-related fractures is well in excess of 50 percent. By age 85, at least 93 percent of the women will have sustained a hip, Colles', humerus, pelvis, or spinal fracture. Fracture and its complications are among the group of leading diseases in the elderly, particularly women. By comparison, about 15 percent of the elderly will have diabetes, 5 percent rheumatoid arthritis, 15 percent hypertension, 10 percent mental problems, and 20 percent cardiovascular disease. In addition, the cost of complications of fractures runs in excess of $4 billion a year in the United States.

Prevention

Physicians engaged in the care of patients, particularly women, must emphasize measures that retard or halt the progress of osteoporosis before irreversible structural defects occur. The mainstay of prevention and management of osteoporosis are a well-structured lifestyle, estrogen, adequate calcium intake, regular exercise, and avoidance of excess protein, alcohol, smoking, and caffeine. It must be emphasized that osteoporosis is an end state of many different possible processes; hence, there is not likely to be a single set of predictive factors.

The RDA of calcium for adults is 800 to 1000 mg. During the menopause the RDA is 1200 to 1400 mg. Milk is the ideal calcium source, Swiss cheese, brick cheese, and cheddar contain more calcium than the soft cheeses. Other foods high in calcium are tofu, red salmon, sardines, nuts, broccoli, and many leafy green vegetables. Many Americans have a lactase deficiency or a lactose intolerance. Since milk, ice cream, puddings, and other milk products contain large amounts of lactose, these people are unable to ingest them without suffering from diarrhea, cramps, and gas. Therefore, people with a lactase deficiency must eliminate all lactose-containing foods from their diet and depend entirely on other food sources for calcium. Another option is to use calcium supplements. This is an easy and reliable way to ensure the ingestion of enough calcium. Another option is to supply the missing enzyme (lactase) by using one of the available commercial enzyme preparations. Of all the calcium preparations, calcium carbonate is usually the least expensive and supplies the highest amount of calcium per tablet. It has been shown that calcium supplements used to protect against bone loss may help to protect against high blood pressure as well. Vitamin D has been referred to as the *sunshine vitamin* and is critical for the creation of new bone after breakdown. The RDA for adults is 400 IU. Vitamin D in the diet is fairly limited: fatty fish, butter, eggs, liver, and milk are the best sources. Milk itself has little vitamin D, but most commercial milk is now fortified with 400 units per quart. Vitamin D increases the absorption of calcium in the intestines and increases the reabsorption of calcium through the kidneys.

Bone Robbers. There are bone robbers, and it is important to control these in the diet. Protein increases calcium excretion more than it increases calcium absorption, resulting in an overall loss of calcium from the body. Salt in the form of sodium chloride results in losing calcium in the urine. The loss is directly related to the quantity of salt ingested; the more sodium in the diet, the greater the excretion of calcium. Other bone robbers include coffee, oxalates, phytates, fiber, and an excess of vitamin A. Diet fads are often the cause of low calcium in the diet. In order to reduce bone loss, a vegetarian diet is best. Red meat not only has protein but is acid and therefore promotes excretion of calcium in the urine. In addition, red meat has phosphorus, which may predispose to bone loss. Certain antacids contain aluminum, which contributes to a negative calcium balance. These antacids are Amphogel, Telcid, Di-Gel, Gaviscon, Gelusil, Maalox, Mylanta, Riopan, Rolaids, and Simeco.

Estrogen Replacement Therapy. Estrogen replacement therapy is highly effective in delaying and possibly preventing osteoporosis in women. Estrogen has been shown to reduce bone resorption and to retard or halt postmenopausal bone loss. Case control studies have shown a substantial reduction in hip and wrist fractures in women whose estrogen replacement has begun within a few years of menopause. Studies also suggest that estrogen reduces the rate of vertebral fractures. Even when therapy is started as late as 6 years after the menopause, estrogen prevents further loss of bone mass, although it does not restore it to premenopausal levels. Oral estrogen protects at low doses, such as 0.625 mg conjugated equine estrogen, 25 mg estranol, or 2 mg estradiol valerate daily. Estrogen replacement therapy is now available by a patch technique. It relieves the patient of taking a pill; furthermore, the first pass is to the general circulation, not through the liver. It has been reported that estrogens delays bone loss by inducing osteoblastic formation of new bone. However, this has proved to be so only in birds. Currently, the primary mechanism of action of estrogen in the bones of mammals is evidently the suppression of osteoclastic bone resorption. Whether the effect of estrogen therapy is direct or indirect is unclear.

Estrogen treatment has been shown to decrease urinary hydroxyproline excretion, decrease serum calcium and phosphate concentrations, and increase serum parathyroid hormone and 1,25(OH)2D concentrations; calcium absorption is increased and urinary calcium excretion is generally decreased. Estrogen increases the efficiency of calcium absorption through the intestine. Estrogen also appears to stimulate the thyroid gland to produce calcitonin, which protects the bones from the dissolving effects of parathyroid hormone and inhibits bone breakdown. Estrogen also stimulates the liver to produce proteins that bind with the adrenal hormones in the blood and prevent the bone-dissolving effects. Progestogens have been shown to augment the effect of calcium in preventing bone loss. The addition of progestogens to estrogen therapy also negates the one negative aspect of estrogen therapy: the association with carcinoma of the endometrium. This association will be discussed in the following chapter.

Prevention for Female Offspring. Genetic factors, as mentioned, play a role in osteoporosis. The osteoporotic syndrome is less common among black women, who tend to have denser bone structure. White women, with a more delicate bone structure, may be at greater risk than those with originally heavy bone structure and thick cortices. It is accepted that women who have osteoporosis have a higher rate of risk to develop osteoporosis in their family history. It is important to look into the family history of these patients. For those seeking advice about whether they are at risk, it is important to point out that if the grandmother, mother, aunt, or sister has osteoporosis, the patient is at very high risk to develop osteoporosis.

Among patients who are at high risk for the development of osteoporosis, it is important to start at an early age with a program for prevention. This includes a well-structured lifestyle, with consumption of alcohol in moderation and the elimination of smoking. A diet that is well balanced, with not too much red meat and an increased amount of vegetables, is important. Calcium supplements are probably well advised. The patient should exercise regularly. Swimming is not a particularly good exercise for the prevention of osteoporosis. Exercise that combines movement, pull, and stress on the long bones of the body is best for protecting against osteoporosis. Walking, jogging, bicycling, hiking, rowing, and jumping rope are all excellent. It must be pointed out that strenuous, prolonged physical training in women may actually have a negative effect on bone mass. It must be pointed out that for women already experiencing the painful signs of osteoporosis, swimming is the exercise of choice. It allows the benefit of activity without placing undue strain on an already weakened and compromised skeleton. All of these practices help to increase the bone mass, and it is important to develop maximal bone mass by age 35. For those patients who may be genetically compromised, it is important at age 35 to start testing with dual-photon absorptiometry. Detection of loss of bone mass at this age calls for an increased and more vigorous preventive program, as well as supplements that have been referred to in this chapter. Patients with a strong history of osteoporosis should have estrogen–progesterone therapy started at the time of menopause and the calcium intake increased, as well as a well-balanced diet and a structured exercise program.

Established Symptomatic Osteoporosis

Advanced osteoporosis may give rise to marked symptoms. When the symptoms are bad, the patient should be placed on rest for 7 to 14 days and given analgesics and muscle relaxants. Moist heat in the form of hot compresses helps to eliminate the symptoms. As soon as the acute phase is passed, the patient should be placed on a regimen of gradual mobilization with assisted ambulation. This should continue for 2 to 5 weeks. Thoracic hyperextension orthosis should be implemented as tolerated. Brushing of the hair, particularly down the neck, is a good exercise. As soon as the pain is controlled, swimming is an excellent rehabilitative exercise.

For those people who have repeated fractures and symptomatic osteoporosis, there is a regimen; it includes sodium fluoride, 1 mg/kg/day for 2 to 5 years, the therapy period determined by the degree of osteoporosis. Vitamin D, 400 units/day, is added, as is calcium carbonate, 3900 mg/day. This regimen, combined with a well-balanced diet, the elimination of factors that deplete bone mass, and a careful program of exercise, will help control the disease.

Calcitonin has recently been approved for clinical usage. It is a useful preparation for women in whom hormone replacement therapy is contraindicated; unfortunately, it must be given by injection. The recommended dose varies from daily to thrice weekly injections of 50 to 100 IU. Calcitonin has analgesic properties, and this is possibly one of its most useful roles in the management of women with established osteoporosis. Calcitonin should not be used for the prevention of osteoporosis.

SUMMARY

Bone is made up of calcium and phosphorus crystals embedded in a matrix of protein fibers. The calcium gives the bone its strength and rigidity, while the protein-collagen makes the bone somewhat flexible. Other materials present in bone include fluoride, sodium, potassium, magnesium, and citrate. These other elements help hold the calcium and phosphorus crystals together.

Bone is a living tissue and is constantly being broken down and reformed. The process begins with bone breakdown. Bone-absorbing cells called *osteoclastic cavities* in the inner surface of the bone can produce microscopic cavities. Next, bone-building cells called *osteoblasts* begin filling in these cavities with new bone cells. These cells begin the bone-rebuilding process by first producing the collagen matrix. This is followed by laying down of the calcium-phosphorus crystals within the matrix, a process called *bone mineralization.* Each year between 10 and 30 percent of the entire skeleton is remodeled this way.

Calcium is essential for bone contraction, blood clotting, and brain and nerve function. It is also a key ingredient in bone mineralization. Poor intake of calcium leads to a negative calcium balance. To correct this problem, the body's hormones release calcium from the skeleton into the bloodstream, making it available for nerves and muscles. If there is a long term deficiency, the skeletal storage deposit can become depleted of its calcium, leaving porous, brittle, breakable bones, a condition known as *osteoporosis.*

There are basically two different types of bone: cortical and trabecular. The cortical bone is a very dense, solid bone; the long, hard bones of the arms and legs are of this type. Trabecular bone is much more porous, honeycombed with many minute spaces. Every bone has both types, with porous trabecular bone on the inside and solid cortical bone on the outside, though in different proportions, depending upon the bone in question. Spinal vertebrae are mostly porous trabecular bone with a thin cortical shell. Since osteoporosis affects trabecular bone more than cortical bone, the spine is one of the first areas to be affected by the disease.

Up to age 35, bone mass usually outweighs the usual loss. After this age there is a gradual loss of bone mass, and after the menopause women lose bone mass much more rapidly than before. This loss is about six times more rapid than that of men. At about age 65, the rate of bone loss slows.

Osteoporosis is epidemic in the United States; one out of four women have or will have it. Fair-skinned women with ancestors from northern Europe, the British Isles, Japan, or China are genetically predisposed to osteoporosis.

Osteoporosis is a painful, disfiguring, and debilitating disease that is often accompanied by psychologic changes. When it is advanced to the point where 30 to 40 percent of the bone mass has been lost, the vertebrae start to collapse, eventually leading to the stooped posture called *dowager's hump.* Loss in height can be as much as 5 to 8 inches. Clothing no longer fits, and the torso is no longer in proportion to the legs and arms. This condition leads to respiratory and gastrointestinal problems.

Bone fractures and broken hips are part of the osteoporosis syndrome. More than 200,000 hips are fractured each year. These fractures are usually preceded by osteoporosis. Approximately 20 percent of the patients die within 3 months.

In the past, it was difficult to make an early diagnosis of osteoporosis. Most diagnostic methods were not definitive. However, sophisticated tests including radionuclide tracer methods, blood and urine calcium levels, and calcium balance determinations are not able to detect bone loss in its early stages. Conventional x-rays do not reveal bone loss until the loss totals approximately 35 percent. However, with the introduction of photon densitometry, it is now possible to make a fairly early diagnosis of osteoporosis.

The best way to prevent osteoporosis is to build strong bones before age 35 and, by so doing, to retain a heavy bone mass through the postmenopausal years. Osteoporosis can be prevented and even perhaps slightly reversed if it is already present. Further progression can usually be slowed or halted. The patient at risk should have a calcium-rich diet, calcium supplements, exercise, and estrogen replacement therapy as the responsible physician deems advisable. The estrogen therapy helps to prevent bone dissolution and aids the digestive system in absorbing calcium more efficiently.

It has been stated that osteoporosis can be prevented. This usually involves a change of lifestyle, including foods, vitamins, and minerals. The diet is important. The patient should have a well-balanced diet including calcium-rich in dairy products. Excess protein or fat intake will accelerate calcium excretion and should be limited. Increased amounts of vegetables in the diet are helpful. Soft drinks, coffee, alcohol, and nicotine cause excessive calcium loss. It should be reemphasized that exercise is the most important consideration. The exercise should involve gravity, movement, and muscle pull on the bones. Therefore, walking or jogging is much better than swimming.

The best sources of calcium are dairy products, including whole or skim milk and cheese. Leafy green vegetables, including broccoli, collards, turnip greens, mustard greens, and spinach, are also good sources. Salmon and raw oysters are high in calcium. Ice cream is not a particularly good source. Increasing the amount of calcium in the diet may increase the risk of kidney stones. However, by drinking enough water and making sure that the calcium intake is not more than 2000 mg daily will reduce this risk. Calcium carbonate is one of the best calcium preparations, is inexpensive, and can be purchased over the counter.

Projects are underway to treat advanced osteoporosis. These treatment protocols include sodium fluoride, vitamin D, calcium carbonate, and estrogen replacement therapy. They must be carefully monitored by a center that is actively working in the field of osteoporosis.

The gynecologist must identify the patient at risk. In addition to counseling, the physician should institute a regimen of estrogen-progesterone therapy if there are no contraindications to the use of these hormones.

REFERENCES

Aloia, J. F., S. H. Cohn. A. Vaswani, et al. 1985. Risk factors for postmenopausal osteoporosis. *Am. J. Med.* 78:95.

Aloia, J. F., A. Vaswani, A. Kapoor, A., et al. 1985. Treatment of osteoporosis with calcitonin, with or without growth hormone. *Metabolism* 34:124.

Avioli, L. 1981. Postmenopausal osteoporosis; prevention versus cure. *Fed. Proc.* 40:2418.

Avioli, L. (ed). 1983. *The Osteoporosis Syndrome.* Grune & Stratton, New York.

Ellis, F. R., et al. 1972. Incidence of osteoporosis in vegetarians and omnivores. *Am. J. Clin. Res.* 25:555.

Ettinger, B., H. K. Genant, and C. E. Cann. 1985. Long term estrogen replacement therapy prevents bone loss and fractures. *Ann. Intern. Med.* 102:319.

Farmer, M. E., L. R. White, J. A. Brody, and K. R. Bailey. 1984. Race and sex differences in hip fracture incidence. *Am. J. Public Health* 74:1374.

Gain, S. M. 1981. The phenomena of bone formation and bone loss, in: *Osteoporosis. Recent Advances in Pathogenesis and Treatment* (H. F. Deluca et al. eds.). University Park Press, Maryland.

Gallagher, J. C., L. J. Melton, B. L. Riggs, B. L., et al. 1980. Epidemiology of fractures of the proximal femur in Rochester, Minnesota. *Clin. Orthop.* July-August, pp. 163.

Gambrell, R. D., et al. 1979. Reduced incidence of endometrial cancer among postmenopausal women treated with progestogens. *J. Am. Geriatric Soc.* 27:389.

Genant, H. K., and C. E. Cann. 1982. Quantitative computed tomography for assessing vertebral bone mineral, in: *Computed Tomography of the Lumbar Spine* (H. K. Genant, N. Chafetz, and C. A. Helmos, eds.). University of California Printing Department, San Francisco, pp. 289–314.

Heaney, R. P. 1976. Estrogens and postmenopausal osteoporosis. *Clin. Obstet. Gynecol.* 19:791.

Horsman, A. P. 1968. The etiology of fractured hips in females. *Am. J. Public Health* 58:485.

Keene, J. S., and C. A. Anderson. 1982. Hip fractures in the elderly. Discharge predictions with a functional rating scale. *JAMA* 248:564.

Lane, J. 1981. Postmenopausal osteoporosis: The orthopedic approach. *Female Patient* 6:43.

Lane, J. M., V. J. Vigorita, and M. Falls. 1984. Osteoporosis: Current diagnosis and treatment. *Geriatrics* 34(4):40.

Lanyon, L. E. 1981. Bone remodelling, mechanical stress and osteoporosis, In: *Osteoporosis. Recend Advances in Pathogenesis and Treatment.* (H. F. DeLuca, et al. eds.). University Park Press, Baltimore.

Linnel, S., J. M. Stager, P. W. Blue, et al. 1984. Bone mineral content and menstrual regularity in female runners. *Med. Sci. Sports Exerc.* 16:343.

Mazess, R. B., W. W. Peppler, R. W. Chesney, et al. 1984. Does bone measurement of the radius indicate skeletal status? Concise communication. *J. Nucl. Med.* 25:281.

McCarthy, D. M., J. A. Hibbin, and J. M. Goldman. 1984. A role for 1,25 dihydroxy-vitamin D3 in control of bone marrow deposition. *Lancet* 8:78.

Nachtigall, L. E., et al. 1979. Estrogen replacement therapy. A 10-year prospective study in the relationship to osteoporosis. *Obstet. Gynecol.* 53:277.

Newcomer, A. D., et al. 1981. Lactase deficiency: Prevalence in osteoporosis. *Ann. Intern. Med.* 89:267A.

Notelovitz, M., and M. Ware. 1984. *Stand Tall. Every Woman's Guide to Preventing Osteoporosis.* Bantam Books, New York.

Osteoporosis. *ACOG Technical Bull. No. 72.* October 1983, pp. 1–5.

Parfitt, A. M. 1984. The cellular basis of bone remodelling: The quantum concept re-examined in light of recent advances in cell biology of bone. *Calcif. Tissue Int.* 36:537.

Recker, R. R. 1985. Non-invasive measurements of bone loss, in: *Non-Invasive Bone Measurement: Methodological Problems.* (J. Dequeker and C. C. Johnston, eds.). IRL Press, Oxford, pp. 1–13.

Recker, R. R. 1985. Calcium absorption and achlorhydria. *N. Engl. J. Med.* 313:70.

Recker, R. R., P. D. Savile, and R. B. Heanney. 1977. Effect of estrogens and calcium carbonate on bone loss in postmenopausal women. *Ann. Intern. Med.* 87:649.

Riggs, B. L., E. N. Seeman, S. F. Hodgson, et al. 1982. Effect of the fluoride/calcium regimen on vertebral fracture occurrence in postmenopausal osteoporosis. *N. Engl. J. Med.* 306:446.

Riggs, B. L., H. W. Wahner, W. L. Dunn, et al. 1981. Differential changes in bone mineral density of the appendicular and axial skeleton with aging; relationship to spinal osteoporosis. *J. Clin. Invest.* 67:328.

Rigotti, N. A., S. R. Mussbaum, D. R. Herzog, and R. M. Neer. 1984. Osteoporosis in women with anorexia nervosa. *N. Engl. J. Med.* 311:1601.

Slovik, D. M., J. S. Adams, R. M. Neer, et al. 1982. Deficient production of 1,25 dihydroxy-vitamin D in elderly osteoporotic patients. *N. Engl. J. Med.* 305:372.

Trotter, M., et al. 1960. Densities of bones of white and negro skeletons. *J. Bone Joint Surg.* 42A:50.

Wasnich, R. D., R. J. Benfante, K. Yano, L. Heilbrun, and J. M. Vogel. 1985. Thiazide effect on the mineral content of bone. *N. Engl. J. Med.* 309:344.

Wasnich, R. D., P. R. Ross, L. K. Heibrun, and J. M. Vogel. 1985. Prediction of postmenopausal fracture risk with bone mineral measurements. *Am. J. Obstet. Gynecol.* 12:745.

Whedon, G. D. 1982. Osteoporosis. *N. Engl. J. Med.* 305:397.

15 Estrogen Therapy and Endometrial Cancer

INTRODUCTION

For more than 40 years, the history of estrogen replacement therapy for menopausal symptoms has been noted for excessive claims of benefits followed by profound fears of possible side effects. The changing accept ability of estrogen replacement has been influenced by the media as much as by sound scientific studies. It is accepted that there is some association between the use of estrogen therapy and endometrial cancer. The important questions are: "What is the relative risk from the use of exogenous estrogen therapy and endometrial cancer?" and "Is estrogen an initiator or a promoter of this cancer?"

Estrogen is a drug. Therefore, like any other drug, it should be given when needed and indicated and should be withheld when it is not needed or if there is a contraindication to its use. A solid body of research is emerging that permits physicians to evaluate patients for the rational use of estrogen and progesterone therapy. If estrogens are to be given, a regimen that includes progesterone should be prescribed.

Estrogen replacement therapy in the peri- and postmenopausal patient is most helpful for those who have flushes, flashes, sweats particularly at night, insomnia, and a dry vagina. Hot flashes are due to hypothalamic dysfunction caused by loss of ovarian feedback signals, with cyclic activation of thermoregulatory pathways resulting in flushing and perspiration. In many patients homeostatic adjustment occurs with time, resulting in spontaneous disappearance of symptoms, although in about 25 percent of cases the hot flushes persist for more than 5 years. Occasionally, after a symptom-free period of time, the flashes and flushes may return. Feedback inhibition of the hypothalamic centers controlling gonadotropin secretion can be partially restored with estrogen and progesterone replacement. The use of both estrogen and progesterone during the time of replacement seems to have a synergistic effect, resulting in better control of the hot flushes and flashes. Estrogen has an effect on the psychologic symptoms and controls the problems of memory, anxiety, and irritability. Estrogen also relieves insomnia and has been shown to decrease sleep latency and to increase the depth and duration of sleep and the amount of rapid-eye-movement (REM) sleep. Hot flashes during sleep have a close temporal relationship to waking episodes and may be the principal cause of sleep disturbances associated with estrogen deficiency. Chronic sleep disturbances can lead to a variety of other symptoms.

ESTROGEN AS A PROTECTION AGAINST OSTEOPOROSIS

To be effective as prophylaxis against the development of osteoporosis, estrogen replacement must be started promptly after cessation of ovarian function. The introduction of dual-photon absorptiometry permits an estimation of bone loss in its earliest stages. It has been recommended that testing start at 35 years of age. CT scanning is probably just as effective but a conventional x-ray examination is not very helpful, since at least 30 percent of the bone mass has to be lost before it can detect this change. Estrogen replacement therapy has been associated with an increase of serum concentrations of 1 alpha, 25-dehydroxy vitamin D [1,25(OH)2D] in postmenopausal women with osteoporosis. Reports that PTH concentrations in these patients also increase suggests that estrogen may act directly by stimulating the production of PTH by the parathyroid gland. Although estrogen was originally thought to delay bone loss by inducing osteoblastic formation of new bone, it is now accepted that the primary mechanism of action of estrogen on the bones of mammals is the suppression of osteoclastic bone resorption. Estrogen has also been shown to decrease urinary hydroxyprolene excretion, decrease serum calcium and phosphate concentrations, and increase serum PTH and 1,25(OH)2D concentrations. Calcium absorption is also increased and urinary calcium excretion is generally decreased. The negative aspect of estrogen replacement in the postmenopausal patient is the possibly increased risk for endometrial cancer when estrogen replacement therapy is employed.

CARCINOMA OF THE ENDOMETRIUM

It has been shown that estrogen is a cell stimulator, but it has never been proved that estrogen can transform a normal cell into a malignant one. Recent work indicates that many cancers are caused by a two-stage process through exposure to one or two different kinds of substances known as *initiators* and *promoters.* Researchers are exploring ways of interrupting the process, thereby preventing the development of cancer. Estrogen therapy has never been shown to be an initiator, but it may serve as a promoter. Jick et al. (1979) reported that the majority of cases of endometrial cancer among estrogen users occurred in women who had taken the drug for at least 5 years. Further evaluation of the data showed that there was a dramatic drop in estrogen use following the initial reports of an association between this drug and endometrial carcinoma in 1975. Six months after discontinuing estrogen therapy, there was an equally dramatic drop in the incidence of endometrial carcinoma. These data suggest that the changes induced by long-term estrogen exposure and the development of endometrial cancer stop or regress shortly after the drug is discontinued. This serves to confirm the role of estrogen as a promoter rather than an initiator.

Iatrogenic Effect

Dunn and Bradbury (1967) and Pacheco and Kempers (1968) used the case control method in studying the relationship of estrogen to endometrial carcinoma. Their reports indicated that there was no increased risk for the development of endometrial cancer when estrogen replacement therapy was given. Following these reports, women were given estrogen freely, some for specific indications and others just as a routine measure.

In 1975, Smith and co-workers and Zeil and Finkle published reports showing a strong association between the incidence of endometrial carcinoma and the use of estrogen replacement therapy in the menopausal and postmenopausal women. Despite the fact that they conflicted with the earlier reports of Dunn and Bradbury and Pacheco and Kempers, both the public and government officials immediately overreacted before first conducting a critical review of the older case studies and the new reports. The news media condemned the medical profession and the pharmaceutical industry for not warning patients sooner about the dangers of estrogen therapy.

Within 2 weeks of the publication of these reports, the Food and Drug Administration's (FDA) Advisory Panel recommended packaged inserts to warn patients about the cancer risk. This warning is still present in the inserts and causes a great deal of concern to patients even when estrogen is prescribed as a vaginal cream. The reason for this warning must be explained to the patient so that she will accept treatment. Biostatisticians, who are the major authors of the studies at issue, exerted enormous influence on the outcome of the hearings. The lesson learned from these hearings may have indirectly set the stage for future clinical research without answering the question of estrogen and its relationship to cancer.

From reading the reports, it was obvious that the statistical analysis of clinical data has become so involved and cryptic that people who know what the statistics and results mean cannot articulate them and, conversely, that people who have the ability to communicate know little about what the statistics mean. Therefore, until recently, the picture has remained clouded.

Prospective Randomized Clinical Trial

How can this controversy be resolved? Technology may provide us with the tools to detect changes within a cell when a certain type of estrogen is given. However, this study belongs to the next decade. At present, a prospective, randomized clinical trial, in which postmenopausal women would be assigned to take or not take estrogen replacement therapy and to receive regular uterine aspiration tests would be the ideal method to determine whether estrogens cause endometrial cancer. This is impossible, however, since most women would not agree to participate in such an experiment. Even if they did agree, such a study would probably be unacceptable to the investigator(s), who would have to assemble some 20,000 women to achieve satisfactory statistical data, since the incidence of endometrial cancer is very low (the expected incidence of new cases for 1987 is 35,000). The project would take years of follow-up examinations and endometrial aspirations or biopsies. Thus, it becomes apparent that the ideal prospective, randomized clinical trial is not practical.

Longitudinal Cohort Study

In the absence of an experimental prospective, randomized trial, a longitudinal cohort study would be the next best way to answer this question. Postmenopausal women who have made their own decision to take or not take estrogens would be followed for a suitably long period of time. To determine the rate at which endometrial cancer develops in the two groups, the members of each group would routinely receive uterine aspirations for diagnostic study. This method has the same disadvantages as the prospective, randomized clinical trial.

Case Control Study

As a result of these difficulties, investigators have turned to an epidemiologic technique, the case control study. This type of research is inexpensive, quick, and easy to perform because it is conducted retrospectively. The investigator begins with a group of cases, that is, women who have already been proved to have endometrial carcinoma. The investigator then arbitrarily chooses a group of controls from among women who have not been shown to have the disease. The two groups are asked about their previous use of estrogen. From these quantitative data, the investigator calculates an *odds ratio.* If this ratio exceeds 1.00 and is statistically significant, the investigator concludes that estrogen use increases the risk of developing endometrial carcinoma. The current controversy rests on the willingness or unwillingness of investigators to accept conventional case control studies as a suitable substitute for clinical trials or longitudinal cohort studies. It is obvious that the important part of this project lies in the controls. Smith et al. (1975) chose patients treated for gynecologic cancer from the Tumor Registry as their controls. It is obvious that many of these patients may not have had a uterus or that the uterus might have been treated with radiation and was not capable of responding to the estrogen.

Alternative Analytic Method

Horwitz and Feinstein (1978) used the alternative analytic method for case control studies and came up with risk ratios far below those reported by Smith et al., Zeil and Finkle, Jick, et al., and others. Horwitz and Feinstein eliminated the community surveillance bias by taking every patient admitted with vaginal bleeding who had received a D&C and obtained their result from the cancers and controls from the same group of patients. Their findings were not dissimilar to those reported by Dunn and Bradbury and Pacheco and Kempers. It is accepted that estrogen has some association with endometrial cancer, but not to the degree reported by Smith et al. and Zeil and Finkle. It has been accepted that the relative risk is about 1.71 instead of the 4 to 10 reported in 1975.

It would seem that long-term unopposed estrogen therapy may produce cancer in patients with a genetic susceptibility to malignancy and has a proliferative effect on estrogen-responsive tumors. It is possible that many tumors that would never normally be diagnosed during a patient's lifetime will be revealed following stimulation with estrogen.

Risk Factors

The risk factors for endometrial carcinoma include a family tendency, race, endometrial hyperplasia, endometrial polyps, leiomyomas, fibroids, menstrual disturbances, metabolic disorders, and other diseases. Atypical adenomatous hyperplasia has been considered a precursor of endometrial carcinoma. Women who have had any of these problems should be kept under careful surveillance even into the geriatric period.

The increased risk of endometrial cancer may be due to a true mutagenic effect, although there is no evidence in humans or animals that the estrogens investigated so far are carcinogenic. Alternatively, this apparent increase may be due to a combination of the following factors: (1) growth of occult endometrial carcinoma, (2) lack of clinical supervision in the form of regular endometrial sampling, (3) use of continuous, often excessive, doses of estrogen, (4) misdiagnosis of hyperplasia of the endometrium, and (5) failure to use progestogens.

It is obvious that by carefully screening patients, it will be possible to identify occult endometrial carcinoma as well as the precursors that may be present. If the precursors are present, estrogen therapy should be stopped so that abnormal cells are not stimulated to progress to frank carcinoma. This is based upon the premise that estrogen is a promoter and not an initiator.

Armed with this data, the physician should be able to give estrogens to the patients who need it. The patient's quality of life is an important consideration in making the decision to use estrogen. Millions of women today are taking estrogen because it gives them relief from many of the symptoms of menopause. It may also arrest osteoporosis or prevent it from forming. There are more than 200,000 hip fractures among postmenopausal patients, with 20,000 deaths, whereas for 1987 there are an estimated 35,000 new cases of carcinoma of the endometrium and only 2900 deaths.

ROLE OF PROGESTERONE

In women in the postmenopausal and geriatric age groups who are using estrogen replacement therapy, it is important to add progesterone. Although Hammond was one of the first to show its protective benefits in a series of cases, Sturdee and his co-workers (1978) expanded on this observation. They showed that there is a protective effect of added progestogens, and that it is the duration rather than the dose of progestogen that is important. They reported that 5 or 7 days of progestogen therapy significantly reduced the incidence of cystic and adenomatous hyperplasia but that 13 days of a small or daily and total dose of progestogens was associated with a 0 percent incidence of hyperplasia, regardless of whether the estrogen was administered orally or by an implant. A practical problem with adding progestogen therapy is that approximately 20 percent of the patients develop symptoms of breast discomfort, nausea, irritability, and water retention, as well as vaginal spotting. These complaints can be reduced by altering the dose of estrogen, and many of the symptoms respond to a mild diuretic.

There is evidence that progestogens promote the formation of intracellular 17-beta-hydroxygenase, which reduces endometrial cell exposure to 17-beta-estradiol. It has been suggested that women at high risk for endometrial carcinoma have a high proportion of estrone precursors, but recent work shows that the estrone is converted in the cell into 17-beta-estradiol. Recent studies have shown that progesterone is capable of diminishing estrogen receptors in endometrial carcinoma patients. Therefore, for women taking estrogen, progesterone should be administered at least once a month or every other month for 10 to 14 days.

Although oral contraceptives are not appropriate for treatment in the postmenopausal and geriatric patient, their relationship to endometrial cancer provides material for making a clinical judgment on the use of estrogen replacement therapy. This relationship has been reported in the literature. However, 82 percent of these patients used Oracon, which contained a very high daily dose of ethinyl estradiol—100 mg—which is 10 times the dose used in the treatment of postmenopausal women, and a weak progestogen, dimethisterone—25 mg daily for 10 days. The question of whether Oracon actually produced endometrial cancer or simply removed an assumed protection given by combined estrogen-progesterone therapy has been solved in an excellent study by Weiss and Sayvetz (1980). The study demonstrated that women taking Oracon had a risk of endometrial carcinoma 7.3 times that of other women and that the users of combined oral contraceptives had only 50 percent of the incidence of endometrial carcinoma of nonusers. Hence the study was a convincing demonstration of both the dangers of excess estrogen stimulation and the protective properties of a balanced daily estrogen-progestogen preparation. Therefore, it serves to provide guidelines for the use of estrogen-progestogen in the postmenopausal and geriatric patient.

It is obvious that in selected patients estrogen replacement not only has a therapeutic value but also adds to the quality of life. It is the responsibility of the clinician to identify those women who need estrogen therapy and those who should avoid it or who will not be helped by it. There are dedicated clinicians and scientists who are able to negate the sensationalism cleverly presented by the media and the entrepreneurs in the medical profession. It is to be reemphasized that women now live one-third of their lives in an estrogen-depleted state and that estrogen is a medicine that should be given as needed.

There has clearly been an overall increased risk in giving straight estrogen therapy, as practiced during the last 40 years. Currently, the task is to quantify the protective effect of different types of progestogen and to clarify the therapeutic dose and duration required for this purpose. The answers will come from current long-term prospective studies supported by evidence from scanning electron microscopic work and receptor site studies.

Since the 1975 reports alleging the increased risk of endometrial cancer for postmenopausal women taking estrogen replacement therapy, there have been many contradictory reports. Several recent studies have commented on the relationship of both endogenous and exogenous hyperestrogenism to the prognosis. Many reports have confirmed that endometrial carcinoma patients who are estrogen users had a better prognosis than those who had not used estrogen. Although the tumors of estrogen users tended to be of a more favorable histologic type and grade than those of nonusers, some reports indicate that the favorable prognosis was independent of these tumor-related factors. Subsequent studies continue to show increased survival among estrogen users, suggesting that the risk benefit ratio for postmenopausal estrogen usage may well swing back to the benefit side.

PROGESTERONE CHALLENGE TEST

The work of Gambrell has made a significant contribution to solving this problem. Gambrell has reported that not all postmenopausal women need estrogen replacement therapy, since some produce sufficient endogenous estrogen to avoid the symptoms to prevent the metabolic changes of later life. During the reproductive years, estradiol secretion by the ovaries is the major source of estrogen production. In addition, both the ovaries and the adrenal glands secrete androstenedione, which is then converted to estrone. When ovarian estradiol secretion diminishes at menopause, and particularly with a surgical menopause, the principal source of estrogens is the peripheral conversion of adrenal androstenedione to estrone.

There are two factors that can increase or maintain endogenous estrogen production after the menopause: (1) increased production rates of androstenedione and (2) increased peripheral conversion of this hormone to estrone. Although the amount of androstenedione produced by normal

213

postmenopausal women is only one-half that of premenopausal women, the percentage conversion of androstenedione to estrone is increased one and a half times over that of the premenopausal subjects. The amount of androstenedione converted to estrone is further increased by aging, obesity, liver disease, hyperthyroidism, compensated congestive heart failure, postoperative convalescence, and starvation. This also explains why some postmenopausal women remain asymptomatic and do not have the metabolic changes of later life such as osteoporosis and atrophic vaginitis.

Within a group of the climacteric, women who are asymptomatic because they are producing sufficient endogenous estrogens may be those at greatest risk for endometrial cancer. This has been confirmed by various reports, since the second highest incidence of endometrial cancer has consistently been found in untreated women. Most of these postmenopausal women were not prescribed estrogen therapy because they were symptom free, and many had evidence of a good estrogen effect on vaginal hormonal cytology. Many were obese and/or nulliparous, but not all had demonstrable predisposing factors. These postmenopausal women produced very little, if any, progesterone. They need to be identified and treated with a progestogen to prevent adenocarcinoma of the endometrium.

Many tests can be performed to identify those postmenopausal women at greatest risk for developing adenocarcinoma of the endometrium. These tests include vaginal hormonal cytology, endometrial biopsy, serum gonadotropins, and serum or urinary estrogen levels. However, the progestogen challenge test is the most reliable test to determine if estrogens, either endogenous or exogenous, are present in sufficient quantity to stimulate growth in the endometrium. All postmenopausal women with an intact uterus should be given a trial of progestogen to see if withdrawal bleeding follows. The progestogen should be continued for 13 days each month for as long as withdrawal bleeding occurs. This includes both estrogen-treated women and those with sufficient endogenous estrogens who do not need estrogen replacement therapy. The progestogen challenge test has been devised to identify postmenopausal women at greatest risk for endometrial cancer. Employment of this test in untreated postmenopausal women has identified many who are at increased risk for adenocarcinoma of the endometrium. It is concluded that the use of this test and the continued use of progestogens in climacteric women who respond with withdrawal bleeding will reduce the risk of endometrial cancer in both estrogen-treated postmenopausal women and those with increased endogenous estrogens. This is a most important point. It is the height of professional integrity to administer estrogen therapy when it is needed and to withhold it if it is not needed or if there is a contraindication to its use.

FACTS ABOUT ESTROGEN REPLACEMENT THERAPY: APPROXIMATE RATE OF DEVELOPMENT OF CANCER OF THE ENDOMETRIUM

Gambrell has reported that women not using estrogen replacement therapy, 2 in 1000 will develop carcinoma of the endometrium; of those using estrogen replacement therapy without progestogen, 4 in 1000; and of those who use estrogen replacement therapy with progestogen, 0.7 in 1000. Progesterone produces a turnaround effect on cancer of the endometrium.

SUMMARY

Over the last three decades, the history of estrogen therapy for the climacteric syndrome has been noted for excessive claims of benefits followed by profound fears of possible side effects. This situation has been influenced as much by journalism as by good scientific studies. However, it is accepted that there is a casual link between exogenous estrogen therapy and endometrial cancer. This link was greatly exaggerated in early reports.

The quality of life is almost as important as the quantity of life. Since women live one-third of their lives in an estrogen-depleted state, estrogen should be given when indicated and when there is no contraindication. The work of Studd, Sturdee, Gambrell, and Hammond has shown that progestogens protect against the development of carcinoma of the endometrium in patients given estrogen replacement therapy. The use of a progestogen that is not metabolized to an androgen even provides protection against cardiovascular accidents. Thus progestogen increases the level of HDL and protects against cardiovascular changes.

Since not only the perimenopausal woman but also the geriatric woman is engaging in intercourse, an estrogenic vaginal cream should be prescribed. Patients should be taught to rub the cream around the introitus, particularly along the posterior and lateral walls and just inside the vagina. This will improve the vaginal mucosa, and bring it to a normal state, and cut down on some of the dyspareunia that may be associated with intercourse.

The use of estrogen and progesterone also adds protection against the development of osteoporosis. Although it will not cure established osteoporosis, it can prevent further progress of the disease. Elderly women are very prone to develop so-called cystitis. In reality this is a distal urethritis. It can be corrected by taking oral estrogen or by using an estrogen cream locally around the urethra and the introitus.

The progestogen challenge test has been devised to identify postmenopausal women at greatest risk for endometrial cancer. It has been reported that the use of this test and the continued use of progestogens in climacteric women who respond with withdrawal bleeding will reduce the risk of endometrial cancer in both estrogen-treated postmenopausal women and those with increased endogenous estrogens.

The proliferative effect of estrogen, whether it be estrone, estradiol, synthetic oral therapy, or an implant or patch, may damage the endometrium and lead to malignancy in susceptible patients. This danger may be prevented by added progestogen. There is a reduced incidence of carcinoma of the endometrium in women treated with estrogen-progesterone than in a control group. The combination of estrogen-progesterone therapy will provide a maximum benefit and a minimal risk. Estrogen-progesterone therapy should be given to the patient when indicated and age per se is not a contraindication.

REFERENCES

Dunn, I. J., and J. T. Bradbury. 1967. Endocrine factors in endometrial carcinoma. A preliminary report. *Am. J. Obstet. Gynecol.* 97:465.

Chang, R. J., H. L. Judd, and R. Horton. 1981. The ovary after menopause. *Clin. Obstet. Gynecol.* 24:181.

Gambrell, R. D., Jr. 1974. Perimenopausal and postmenopausal bleeding: Mechanism, pathology, management with progestational agents, in: *The Menopausal Syndrome.* (R. B. Greeblatt, V. B. Mahesh, and P. G. McDonough, eds.). Medcom Press, St. Louis, pp. 147–156.

———. 1977. Postmenopausal bleeding. *Clin. Obstet. Gynecol.* 4:129.

———. 1978. The prevention of endometrial cancer in postmenopausal women with progestogens. *Maturitas* 1:107.

———. 1980. Use of the progestogen challenge test to reduce the risk of endometrial cancer. *Obstet. Gynecol.* 55:732.

———. 1982. The menopause: Benefits and risks of estrogen-progestogen replacement therapy. *Fertil. Steril.* 37:457.

———. 1982. Clinical use of progestins in the menopausal patient: Dosage and duration. *J. Reprod. Med.* 27:531.

Gambrell, R. D. Jr., R. M. Massey, T. A. Castaneda, et al. 1979. Reduced incidence of endometrial cancer among postmenopausal women treated with progestogens. *J. Am. Geriatric Soc.* 27:389.

Hammond; C. B., F. R. Jelovsek, K. L. Lee, W. T. Greasman, and R. T. Parker. 1979. Effects of long-term estrogen replacement therapy. I. Metabolic effects. *Am. J. Obstet. Gynecol.* 133:525.

———. 1979. Methodologic standards and contradictory results in case-control research. *Am. J. Med.* 66:556.

Horwitz, R. I., and A. R. Feinstein. 1978. Alternative analytic methods for case-control studies of estrogens and endometrial cancer. *N. Engl. J. Med.* 299:1089.

Jick, H., et al. 1979. Replacement estrogens and endometrial cancer. *N. Engl. J. Med.* 300:218.

Lindsay, R., D. M. Hart, and D. M. Clark. 1984. The minimum effective dose of estrogen for prevention of postmenopausal bone loss. *Obstet. Gynecol.* 63:759.

Pacheco, J. C., and R. D. Kempers. 1968. Etiology of postmenopausal bleeding. *Obstet. Gynecol.* 32:40.

Silverberg, S. G. 1984. New aspects of endometrial carcinoma. *Clin. Obstet. Gynecol.* 11(1):189.

Silverberg, S. G., and E. L. Makowski. 1980. Endometrial carcinoma in young women taking oral contraceptive agents. *Obstet. Gynecol.* 55:732.

Smith, D. C., et al. 1975. Association of exogenous estrogen and endometrial carcinoma. *N. Engl. J. Med.* 293:1164.

Studd, J. 1976. Oestrogens as a cause of endometrial carcinoma. *Br. Med. J.* 1:1276.

———. 1981. Oestrogens and endometrial cancer, in: *Progress in Obstetrics and Gynecology,* Vol. 1. (J. Studd, ed.). Churchill Livingstone, Edinburgh, chap. 14.

Studd, J., and M. H. Thom. 1979. Oestrogen use and endometrial cancer. *N. Engl. J. Med.* 100:922.

Studd, J., M. R. Thom, M. Paterson, and T. Wade-Evans. 1980. *The prevention and treatment of endometrial pathology in Postmenopausal Women Receiving Oestrogens.* MTP Press, Longdon, pp. 127–139.

Sturdee, D. W., T. Wade-Evans, M. Paterson, M. H. Thom, and J. Studd. 1978. Relations between bleeding pattern, endometrial histology and oestrogen treatment in menopausal women. *Br. Med. J.* 1:1575.

Utain, W. H. 1980. *Menopause in Modern Perspective.* Appleton-Century-Crofts, New York.

Weiss, N. S. and T. A. Sayvetz. 1980. Incidence of endometrial cancer in relation to the use of oral contraceptives. *N. Engl. J. Med.* 302:551.

Ziel, H. K., and W. D. Finkle. 1975. Increased risk of endometrial carcinoma among users of conjugated estrogens. *N. Engl. J. Med.* 293:1167.

16 Urologic Changes and Problems in the Elderly

INTRODUCTION

Incontinence of urine is the involuntary loss of urine. The urine may escape continuously both by day and by night, or it may escape intermittently. The causes of each variety of incontinence need to be understood if treatment is to be successful. Incontinence is a most distressing and degrading disability, and failure of treatment is often the result of inadequate investigation.

There are four common types of urinary incontinence: (1) stress incontinence, (2) total incontinence, (3) urge incontinence, and (4) overflow incontinence.

OTHER URINARY DYSFUNCTIONS

Increased frequency of micturition is defined as the passage of urine seven or more times during the day and twice or more during the night. It may arise from any source of irritation, including infection, detrusor instability, tumor, and incomplete emptying. It is usually diurnal (during waking hours only), but in severe cases it will awaken the patient from sleep. In one survey, inappropriate leakage of urine in women between the ages of 35 and 64 occurred in 10 percent. It is more common after childbearing, but also occurs in the nulliparous woman who is more prone to detrusor instability than to genuine stress incontinence. The shortness of the female urethra may be a factor.

STRESS INCONTINENCE

When a sudden increase in intravesical pressure is caused by a contraction in the detrusor muscle or by an increase in intraabdominal pressure, such as by coughing or straining, the stimulus is usually applied to the intraabdominal urethra as well, and there is no leakage of urine. If urine does escape, the condition is called *stress incontinence.*

Genuine stress incontinence is the involuntary leakage of urine occurring in the absence of a detrusor contraction. This leakage is attributed to some displacement of the bladder neck so that it cannot respond normally to a sudden increase in intraabdominal pressure. The cause is likely to be a pelvic floor weakness as a result of parturition, prolapse, aging, or a combination of all three. Detrusor instability is defined as a contraction exceeding 15 cm of water in pressure, occurring during filling of the bladder or when standing erect or coughing and straining. It may also cause involuntary incontinence, but the mechanism is altogether different from that of genuine stress incontinence. Both of these causes of involuntary or stress incontinence can exist together, making diagnosis difficult.

The open Allis clamp at the urethro-vesical junction elevates the junction, and when the patient is asked to cough, there is no loss of urine. Other tests that may be performed are the cotton tip applicator test, urethrocystoscopy, cystometrography, urethral pressure measurements, voiding cystourethrography, and B chain cystourethrography.

URGE INCONTINENCE

Urge incontinence is defined as a desire to void urine before the bladder contains 50 mL of urine. True urgency occurs in the absence of detrusor contraction and is often associated with infection. Severe urgency leads to urge incontinence. Dysuria, pain associated with micturition, indicates infection of the bladder and urethra or of the vulvar and perineal epithelium, which is irritated by the dribbling of urine.

Urge incontinence refers to the inability to hold urine long enough to reach a toilet. It is often associated with conditions such as stroke, senile dementia, Parkinson's disease, and multiple sclerosis, but it can also occur in otherwise normal elderly persons. Many older people with normal urinary control have difficulty reaching a toilet in time because of arthritis or other crippling disorders. A person who is not always able to reach a toilet in time to avoid wetting should not be considered incontinent. Instead, every effort should be made to make it easier to reach the toilet. Urinary tract infection is a common cause of urge incontinence and must always be ruled out.

The patient experiences an irresistible desire to micturate. Detrusor muscle instability is the most common cause, but the condition may also be due to inflammatory disease of the bladder without detrusor contraction. All forms of bladder pathology must be considered, including calculus and carcinoma. There is usually an associated complaint of frequency.

OVERFLOW INCONTINENCE

Overflow incontinence describes the leakage of small amounts of urine from a constantly filled bladder. A common cause in older men is blockage of urine outflow from the bladder by an enlarged prostate. Another cause is loss of normal contraction of the bladder in some people with diabetes. The patient may not feel any urge to urinate. Finally, overflow incontinence may be associated with deterioration of the nervous system, drug therapy, or emotional factors. Neither stress nor the patient's usual ability to control the bladder plays a part.

Sudden urine retention is rare in women except after pelvic floor operations. Spasmodic detrusor contractions force a little urine into the urethra, and the overdistended muscle takes several days to regain its tone. When obstruction to overflow occurs gradually, as from pressure by a pelvic tumor or an incarcerated gravid uterus, the detrusor has time to hypertrophy and for a time forces urine out. Eventually, however, the bladder becomes atonic and painless, and urine dribbles out only when the intraabdominal pressure is raised.

NEUROLOGIC DISEASE

Failure of detrusor inhibition is the most common symptom and is the cause of senile incontinence. It is also a symptom, although not usually the presenting one, of multiple sclerosis. Full sensation is present, but the incontinence is of the urge type and cannot be resisted. Failure of bladder sensation is a result of diseases that interrupt the posterior column of the cord, such as tabes, syringomyelia, and occasionally multiple sclerosis. Chronic overdistention leads to an atonic bladder and overflow incontinence. Infection is a common complication.

NORMAL CONTROL OF MICTURITION

Embryologically, anatomically, and functionally, the lower urinary tract and the female genital tract are intimately related. The clinical problems in female patients primarily concern the bladder neck and the urethra. The use of effective endoscopic procedures by gynecologists to view the urethra and bladder neck puts them in a very good position in the management of urinary incontinence in women, a position that is strengthened by their familiarity with the medical and surgical management of other problems in the region.

The mechanisms responsible for urinary incontinence in the female are still not completely understood. Three factors will be considered: (1)

muscular control, (2) external pressure on the urethra, and (3) reflex control.

Physiology of Micturition

The involuntary voiding of small amounts of urine is very common in women. It is known, perhaps wrongly, as stress incontinence, and its treatment calls for an understanding of bladder and urethral physiology.

The bladder is capable of adapting to an increased urinary volume. Pressure remains below 10 cm water until over 500 ml of urine is contained.

Urethral pressure is maintained by the internal sphincter, which is made up of longitudinal and circular plain muscle and elastic tissue, and an external sphincter, which contributes striated muscle. A urethral pressure profile shows the changes and pressure along the length of the urethra. This is normally much greater than the intravesical pressure, thus ensuring continence.

The innervation of the bladder and urethra is outlined to clarify the reader's understanding of the physiology of micturition. There is an intercommunicating sympathetic, parasympathetic, and somatic supply. The parasympathetic nerves stimulate detrusor contraction, and the sympathetic fibers (chiefly through the alpha receptors) stimulate contraction of the bladder neck and urethra. There is thus some degree of reciprocal activity, but the precise function of each type of nerve and the exact control of the mechanism of the bladder neck opening are not yet known.

The striated muscle has been shown to have a dual autonomic/somatic supply via the pelvic plexus, and the long-held concept of pudendal innervation is now being questioned. For a normal urethral closure, all the components of the sphincter mechanism must function together, and the striated muscle has more to do than merely contract voluntarily when the desire to micturate must be resisted.

Mechanism of Voiding. Cystometry recording demonstrates the timing of events. These include (1) intraabdominal pressure increase (measured per rectum), (2) detrusor contractions (intravesicle pressure increase), (3) sphincter relaxation (electromyogram of anal sphincter) and the start of urine flow.

The urethra and the bladder neck are maintained in the closed state by the trigonal condensation of muscle (the base plate) and the urethral sphincter (plain and striated muscle). When cortical inhibition is withdrawn, the detrusor contracts and the bladder and neck relax (funneling). The sphincter also relaxes and the urine is voided. As the flow continues, the bladder neck moves downward and backward and the urethrovesical angle is obliterated.

Bladder. The bladder is a hollow, muscular organ lined with mucous membrane. The muscle wall is composed of a rich framework of plain muscle fibers. The submucosa is very loose. This looseness causes the mucous membrane of the greater part of the contracted organ to be thrown into a series of folds, giving it a trabeculated appearance. The bladder varies in size, is smaller in the female than in the male, and is capable of undergoing considerable distention. When empty, it lies immediately in front of the uterus and vagina and behind the bodies of the pubis. As it fills, it rises above the pelvic brim into the abdominal cavity between the fascia transversalis and the peritoneum.

The full capacity of the bladder is, on average, about 450 mL, and the average normal voiding is about 300 mL. It is possible to distend the bladder gradually to a capacity of 3 to 4 L without rupture. It has been shown that an intravesical pressure greater than 10 mm Hg results in the desire to micturate. Emptying of the bladder is accomplished by a sudden strong contraction of the whole detrusor muscle (the musculature of the lateral walls and dome), which creates an intravesical pressure of 40 mm Hg or more. This pressure is maintained throughout the act of micturition.

The lateral wall chiefly consists of interlacing smooth muscle fibers of the involuntary detrusor muscle. Inferiorly there are two horseshoe-shaped concentrations of smooth muscle that surround the vesicourethral junction. They are continuous with the intrinsic muscle fibers of the urethra and act as an internal sphincter. When the detrusor muscle actively contracts, these sling-like bands of muscle relax, allowing the bladder neck to widen into a funnel shape so that urine flows into the urethra. Therefore, the bladder detrusor is a smooth muscle appearing as a meshwork of fibers that are recognizable only at the bladder outlet as three distinct layers—the outer longitudinal, the middle circular, and the inner longitudinal.

The internal sphincter is supported by striped muscle fibers from the medial edge of the pubococcygeus part of the levator ani, which also forms a sling around the bladder neck posteriorly. Below this, between the two layers of the urogenital diaphragm (triangular ligament), is the deep transverse perineal muscle (compressor urethra), which can compress the urethra strongly at that level. Contractions of these voluntary muscles of the pelvic floor can prevent the escape of urine; even if micturition is in progress, a normal woman can stop the stream voluntarily by activating them, and since the pelvic floor muscles contract reflexively during coughing, they will also prevent any escape of urine from the rise of intraabdominal pressure on coughing.

Urethra

The female urethra extends from the neck of the bladder to the external orifice. Its length ranges from 3 to 5.5 cm, with an average of 4.1 cm. A feature of the adult female urethra is the ease with which it can be dilated, sometimes to a diameter of 10 mm. The mucous membrane of the meatus, which is the narrowest part of the canal, may, however, split before such a limit is reached. The female urethra is lined approximately with transitional epithelium and distally with stratified squamous epithelium. It is surrounded mainly by smooth muscle. The striated muscle urethral sphincter, which surrounds the middle third of the urethra, contributes about 50 percent of the total urethral resistance and serves as a secondary defense against incontinence. It is also responsible for the interruption of urine flow at the end of micturition.

The upper half of the urethra is separated from the anterior vaginal wall by connective tissue, but the lower half is actually adherent to the musculature of the vaginal wall. The urethra pierces both layers of the urogenital diaphragm where it is surrounded by the sphincter urethra membranacea. The urethra is surrounded by a number of rudimentary glands of the compound racemose variety. These glands open into the paraurethral ducts of Skene, which descend in the wall of the urethra and open into its interior near its termination. They are liable to become the sites of a gynecoccal infection that can be extremely troublesome. The glands are believed to be homologues of the prostate gland.

The two posterior pubourethral ligaments provide a strong suspensory mechanism for the urethra and serve to hold it forward in close proximity to the pubis under conditions of stress. They extend from the lower part of the pubic bone to the urethra at the junction of the middle and distal thirds.

The external urethral orifice opens into the vestibule and has an everted edge that sometimes forms two or three overhanging lips, which may make it difficult to locate. It can be traced by separating the labia minora and is found an inch below and behind the clitoris.

There is a feeling that continence is also assisted by external pressure on the intraabdominal part of the urethra (above the urogenital diaphragm) that is equal to the pressure on the fundus of the bladder. It is suggested that if the pelvic floor muscles are relaxed, or if there is prolapse of the bladder neck as a result of trauma during delivery, any increase in intraabdominal pressure will act on the bladder alone, so that urine will escape into the urethra.

Innervation: Reflex Control

Afferent impulses pass from the bladder to the cord, where there is a reflex center, but micturition is a reflex act only in the infant. Later this reflex center becomes controlled by the higher centers in the brain stem. Micturition has, therefore, been aptly and neatly described as a release of lower reflex centers from higher inhibition.

The bladder has a sympathetic supply from the hypogastric nerves and a parasympathetic supply from the nervi erigentes, while part of the external sphincter is supplied by pudendal nerves. When the bladder fills with urine, it accommodates the increasing volume with a gradual rise in intravesical pressure, until the sensory stretch receptors are stimulated to trigger detrusor contraction and relaxation of the internal sphincter. The sympathetic and parasympathetic controls are delicately balanced, there being a reciprocal arrangement of adrenergic alpha and beta receptors in the fundus and bladder-neck regions, which act so that when one area contracts the other relaxes, and vice versa. If it is inconvenient to micturate, this reflex mechanism can normally be overriden by voluntary cortical control, so that the desire to micturate caused by increased intravesical pressure and detrusor contraction can be suppressed by active contraction of the pelvic floor muscles. Continence therefore depends on multiple factors, requiring both an intact urethral closure mechanism and normal reflex action.

A great deal of attention has been directed to the innervation of the urinary tract. It has been shown that the urinary tract is under the control of both parasympathetic and sympathetic fibers. The parasympathetic fibers originate in the sacral spinal canal segments S2–3 through S4. Stimulation of the pelvic parasympathetic nerves and administration of cholangeric drugs cause the detrusor muscle to contract. Anticholangeric drugs reduce vesical pressure and increase bladder capacity.

The sympathetic fibers originate from thoracolumbar segments (T10–L2) of the spinal cord. The sympathetic system consists of alpha- and beta-adrenergic components. The beta fibers terminate primarily in the detrusor muscle, while the alpha fibers terminate principally in the urethra. Alpha-adrenergic stimulation contracts the bladder neck and urethra and relaxes the detrusor. Beta-adrenergic stimulation relaxes the urethra and the detrusor muscle. The pudendal nerve (S2–4) provides motor innervation to the striated urethral sphincter.

When the sympathetic nerves are sectioned, the internal sphincter remains closed. Bladder pain is diminished but not entirely abolished when the presacral nerve is cut, and these afferent fibers in the sympathetic reach the spinal cord at least as high as the ninth thoracic segment and probably as low as the fourth lumbar segment. Within a few days of sympathetic neurectomy, the control of micturition returns to normal; therefore, the sympathetic nerves are not essential for the act of micturition. Bilateral neurectomy of pudendal nerves in the female has no effect on bladder control. When the sympathetic nerves are cut, the patient is unable to pass urine voluntarily and the musculature of the bladder becomes paralyzed. It has been concluded that the parasympathetic contains fibers that convey messages to the higher centers regarding the degree of distention of the bladder and that some pain fibers travel by this route. It has been stated that the parasympathetic alone is necessary for the act of micturition.

DIAGNOSIS

The first and most important step in treating incontinence is to obtain a detailed history of the patient's health and related problems, as well as a physical examination that focuses on the urinary and nervous systems and reproductive organs. The physician must initially do an analysis of urine samples.

The best method of assessing patients with incontinence is by simultaneous radiologic cystourethrography and measurement of the intravesical pressure in urine flow, which gives a video cystogram. A rectal catheter is used to record the intraperitoneal pressure. Another catheter in the bladder records the total bladder pressure, and subtraction of the intraperitoneal pressure gives the intrinsic bladder pressure. While the bladder is being filled with contrast medium and during voiding, the intrinsic bladder pressure and flow rate are recorded, while a camera simultaneously observes the radiologic changes in the bladder and urethra. The apparatus is expensive, and interpretation of the results requires experience. However, special centers have been set up to study bladder function, and it is important to refer them for evaluation. This will prevent many unsuccessful operations.

Investigation of Incontinence

It is necessary to distinguish between urethral and bladder dysfunction, since their treatment is different. This cannot be done with certainty on the basis of the history and clinical examination alone. Stress incontinence may be due to bladder neck incompetence (genuine stress incontinence). There is a gradual onset after one or more pregnancies. Urine appears only after effort (stress) such as coughing, laughing, running, or jumping. Small quantities of urine are passed, whether the bladder is full or not. Another type of stress incontinence is due to detrusor instability. There is a history of a weak bladder even before pregnancies, if any. There is also a history of enuresis, especially in childhood. The patient complains of urge incontinence and frequency, especially at night (nocturia).

Stress incontinence combined with urge incontinence due to bladder infection or a cystocele is quite common. Continuous incontinence suggests a fistula. The degree of severity is indicated by the extent to which the patient feels socially restricted.

Tests of Bladder Function and Urodynamic Investigation of Bladder Function

In most instances, it is not necessary to subject the elderly patient to an extensive workup. However, if there is a question about the cause of bladder dysfunction, it is important to make an accurate diagnosis.

The Nappy is a pad containing aluminum electrodes and impregnated with a dry electrolyte that dissolves in any urine that may be passed. It is energized by low-voltage current, and the capacitance is shown on a dial calibrated in milliliters of urine. The Nappy is applied to the vulva inside tight-fitting pants, and the patient than makes movements such as bending, coughing, and straining, which she states to be the cause of stress incontinence. This system is useful in making an objective measurement of the amount of urine lost, especially in those patients in whom no incontinence can be demonstrated.

Cystometry

Urodynamics is an investigation of bladder movement and tension during different levels of filling. It involves the movement of bladder activity (cystometry) and urethral flow (uroflowmetry). This apparatus is expensive. Cystometry measures bladder pressures; they are continuously recorded as the bladder is filled. Single-channel cystometry does not record intraabdominal pressure. Twin-channel cystometry is designed so that the rectal pressure that represents intraabdominal pressure is simultaneously recorded by a transducer in the rectum. Electronic circuitry subtracts one channel from the other, thus recording the true intravesical pressure. Modern urodynamic apparatus also measures detrusor pressure and urethral activity.

Videocystourethrography (VCU)

This complicated technique demonstrates bladder neck activity by means of cineradiography and, at the same time, measures changes in intravesical pressure. It gives the most reliable evidence of the presence or absence of detrusor instability, but it is costly and should not be used for routine screening. The VCU is carried out as follows: the bladder is filled with contrast medium and is seen on a screen. Bladder neck incontinence is diagnosed by the presence of an open bladder neck at rest or on coughing.

Two electrodes in the bladder and rectum record the required pressures. A flowmeter records the rate at which urine is voided.

This test should be carried out in the elderly only after very careful consideration because there is a 2 percent risk of infection. However, it is justified in the presence of the following conditions: (1) continuing difficulty in distinguishing genuine stress incontinence from detrusor instability, (2) after the failure of surgery to relieve a complaint of incontinence, (3) where there are other complicating factors such as neurologic disease, or (4) where difficulty in voiding is complained of or is suspected. The last condition may occur after pelvic surgery and may lead to incomplete emptying and perhaps retention overflow.

Other Investigations

Bacteria culture of the urine must be carried out in every case. The possibility of neurologic disease must be eliminated. This may be present, and the gynecologist should test for reflexes in the usual manner. The integrity of the sacral reflexes is demonstrated by contraction of the anal sphincter in response to a perineal skin prick. Where there is doubt, the patient must be referred to a neurologist. Endocrine disease such as diabetes mellitus and insipidus may be present and may be accompanied by urinary frequency. Therefore, hormonal assays may be required. X-ray urethrocystography may be undertaken independently of urodynamic investigations. In these studies, the bladder is filled with contrast medium and radiographs are taken at rest, during straining, and during micturating. This investigation can be carried out with normal x-ray facilities, but it does not distinguish between sphincter weakness and detrusor instability. The relationship between incontinence and urethrovesical angles, as shown by this technique, is unpredictable. In the normal resting x-ray there is a well-formed urethrovesical angle, and on normal micturition there is funneling, downward displacement, and flattening of the angle.

MANAGEMENT

General

The treatment of urinary incontinence should be tailored to each patient's needs. A number of medications can be used. However, these drugs may cause such side effects as dry mouth, eye problems, and a buildup of urine; therefore, they must be used carefully under a physician's supervision.

Biofeedback. *Behavior therapy* is a term that is about 15 years old; however, its methods have been used for a much longer period. It is an attempt to change human behavior in a beneficial way, using the laws of modern learning theory (for example, the principles of conditioning). *Biofeedback* refers to a term and a technique that is less than 10 years old. It is the process by which data obtained from a specific body function are given back to the subject through visual or auditory displays. It is currently receiving a great deal of attention.

Certain behavioral management techniques, including biofeedback and *bladder retraining,* have proven helpful in the control of urination. These can help the person sense bladder filling and delay voiding until he or she can reach a toilet.

Behavioral therapy (biofeedback) in the treatment of medical problems has been used for a long time—for example, in the treatment of obesity and excessive smoking. In behavioral therapy, a specific problem that may involve several bodily functions is treated. Biofeedback is a kind of behavior therapy in which one specific bodily function is treated. It has been used to control heart rate and lower high blood pressure. However, most of the studies on the applications of biofeedback to medicine are still at the laboratory stage. Two applications of significance in treating medical problems of the elderly are now practical and have been successfully used. In the first, patients with neurologic disorders caused by stroke have been rehabilitated through the use of biofeedback. A second application of biofeedback is in treating incontinence; it has been quite successful. A significant number of older people are probably put into nursing homes not because they are incompetent, but because they are incontinent. Although urinary incontinence is more common, fecal incontinence is a significant problem and is very debilitating socially. Biofeedback has added another dimension to the treatment of incontinence.

Other Methods. Exercises can be used to strengthen the muscles that help close the bladder outlet.

Several types of surgery can improve or even cure incontinence that is related to a structural problem such as an abnormally positioned bladder or blockage due to an enlarged prostate.

Artificial devices that replace or aid the muscles that control urinary flow have been tried in the management of incontinence. Many of these prosthetic devices require surgical implantation.

Sometimes incontinence is treated by inserting a flexible catheter into the urethra and collecting the urine in a container. However, long-term catheterization, although sometimes necessary, creates many problems, including urinary infection.

Specially designed absorbent underclothing is available. Many of these garments are no bulkier than normal underwear, can be worn easily under everyday clothing, and free the person from the discomfort and embarrassment of incontinence.

It must be emphasized that incontinence can be treated and often cured. Further, even incurable problems can be managed to reduce complications, anxiety, and family stress.

Stress Incontinence Management

In patients with a mild degress of stress incontinence, perineal exercises such as those suggested by Kegel (1956) often relieve the symptoms. The patient is instructed to tighten her anal sphincter as if to stop a bowel movement or the passage of gas. The patient is told to keep the sphincter tight for a count of five and then relax. The next exercise is to tighten her urinary and vaginal muscles as if to stop the flow of urine. The patient is told to keep the muscles tight for a count of five and then relax. These exercises should be carried out approximately four times a day for 2 minutes at a time. It takes approximately 6 to 8 weeks before improvement is noted.

Drug Therapy. A variety of drugs have been tried for stress incontinence. This form of incontinence is quite likely to be due in part to functional causes; if so, the drug therapy will have a beneficial effect. Two of these drugs are the muscle relaxants propanithelene bromide (Pro-Banthine) and flavoxate HCL (Urispas). When given in therapeutic doses, they can induce an atropine-like effect. However, although widely used, they are unsuccessful except in the mildest cases. It is important to make sure that the patient does not have glaucoma when using these drugs. Another group of drugs are the beta-adrenergic stimulators and vasodilators, including Didenyline, metaprotenenol (Alupent), and ritordine hydrochloride (Yutopar). These sympathomimetic drugs tend to cause tachycardia when used in large doses, enough to inhibit detrusor contractions. It is particularly important to monitor these drugs carefully if the patient has any type of or tendency toward cardiac arrhythmias. Calcium antagonists such as Flunarizine may also be helpful in treating incontinence. These drugs inhibit calcium influx in smooth muscles. Prostaglandin synthetase inhibitors, such as Endocin or Flurbiprofen often have a favorable effect in controlling or eliminating incontinence. Although these drugs are successful in many cases, their dosage is limited by their tendency to cause nausea and gastric symptoms. Another group of drugs that have some effect are the tricyclic antidepressants such as imipramine (Tofranil). This drug is principally used for its antidepressant properties; it tends to cause hypotension and atropine-like side effects (blurring of vision, dryness of the mouth, and constipation). Although these drugs may be helpful, none of them are specific and predictable in their action.

Surgical Management

Surgical procedures are divided into those that are done vaginally, abdominally, and by a combination of vaginal-abdominal approach. In cases of cystocele, the operation that is usually chosen is an anterior vaginal repair. It is important to tighten and draw together the tissues under the bladder neck. This cures a great number of cases.

When no cystocole is present, the Marshall-Marchetti-Krantz operation is most often selected as the treatment for these patients. In this operation, the prevesical space is approached by a suprapubic incision without opening the peritoneal cavity. Then the urethro-vesical junction is drawn upward and fixed with stitches to the fascia on the back of the pubic bone and abdominal wall. Burch modified this procedure by attaching the sutures to Cooper's ligament. This restores the normal intraabdominal position of the urethra.

An alternative but more difficult operation is to support the vesicourethral junction with a sling. The sling may be fashioned from external oblique aponeurosis when it is passed around the urethra from an abdominal approach, or fascia lata or nylon may be used and inserted from the vaginal aspect. The sling is arranged to pass under the urethra and is fixed above the rectus sheath.

The modified Pereyra procedure consists of suspension of the vesical neck, as in the retropubic procedures, but the operation is done primarily through the vagina. Nylon sutures are placed in the endopelvic fascia on either side of the urethra through a vaginal incision at the level of the bladder neck. The sutures are threaded through the space of Retzius with a special needle and are tied to the anterior rectus fascia through a small suprapubic incision. In the Syme's procedure, a 1-cm sleeve of 5-ml Dacron is threaded under the urethra at the bladder neck to provide additional support. These two operations are often accompanied by a long delay in spontaneous voiding.

Adjuvant measures are sometimes helpful. These include a strict diet for women who are overweight, instructions by physiotherapists, and pelvic floor exercise. It is also important to keep these patients on a urinary antiseptic for a period of time after the operation so that cystitis does not develop. After the menopause, the muscles of the pelvic floor are atonic and the submucosal venous plexus is less vascular; some benefit has been claimed for treatment with estrogens.

URETHRAL SYNDROME

Symptoms

The symptoms of the urethral syndrome include frequency, urgency, dysuria, incontinence, pelvic pressure, pain, discomfort, back pressure, hesitancy, weak stream, small voided amounts, feeling of incomplete emptying, malaise, and dyspareunia.

Complaints generally focus on the urinary tract (as opposed to the genital or musculoskeletal tract), and patients generally state that they were all right until the menopause.

Positive findings include infection (70 percent), involuntary bladder contractions (up to 28 percent), anatomic outlet obstruction (0 to 100 percent), functional outlet obstruction (dyssynergia) (up to 100 percent), interstitial cystitis, urethral instability, and emotional instability as contributing causes.

Urinary infection is strictly defined as being present only when 10 or more typical urinary pathogens are grown per milliliter of freshly voided midstream urine. It may be that the urethral syndrome is simply a condition caused by fewer than the usual number of organisms, or by organisms that cannot be cultured in the media used for conventional organisms. Clinically these patients must be regarded as suffering from a urinary tract infection, and an investigation must be done. Even if no evidence of an infection is obtained, some empirical treatment should be given.

Estrogen-dependent women often have an atrophic distal urethritis that results in a thickened, nondistensible distal urethra with partial bladder outlet obstruction. The condition is amenable to estrogen therapy or urethrotomy and, less frequently, to urethral dilatation. This mechanism may account for the urethral syndrome (recurring abacterial urethritis) that frequently plagues the postmenopausal patient.

The urethral syndrome occurs in a patient with various lower urinary tract symptoms in the absence of obvious bladder or urethral abnormality and with no evidence of urinary tract infection. The diagnosis is based on a detailed history and a physical examination, negative urine culture, dynamic cystourethroscopy, and urodynamic studies.

These patients are often difficult to manage. Serial urethrodilatation and urethral massage are the most commonly employed methods for treating chronic urethritis. The application of estrogen cream, particularly if it is rubbed into the urethra, especially at the external meatus, has a very good effect. Although these patients are probably overtreated with sulfa and antibiotic drugs, some do improve with the use of tetracyline administered for 14 days.

Urinary Tract Care

There are a variety of apparatuses designed for male incontinence. However, the female patient presents a different problem. The question is, how can she be protected from the embarrassment and discomfort of incontinence without resorting to catheterization?

If the patient experiences only intermittent dribbling incontinence, sanitary pads designed for menstrual flow may be adequate. To protect her against heavier urine flow, however, the physician should consider using a commercially made incontinent pant, for example, the Dignity Pant made by Humana Care International, Inc.

The Dignity Pant is made of a machine-washable polyester knit for the patient's comfort and convenience. It is available in six sizes. Its disposable inner pad (available in regular or heavy-duty sizes) fits inside the pant's crotch pocket. For a nonambulatory patient, Dignity Pants are also available with side openings joined by Velcro strips. The Dignity Pant is only one example of the many incontinent pants and diapers on the market. Pampers are also successfully used in some patients. According to the patient's need and preference, it is possible to choose a plasticized incontinent pant with either a disposable or reusable inner pad or a completely disposable adult diaper.

No matter what type is selected, it is important to remember to check the inner pads and diapers frequently and to change them as needed. Prolonged skin contact with urine increases the risk of infection and contributes to skin irritation and breakdown. It is important to perform routine perineal and skin care each time a pant or diaper is changed. The patient's skin should be protected with a skin barrier such as Bard moisture barrier ointment.

Although urinary incontinence is not a typical change associated with aging, it is one of the more common and upsetting conditions that can occur. By one estimate, up to 40 percent of all people older than age 62 suffer from urinary incontinence. The use of an indwelling catheter should be avoided if possible. The risk of repeated bladder and kidney infections is high among catheter users.

DETRUSOR INSTABILITY

In this condition, there is a history of a weak bladder even before pregnancies, if any, have occurred. The patient often has a history of enuresis, especially in childhood. There are complaints of urge incontinence and frequency, especially at night (nocturia).

Bladder training (bladder drill) is advocated as the first treatment. This is a psychologic approach to a condition the cause of which is often in doubt. Although it involves about 10 days' stay in the hospital and much supervision, it is well worth a trial in resistant cases.

After a full explanation, the patient is instructed to pass urine only at hourly intervals, which are gradually increased to every 3 hours if possible. Fluid balance and times of micturition are recorded. The patient must be motivated to persist with the treatment. This drill is followed only during the day. However, it is continued in modified form after the patient has been discharged from the hospital.

SUMMARY

The involuntary voiding of small amounts of urine is very common in women. It is known, perhaps wrongly, as *stress incontinence,* and its treatment calls for an understanding of bladder and urethral physiology.

The bladder is able to adapt to increased urinary volumes. Pressure remains below 10 cm of water until more than 500 mL of urine is collected.

Urethral pressure is maintained by the internal sphincter, made up of the longitudinal and circular plane muscle and elastic tissues, and an external sphincter, which contributes striated muscle.

A urethral pressure profile along the length of the urethra demonstrates much greater pressure than the intravesical pressure, thus ensuring continence.

Cystometry recording demonstrates the timing of events and the mechanism of voiding. First is an intraabdominal pressure increase, which is measured per rectum. The detrusor muscle contracts and increases the intravesical pressure. The anal sphincter then relaxes; this is measured by an electromyogram of the sphincter. At this point the urine starts to flow.

It has been demonstrated that the urethra and bladder neck are maintained in a closed state by the trigonal condensation of muscle in the urethral sphincter. When cortical inhibition is withdrawn, the detrusor contracts and the bladder neck relaxes (funneling). The sphincter also relaxes and urine is voided. As the flow continues, the bladder neck moves downward and backward and the urethrovesical angle is obliterated. The symptoms and signs of incontinence include frequency, urgency, dysuria, and stress incontinence.

Urodynamic investigation of bladder function consists of a study of bladder movements and tension during different levels of filling, and involves measurement of bladder activity (cystometry) and urethral flow (uroflowmetry). Bladder apparatus is sophisticated and expensive.

The indications for urodynamic assessment are (1) continuing difficulty in distinguishing genuine stress incontinence from detrusor instability, (2) after failure of surgery to relieve a complaint of incontinence, (3) where there are other complicating factors such as a neurologic disease, and (4) where difficulty in voiding is complained of or suspected. The last condition may occur after pelvic surgery and may lead to incomplete emptying and perhaps retention overflow.

Until recently, incontinent people have typically withdrawn from family, friends, and active living for fear of accidents and public embarrassment. They have become prisoners in their own home. The elderly are often abandoned by their family and sent off to a nursing home without proper evaluation to see whether the problem of incontinence can be corrected. Urinary incontinence has been called the last taboo. When an elderly person is incontinent, it is the responsibility of the physician in charge to make certain that the reason for the incontinence is documented and, if possible, to correct it. All too often elderly patients are placed in a nursing home because they are incompetent when indeed they are only incontinent.

The incontinent patient should have a thorough workup including urine cultures and a urodynamic evaluation. Once a diagnosis is made, the patient should be given the appropriate treatment to correct the problem. This may require medication, Biofeedback training, perineal exercise, and, less often, surgery.

REFERENCES

Altman, B. L. 1976. Treatment of urethral syndrome with triamcinolone acetonide. *J. Urol.* 116:583.

Barber, H. R. K. 1986. Geriatric gynecology, in: *Clinical Geriatrics,* 3rd ed. (I. Rossman, ed.). J.B. Lippincott Co., Philadelphia, pp. 364.

Brocklehurst, J. C., and J. B. Dillane. 1966. Studies of the female bladder in old age. I. Cytometrograms in nonincontinent women. *Gerontol. Clin.* 8:285.

Brocklehurst, J. C., J. B. Dillane, L., Griffiths, and J. Fry. 1968. The prevalence and symptomatology of urinary infection in an aged population. *Gerontol. Clin.* 10:242.

Brocklehurst, J. C., J. Fry, C. C. Griffiths, and G. Kalton. 1972. Urinary infection and symptoms of dysuria in women age 45–64 years: Their relevance to similar findings in the elderly. *Age Ageing* 1:41.

Brown, A. D. G. 1977. Postmenopausal urinary problems. *Clin. Obstet. Gynecol.* 4:181.

Cantor, T. J., and C. P. Bates. 1980. A comparative study of symptoms and objective urodynamic findings in 214 incontinent women. *Br. J. Obstet. Gynaecol.* 87:889.

Castleden, C. M., H. M. Duffin, and M. J. Ashner. 1981. Clinical and urodynamic studies in 100 elderly patients. *Br. Med. J.* 282:1103.

Corlett, R. C. Jr. 1979. Urologic problems in menopause. *Female Patient* 4:30–34.

Drutz, H. P., and F. Mandel. 1979. Urodynamic analysis of urinary incontinence symptoms in women. *Am. J. Obstet. Gynecol.* 134:789.

Eastwood, H. D. H. 1979. Urodynamic studies in the management of urinary incontinence in the elderly. *Age Ageing* 8:41.

Elder, D. D., and T. P. Stephenson. 1980. An assessment of the Frewen regime in the treatment of detrusor dysfunction in females. *Br. J. Urol.* 52:467.

Faber, P., and J. Heidenreich. 1977. Treatment of stress incontinence and estrogen in postmenopausal women. *Urol. Int.* 32:221.

Farrar, D. J., C. J. Whiteside, J. L. Osborne, and R. T. Tuner-Warwick. 1975. A urodynamic analysis of micturition symptoms in the female. *Surg. Gynecol. Obstet.* 141:875.

Frewen, W. 1979. Role of bladder training in the treatment of the unstable bladder in the female. *Urol. Clin. North Am.* 6:273.

Gartley, C. B. (ed). 1985. *Managing Incontinence.* Jameson Books, Ottawa, Ill.

Gowan, A. D. T., C. Hodge, and R. Callander (eds.). 1985 *Gynaecology Illustrated,* 3rd ed. Churchill Livingstone, Edinburgh.

Green, T. H. Jr.: Urinary stress incontinence. Differential diagnosis, pathophysiology and management. *Am. J. Obstet. Gynecol.* 122:368.

Hilton, P., and S. L. Stanton. 1981. Algorithmic method for assessing urinary incontinence in elderly women. *Br. Med. J.* 282:940.

Hodgkinson, C. P., and B. H. Drukker. 1977. Infravesical nerve resection for detrusor dyssynergia. *Acta Obstet. Gynecol.* Scand. 56:401.

Jarvis, G., and D. R. Millar. 1980. Controlled trial of bladder drill for detrusor instability. *Br. J. Urol.* 281:1322.

Johnson, W. 1960. *The Older Patient.* Hoeber, New York, pp. 467–512.

Kegel, A. 1956. Stress incontinence of urine in women: Physiologic treatment. *J. Int. Coll. Surg.* 25:487.

Khanna, O. P. 1976. Disorders of micturition: Neuropharmacologic basis and results of drug therapy. *Urology* 8:316.

Lipsky, H. 1977. Urodynamic assessment of women with urethral syndrome. *Eur. Urol.* 3:202.

Mahony, D., R. Laferte, and D. Blais. 1977. Integral storage and voiding reflexes. *Urology* 9:95.

Osbourne, J. L. 1976. Postmenopausal changes in micturition habits and in urine flow and urethral pressure studies, in: *The Management of the Menopause and Post-Menopausal Years.* (S. Campbell, ed.). Lancaster, PA, p. 285.

Ostergard, D. R. 1979. Lower urinary tract symptoms: The role of the urethra. *Female Patient* 4:30.

Ouslander, J. G., R. L. Kane, and I. B. Abrass. 1982. Urinary incontinence in elderly nursing home patients. *JAMA* 284:1194.

Overstall, P. W., K. Rounce and J. H. Palmer. 1980. Experience with an incontinence clinic. *J. Am. Geriatric Soc.* 28:535.

Pengelly, A. W., and C. M. Booth. 1980. A prospective trial of bladder training as treatment for detrusor instability. *Br. J. Urol.* 52:463.

Plante, P., and J. Susset. 1980. Studies of female urethral pressure profile. I. The normal urethral pressure profile. *J. Urol.* 123:64.

Raz, S. 1978. Pharmacological treatment of lower urinary tract dysfunction. *Urol. Clin. North Am.* 5:323.

Rud, T. 1980. The effects of estrogen and gestagens on the urethral pressure profile in urinary continent and stress incontinent women. *Acta Obstet. Gynecol. Scand.* 59:265.

Smith, P. 1976. Postmenopausal urinary symptoms and hormonal replacement therapy. *Br. Med. J.* 2:941.

Susset, J., and P. Plante. 1980. Studies of female urethral pressure profile. II. Pressure profile in female incontinence. *J. Urol.* 123:70.

Tanagho, E. A. 1980. If the complaint is incontinence, determine pressure profile. *Contemp. Obstet. Gynecol.* 15:105.

Tanagho, E. A., and E. Miller. 1973. Functional consideration of urethral sphincter dynamics. *J. Urol.* 109:273.

Tanagho, E. A., E. Miller, F. Meyers, and H. R. Corbett. 1966. Observation on the dynamics of the bladder neck. *Br. Urol.* 38:72.

Wein, A. J., and D. M. Raezer. 1979. Physiology of micturition, in: *Clinical Neuro-Urology* (R. J. Krane and M. D. Siroky, eds.). Little, Brown & Co., Boston, pp. 1–34.

Williams, M. E. 1983. A critical evaluation of the assessment technology for urinary continence in older persons. *J. Am Geriatric Soc.* 31:657.

Williams, M. E., and F. C. P. Pannill. 1982. Urinary incontinence in the elderly. *Ann. Intern Med.* 97:895.

Yarnell, J. W. G., and A. S. St. Leger. 1979. The prevalence, severity and factors associated with urinary incontinence in a random sample of the elderly. *Age Ageing* 8:81.

17 Sexuality in Aging Women

INTRODUCTION

Roland's Illustrated Medical Dictionary (26th edition) defines *sexuality* as a characteristic quality of male and female reproductive elements and as the constitution of an individual in relation to sexual attitudes or activity. Thus, *sexuality* is a broad term; it is not limited to the narrow concept of coitus

With better nutrition, more cholesterol in their diet, more rest, and better health, women are maintaining an interest in sexual function well into their postmenopausal years. Continued sexual outlets and functioning are the most important factors in maintaining sexual interest and capacity in the geriatric woman. If for any reason a woman is sexually inactive for several years in the postmenopausal period, there may be difficulty with reinstitution of sexual function.

There are many stories about famous people who possess a strong libido and sex drive. Among these is Catherine the Great, a German princess with a French education, who ruled the vast Russian Empire as an autocrat for 34 years. Catherine had numerous men throughout her life. However, growing old at last, the 60-year-old empress succumbed to the wiles of 22-year-old Platon Zubov, an officer of the Horse Guards, who was very ambitious. Zubov was her main sexual interest until her death at age 67. It is interesting to note that at this time there were no systemic or local estrogen hormones that could be used to augment her libido.

An overview of sexuality in the older person implies the capacity for involvement in all of life. This includes the physiologic response of sexual tension, the psychologic expression of emotions and commitment to others, and social identification of gender and roles in life. It is obvious that sexuality is more than the physical act of sexual union. There are a great number of myths about sexuality in the postmenopausal and geriatric patient that must be dispelled. Several sexologists have reported that older people remain interested in sex and that sexual activity is possible well into the last years of life. The idea that older people do not find each other attractive is wrong. There is a great deal of individual variation as far as sexual desirability is concerned. Healthy sexual expression in this age group usually means a healthy body and mind and indicates that sexuality may contribute to overall well-being rather than being dangerous. Therefore, it is quite evident that in the postmenopausal and geriatric years, sexual union may continue with mutual gratification.

LIBIDO

In 1953 Kinsey reported that the sexual activity of unmarried women remains relatively constant until age 55, whereas that of unmarried men declines progressively from adolescence. Among married couples as well, the frequency of sexual intercourse appears to decline in a similar fashion with aging. Kinsey concluded from these observations that in women age has no effect on sexual activity until very late in life, and he suggested that the subsequent reduction in sexual activity may be due primarily to diminution in the sexuality of the male partner. It is a quirk of nature that women are not able to bear children after the menopause but can continue a very active sex life, whereas men are able to impregnate a woman throughout their lives but with advancing age have difficulty in completing the sexual act.

A study of the sexual activity of single women between 50 and 69 years of age compared previously married subjects to those who had never been married. Both groups reportedly maintained sexual activity, including masturbation (59 percent of the previously married and 44 percent of those never married), coitus (37 and 25 percent), and orgasmic dreams (35 and 52 percent).

HISTORY

Sexuality is a delicate subject. Older women are embarrassed by talking about it, but they welcome a professional approach in exploring this part of their lives. It is important to start off slowly with general questions, and it is particularly important to allow the patient to talk if she chooses. Some will talk freely, while others require a period of time before confidence and the patient–physician relationship is established. It is important to impress

236

upon the patient that this is only one aspect of providing overall care to her. It is also important to appreciate the level of education of the patient, as well as her religious, ethnic, and social background. It is often necessary to use medical terms with certain groups, while with others, it is important to use terms that they have been accustomed to using.

Ideally, the history should be directed toward opening up the subject and then allowing the patient to set the pace. However, for those who have difficulty expressing and defining their own role in this delicate problem, carefully worded questions are important. It is important to find out what the patient's past history has been, what is currently going on in her life, and what expectations she has for the future. It is interesting to note that in the geriatric patient, unlike the patient in the reproductive years, there are different types of intimate relationships that are pleasurable. These include touching, physical closeness, stroking, and petting; others want a more aggressive approach that ends in intercourse. Some women explain that they have an interest in intercourse but that there is pain because of dryness. The patient should be carefully counseled that this is a physiologic response and that there are pharmacologic treatments that can counteract this problem.

When taking the history, it is important to try to identify the patient's self-image. Some women who have had a mastectomy or hysterectomy feel that they are totally unattractive or that they have been robbed of their so-called femininity. Careful explanation will usually allay their fears and improve their self-image.

It is important to discuss with them any medical or metabolic disorders that may interfere with their libido. Diabetes, infections, and other medical problems may so preoccupy them that they may be frightened by any expression of sexuality. This should be explored with the patient and help offered. The use of drugs is often implicated in the decrease in libido. These drugs should be carefully reviewed with the patient. Anticholinergic, antispasmodic, antihypertensive, and antianxiety agents, tranquilizers, and sedatives may decrease libido. Some women resort to alcohol in the hope that it may improve their sexuality. It must be carefully explained that alcohol has a sedative rather than a stimulatory effect and that it is very important to limit their alcohol intake.

Last but not least, it is important to review with the patient her past history and try to explore the impact of the personal, moral, and religious values that play a role particularly in the elderly. Myths should be dispelled, and the patient should be encouraged to achieve the level of gratification that she feels necessary for a stable lifestyle. The fact that the physician has the empathy and understanding to explore this part of the geriatric patient's life gives her the confidence to ask questions and to proceed to achieve the lifestyle that she hopes for and often fantasizes about.

It is important for the physician to impress upon the patient that sexual health is an important component of her overall well-being and should be explored during the history and physical examination. The changing attitude of society about sexuality is bringing these problems into focus, and the physician dealing with the geriatric patient must be prepared to offer help, guidance, and counseling on these important matters.

ANATOMIC CHANGES IN THE REPRODUCTIVE ORGANS

Alterations in sexual response associated with aging are a result of a generalized decrease in the tone, strength, and elasticity of tissues and the lengthening of response time. The aging woman's vagina undergoes specific involuntary changes, and changes may also occur in the labia, uterus, and breast. There is a loss of length and width in the vagina during the aging process. This organ also loses some of its expansive ability, as might be anticipated from the reported loss of vaginal wall thickness. The involuntary neuromuscular response to sexual tension that results in expansion in vaginal length and transcervical width obviously is influenced by the states of sex hormone withdrawal. It has been reported that the clitoris and the minor and major labia vary in their responsiveness to sexual tensions as the human female ages. The clitoral response continues into the seventies in patterns similar to those of the premenopausal female. On the other hand, reactions of the minor and major labia reflect involuntary changes that appear to be inherent in the aging process. The major labia lose fatty tissue deposits in the postmenopausal years. The loss of major labial body content is accompanied by some loss of elastic tissue. There is a flattening and separation as well as elevation of the major labia that develop in response to elevated sexual tension; these responses are lost as the woman ages. The small labia undergoes a reduced vasocongestive reaction in the older female. The sex skin reaction of the small labia, which is pathognomonic of the pending orgasm in the premenopausal female, is usually lost in the older woman. Secretory activity of the Bartholin's gland is somewhat slowed by the aging process, but not until the female is well into the postmenopausal years. In the older woman, secretory activity is decreased.

Alterations in sexual response associated with aging are a result of a generalized decrease in the tone, strength, and elasticity of tissues and the lengthening of response time. In older women, it may take 3 to 5 minutes for vaginal lubrication to occur, whereas in the young woman it takes only 15 to 20 seconds. At the same level of arousal, the older woman will have a smaller volume of lubrication. Again, provided that she is in good health, and especially if there has been continuing sexual functioning, lubrication for intercourse will be adequate. Use of commonly available lubricants may be helpful. Currently, Upsher-Smith Laboratories has introduced Lubrin, a vaginal lubricating insert, which is unscented, colorless, convenient, and provides long-lasting lubrication for sexual intercourse.

Most older women want and are able to lead an active, satisfying sex life. With age, women do not ordinarily lose their physical capacity for orgasm or men their capacity for erection and ejaculation. There is, however, a gradual slowing of response, especially in men, a process currently considered part of normal aging but perhaps eventually treatable or even reversible. A pattern of regular sexual activity (which may include masturbation) helps to preserve sexual function. When problems occur, they should not be viewed as inevitable but rather as a result of disease, disability, drug reaction, or emotional upset and as requiring medical care. Women generally experience little serious loss of sexual capacity due to age alone. Those changes that do occur, mainly in the shape, flexibility, and lubrication of the vagina, can usually be traced directly to lower levels of the hormone estrogen during and after menopause. Women who have severe problems are sometimes treated with estrogen.

However, all too often, the menopausal woman complaining of sexual inadequacy is often told by her physician that loss of sexual function is to be expected with the change of life and that nothing can be done about it. Although sexual behavior is the sum total of the individual's makeup, including chromosomal sex, gender identification, gonadal adequacy, childhood rearing, environmental influences, and possibly hypothalamic sensitizing and hormone factors, there is a definite role for hormone therapy in modifying sexual responsiveness. Combinations of estrogen and androgen are often beneficial.

HORMONE THERAPY

Equine conjugated estrogen or its equivalent in a dose of 0.625 mg with 5 mg methyltestosterone is recommended. In some women, methyltestosterone 10 mg three times a day for 2 weeks will often increase their libido, and if the patient engages in intercourse, the desire will continue without the need for stimulation from hormonal therapy. Testosterone apparently has a fairly predictable potential for increasing libido among women. Experiments have been conducted with women suffering from terminal metastatic breast cancer. Among one group that received testosterone as palliative therapy, more than half complained of an almost intolerable increase in sexual desire. Several stated that they had experienced orgasm for the first time in their lives. In another experiment, a group of women with secondary frigidity were given a variety of steroidal hormones. Estrogens were effective in improving libido and sex drive in about 30 percent, androgens in more than 75 percent; progesterone, cortisol, and placebos were wholly ineffective. No more than 100 mg testosterone compound should be administered per month, and it is important to provide this therapy only intermittently.

In woman in whom intercourse is difficult because of the shrinkage secondary to estrogen withdrawal, hormonal cream is often beneficial. This should be applied locally on the outside around the inside lip of the small labia, up around the clitoris, and around the fourchette. It is important to treat the area carefully where penetration occurs during intercourse. The treatment should be carried out two to three times a week until the tissue has undergone a period of rejuvenation. The treatment should then be continued at less frequent intervals. A quarter of an applicator of estrogen cream inserted into the vagina every 2 to 3 weeks usually keeps the upper part of the vagina pink and moist.

Some women seek advice about masturbation. Since they are elderly, they feel that it is a sign of some abnormal psychologic condition. The patient must be instructed that it has no harmful physical effects and is within normal limits. However, if the patient considers masturbation to be a moral issue, it is best to refer her to a sex counselor or a clergyman.

Masters and Johnson (1966) have demonstrated with a small sample of older people that sexual ability and interest can be maintained until old age. Their subjects were in their late seventies and eighties. Those who had been sexually active throughout their lives had fewer sexual dysfunctional symptoms and also had less trouble resulting from the decrease in estrogen that many women experience. Masters and Johnson were cautious not to draw any conclusions from the small subsample of women. However, they inferred that women who have had an active sex life with orgasm from an early period do not develop the vaginal changes that decrease the ability to lubricate that other aging women in their study experienced.

PHYSIOLOGIC CHANGES IN ELDERLY WOMEN

Masters and Johnson (1966) have shown that all four stages of the response cycle (excitement, plateau, orgasm, and resolution) are somewhat diminished with increasing age. In the excitement stage, the breasts are less engorged and the sexual flush may be absent. The clitoris enlarges normally. The flattening, separation, and elevation of the major labia that develop in response to elevated sexual tension, particularly in the nulliparous woman, are lost as the woman ages. This reaction normally separates and elevates the labia in an upward and outward direction away from the vaginal outlet. The geriatric patient loses the major labial body content and also some of the elastic tissue. Therefore, it is not unexpected that the major labial elevation reaction would be basically altered in advanced years. In females, lubrication time is delayed from 15 to 30 seconds to 5 minutes, and the expansion capacity of the vagina is reduced. Vaginal burning, however, can occur later in the plateau phase and often is marked. Vaginal lubrication is reduced. In the plateau stage, uterine elevation is reduced. However, the clitoral response remains similar to that of younger women. The orgasmic phase is characterized by a decrease in the number of contractions, and the contractions are of shorter duration. They may be spastic rather than rhythmic in nature. Sometimes the uterine spasms may render orgasm painful. However, the severity, duration, and degree of recurrence of these contractions vary tremendously from individual to individual and within the same individual, depending upon the intensity of the orgasm. At present, there is no definite information available on the physiologic response of the senile uterus to effective sexual stimulation. The resolution phase is rapid in elderly women, and, occasionally because of urethral trauma, is accompanied by a desire to void. However, the elderly female remains multiorgasmic. A decrease in the strength of vaginal contractions with orgasm is another change that occurs in elderly women. This effect is recordable and has been documented. However, older women may report no diminution in the experience of pleasure or the gratification of release (Fig. 17-1).

SOCIAL-CULTURE FACTORS

There are far more elderly women than elderly men. Therefore, the elderly female does not always have a socially acceptable partner. These women are often widowed or are caring for a husband who is ill or disabled.

Public acceptance of sexuality in the elderly is gradually increasing. It is anticipated that the special aspects of sexuality in old age will become generally understood, and that when diagnosis and treatment of sexual

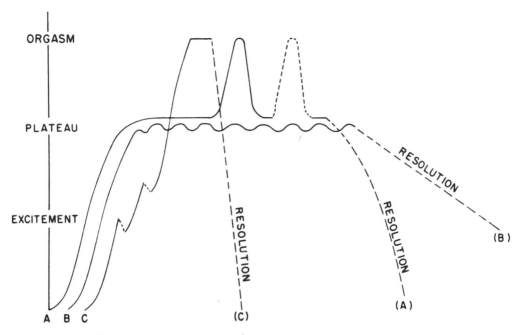

Figure 17-1. The female sexual response cycle.

problems are refined to a much greater degree, there will be greater sexual participation among the elderly. In some societies, postmenopausal women are respected and looked up to; however, in youth-oriented societies, they do not enjoy this position. This fact has a major impact on how women cope during the postmenopausal years. Women in a society experiencing cultural gains following the menopause will have an easier adjustment than those in a youth-oriented society. Deutsch (1945) referred to the loss of reproductive capacity as a partial death. In addition to the loss of youthful attractiveness, there are numerous social adjustments that may be stressful. The postmenopausal woman may have to adjust to seeing her children leaving home, getting married, and having their own children, as well as the increasing physical ill health that may occur either to her or her partner. The patient who has made her family her entire life may find the departure of her children to seek their own lives, or her husband's need to spend time away from home in order to advance his own career, traumatic. Women very often feel lonely and depressed, and lack interest in all pleasurable activities, including sex. Therefore, it is important for women to have hobbies or outside interests, as well as a positive and secure marital relationship.

EFFECTS OF ILLNESS OR DISABILITY

The incidence of illness and disability increases with age. However, although these problems can affect sexuality in later life, even the most serious diseases rarely warrant stopping sexual activity. Multiple physical illnesses are the rule rather than the exception in the elderly and, therefore, may have an adverse effect on sexuality.

Decreased sexual desire may be secondary to an endocrinopathy such as hypothyroidism. In this case, thyroid replacement therapy may be very rewarding.

Heart disease, especially if a heart attack has occurred, leads many older people to give up sex altogether for fear of causing another attack. Yet the risk of death during sexual intercourse is very low. Although a doctor's advice is needed, sex usually can and should be resumed an average of 12 to 16 weeks after a heart attack, depending on one's physical condition. An active sex life may in fact decrease the risk of a future attack.

Diabetes in the male is one of the few diseases that can cause impotence. Once diabetes is diagnosed and controlled, however, potency may be restored. When impotence persists in well-controlled diabetics, it may be permanent. Replacement of a severely damaged aorta secondary to arteriosclerosis can increase the blood supply to the pelvis and often restores sexual function. Diabetes does not cause as severe a problem in the woman as in the man.

Stroke rarely damages the physical aspects of sexual function, and it is unlikely that sexual exertion will cause another stroke. Using different positions or medical devices that assist body function can help make up for any weakness or paralysis that may have occurred.

Joint pain due to rheumatoid arthritis can limit sexual activity. Surgery and drugs can relieve these problems, but in some cases the medicines used can decrease sexual desire. Exercise, rest, warm baths, and changes in the position and timing of sexual activity (such as avoiding evening and early morning hours of pain) can be helpful.

MENTAL ILLNESSES

Psychologic stresses also may be expressed by sexual dysfunction. Most observers agree that there is no difference in psychologic history between women who maintained sexual activity after the menopause and those who do not. The most common mental illness causing a loss of sexual interest is depression. Additional factors that may have a role in the loss of sexual interest include a stressful relationship with the partner, a change in marital status, a reduction in self-image, and other intrapersonal and environmental factors. The impact of mania, schizophrenia, and paranoid disorders on the sexual behavior of the elderly female is undergoing continuous study. In rare cases, organic brain disorders such as presenile dementia (Alzheimer's type) or neurosyphilis may present as depressive states, with an associated decrease in sexual interest and activity.

INFLUENCE OF DRUGS

Excessive use of alcohol, which reduces potency in men and delays orgasm in women, is probably the most widespread drug-related cause of sexual problems. Tranquilizers, antidepressants, and certain high blood pressure drugs can cause impotence; other drugs can lead to failure to ejaculate in men and reduce sexual desire in women. Such effects are reversed when the medication is stopped. A doctor may prescribe a drug with less effect on sexual function if he or she realizes that this is important to the patient. Lithium usually decreases the hypersexuality of manic behavior. There have been reports of impairment in the orgasmic phase in females with the use of monamine oxidase inhibitors. It has been stated that various antihypertensive and cardiac drugs decrease sexual desire. However, the effects of these agents on the sexual response cycle of females are not well understood.

LONG-TERM CARE FACILITIES

Many elderly women spend their last years in adult nursing homes. In considering the total care of the elderly in long-term facilities, sexual and intimacy needs must not be avoided. A holistic view of sexuality embraces three major areas: the physiologic release of sexual tension, the psychologic expression of emotions and commitment to others, and the social identification of gender and roles in life. Therefore, sexuality is more than an act of physical union.

As long as good general health is maintained, sexual behavior can continue into old age. Some elderly patients have health problems and are so debilitated that they may not be able to engage in sexual activity. However, within the broad definition of sexuality, intimacy and closeness, coupled with skin contact or touching, are considered essential for survival. Yet, they are not necessarily substitutes for, or limited to, a heterosexual relationship. These needs do not disappear with old age. Persons who are physically disabled can still show certain behaviors that express sexual feeling such as holding hands, exposing, masturbation, sex talk, and interest in any human contact. These factors of sexuality, intimacy and touch and hand communication, enhance the quality of life for the geriatric patient.

It is vital to understand what the elderly woman is trying to express, and it is important not to be judgmental. These patients are human beings, and it is the responsibility of those taking care of them to provide privacy as an essential part of the environment, including living space as well as during health care procedures. Privacy also allows them to express appropriate sexual desires. The medical and nursing staff and ancillary aides must be supportive and treat the elderly as individuals who have the capacity for love, affection, intimacy, and closeness to other human beings. Sexual counseling, therapy, and specific treatments should be available to these patients. They may help alleviate the sexual problems in the geriatric population in an institutional environment.

SUMMARY

Public acceptance of sexuality in later life is gradually increasing. In the future, the special aspects of sexuality in old age will become generally understood and the diagnosis and treatment of sexual problems will be greatly refined.

Sexuality is more than intercourse. Every aspect of pleasuring, holding, and skin contact is important. Clinicians should be conscious of the social, psychologic, and culture factors and consider them to be as important as the organic ones.

A careful sexual history and gynecologic examination are very important in treating the elderly patient. They often establish a close patient –physician relationship and facilitate the care of the geriatric patient. There is no evidence to support the view of hormonal deprivation as the primary cause of a reduction in sexual activity. It has been adequately demonstrated that sexual decline is a matter of circumstance, not of potential.

REFERENCES

Anderson, C. J. 1980. Sexuality in the aged, in: *Readings in Gerontological Nursing* (E. M. Stilwell, ed.) C. B. Slack, Thorofare, N.J., p. 105.

Burnside, I. M. 1973. Touching is talking. *Am. J. Nurs.* 73(12):2060.

Butler, R., and M. Lewis. 1976. *Sex After Sixty: A Guide for Men and Women in Their Later Years.* New York, Harper & Row.

Christenson, C. V., and A. B. Johnson. 1973. Sexual patterns in a group of older, never-married women. *J. Geriatric Psychiatry* 7:80.

Comfort, A. 1974. Sexuality in old age. *J. Am. Geriatric Soc.* 22:440.

————. 1978. *Sexual Consequences of Disability.* George F. Stickley Co., Philadelphia, pp. 186–187.

Dean, S. R. 1972. Discussion (of the paper by Pfeiffer, Berwoerdt and Vans 1972). *Am. J. Psychiatry* 128:1267.

Deutsch, H. 1945. *The Psychology of Women. Motherhood,* vol. 2. Grune & Stratton, New York, pp. 456–485.

Dinnerstein, L., and S. Burrows. 1982. Hormone replacement therapy and sexuality in women. *Clin. Endocrinol. Metab.* 2:3.

Ebersole, P., and P. Hess. 1981. *Toward Healthy Aging: Human Needs and Nursing Response.* C. V. Mosby Co., St. Louis, p. 325.

Flint, M. 1975. The menopause: Reward or punishment. *Psychosomatics* 16:161.

Friedman, J. 1979. Development of sexual knowledge inventory for elderly persons. *Nurs. Res.* 28:374.

Glover, B. H. 1978. Sex counseling, in: *The Geriatric Patient* (W. Reichel, ed.). H.P. Publishing Co., New York, p. 125.

Gruis, M. L., and N. N. Wagner. 1979. Sexuality during the climacteric. *Postgrad. Med.* 65:197.

Hallstrom, T. 1977. Sexuality in the climacteric. *Clin. Obstet. Gynaecol* 4:227.

Hollinger, L. M. 1980. Perception of touch in the elderly. *J. Gerontol. Nurs.* 6(12):741.

Ludeman, K. 1981. The sexuality of the older person: Review of the literature. *Gerontologist* 21(2):203.

Kinsey, A. C., W. B. Pomeroy, C. R. Marten, et al. 1948. *Sexual Behavior in the Human Male.* W. B. Saunders Co., Philadelphia.

————. 1953. *Sexual Behavior in the Human Female.* W. B. Saunders Co., Philadelphia.

Kolodny, R. C., W. Masters, and V. Johnson. 1979. *Textbook of Sexual Medicine.* Little, Brown & Co., Boston.

Krystal, S., and D. A. Chiriboga. 1979. The empty nest process in mid-life men and women. *Maturitas* 1:215.

Kuhn, M. E. 1975. Sexual myths surrounding the aging, in: *Sex and the Life Cycle.* (W. Oaks, G. Melchiode, and I. Fischer, eds.). Grune & Stratton, New York, p. 117.

Masters, W. H., and V. E. Johnson. 1966. *Human Sexual Response.* Little, Brown & Co., Boston.

————. 1970. *Human Sexual Inadequacy*. Little, Brown & Co., Boston.

————. 1981. Sex and the aging process. *J. Am. Geriatric Soc.* 29:385.

McCorkle, R. 1974. Effects of touch on seriously ill patients. *Nurs. Res.* 23(2):125.

Munjack, D. J., and L. J. Oziel. 1980. *Sexual Medicine and Counseling in Office Practice: A Comprehensive Treatment Guide*. Little, Brown & Co., Boston.

Notelovitz, M. 1978. Gynecologic problems in menopausal women: I. Changes in genital tissue. *Geriatrics* 33(8):24.

————. 1978. Gynecologic problems in menopausal women: II. Treating estrogen deficiencies. *Geriatrics* 33(9):35-4227:73.

Mewman, G., and C. R. Nichols. 1960. Sexual activities and attitudes in older persons. *JAMA* 173:33.

Parsons, V. 1981. Assessment of older clients' sexual health, in: *Nursing and the Aged*, 2nd ed. (I. M. Burnside, ed.). McGraw-Hill, New York, p. 374.

Pfeiffer, E., A. Verwoerdt, and H. S. Wang. 1968. Sexual behavior in aged men and women: I. Observations on 254 community volunteers. *Arch. Gen. Psychiatry,* 19:753.

————. 1969. The natural history of sexual behavior in a biologically advantaged group of aged individuals. *J. Gerontol.* 24:193.

Scheingold, L. D., and N. N. Wagner. 1974. *Sound Sex and the Aging Heart*. Human Sciences Press, New York, p. 44.

Semmens, J. P., C. C. Tsai, E. C. Semmens, et al. 1985. Effects of estrogen therapy on vaginal physiology during menopause. *Obstet. Gynecol.* 66:15.

Shoemaker, D. M. 1980. Integration of physiological and sociocultural factors as the basis for sex education in the elderly. *J. Gerontol. Nurs.* 6:311.

Shortle, B., and R. Zewelewics. 1986. Psychogenic vaginismus. *Med. Aspects Human Sexuality* 20(4):32.

Sparrow, D., R. Bosse, and J. W. Rowe. 1980. The influence of age, alcohol consumption and body build on gonadal function in men. *J. Clin. Endocrinol. Metab.* 51:508.

Tobiason, S. J. B. 1981. Touching is for everyone. *Am. J. Nurs.* 81(4):728.

Traupman, J., E. Eckels, and E. Hatfield. 1982. Intimacy in older women's lives. *Gerontologist* 2:493.

Wharton, G. F. 1978. *A Bibliography on Sexuality and Aging*. Rutgers University Press, New Brunswick, N.J.

Woods, N. F. 1979. Sexuality and aging, in: *Current Practice in Gerontological Nursing* (A. M. Reinhardt and M. D. Quinn, eds.). C.V. Mosby Co., St. Louis.

18 Major Gynecologic Surgical Procedures In The Aging Woman

INTRODUCTION

"Surgery (sur'jer e) (L. *chirurgia* from Gr. *cheir,* the hand + *ergon,* work)—That branch of medicine which treats diseases, injuries and deformities by manual or instrumental operative methods" as defined by Dorland's Illustrated Medical Dictionary Twenty-sixth edition.

The menopausal and geriatric patient can have any non-pregnancy-related surgical problem that occurs in the premenopausal patient. However, often the presenting clinical picture in these two groups of patients is slightly different. Those who reach age 65 or more are subject to a wide range of disorders, many of which are best treated by surgery. In the last three decades, indications for surgery in this age group have been expanded because of the advances in technology, pharmacology, and an understanding of physiologic changes in the aging.

A comparison of the older literature with current writings indicates that the most important therapeutic advances are related to anesthesia, water and electrolyte balance, methods of measuring impaired function to determine the individual's capacity to withstand the surgical procedure, and the expanded use of monitoring devices such as the Swan-Ganz catheter.

Replacement of organs and transplantation, as well as the use of mechanical devices, have also expanded considerably. Unless the patient shows dementia, age is not considered a contraindiction to the use of surgical procedures. Many systemic changes occur with aging. The nervous, cardiovascular, and respiratory systems, the gastrointestinal and urinary tracts, and the musculoskeletal system do show changes. However, there is no reason to consider most women at age 60 old. It is probably more realistic to put 80 years of age as the upper limit for considering the patient old because it is at this point that geriatric aspects are predominant. In this category of patients, approximately 7 percent over the age of 60 undergo gynecologic surgery. The surgical procedure itself should be part of the continuum of management. Considered alone, the procedure may represent a triumph of technique over reason. It is important to evaluate the operative risk for a given patient in terms of invalidism, morbidity, and mortality, as well as the salvage rate and the potential to achieve rehabilitation with an acceptable quality of life.

There are increased risks for the geriatric patient undergoing surgery. However, chronologic age per se should not be a contraindication. The patient must be evaluated completely. Geriatric patients present many different types of systemic aging; some have impairment of heart function with good kidney function, or impairment of respiratory function with a fairly good endocrine system reserve. The amount of surgical stress that the patient can tolerate is limited by the functional reserve capacity of her organ systems. This capacity diminishes with age and can be further deteriorated by chronic or endocrine disease. The distinction must be made between emergency and elective surgery. In emergency surgery, a greater risk may be taken than is permissible with elective and corrective surgery.

Three systems are particularly important in evaluating a geriatric patient for surgery: the cardiovascular, pulmonary, and renal systems. Each merits an in-depth discussion. However, for the purposes of this presentation, it is important to address the most important changes.

CARDIOVASCULAR FUNCTION

The heart tends to become smaller in the aged person unless there is some pathology that leads to cardiomegaly. The aorta and coronary vessels lose their elasticity and show signs of arteriosclerosis. The valves become more rigid, the stroke volume decreases, and the cardiac output in the geriatric patient is about one-third that of a person in his twenties. The most important changes are a reduction of peripheral tissue perfusion, decreased velocity of blood flow, redistribution or reduced cardiac output, and reduction of cardiac reserves. A myocardial infarction within 3 months preceding surgery is associated with either another myocardial infarction or cardiac death in 30 percent of these patients. As the interval from the time of infarction increases, the percentage of heart attacks and risks drops. The risk can be kept to an acceptable minimum due to advances in anesthesia, preoperative assessment and perioperative monitoring, and treatment of arrhythmias and hemodynamic problems. The cardiologist is a very important member of the team preparing the elderly patient for surgery (Fig. 18-1).

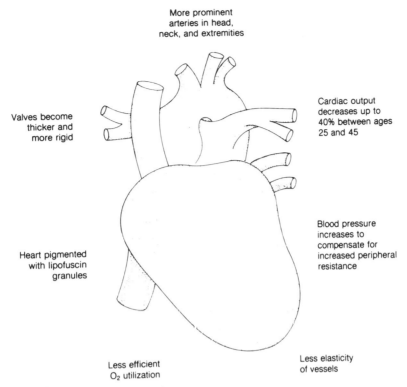

More prominent
arteries in head,
neck, and extremities

Cardiac output
decreases up to
40% between ages
25 and 45

Valves become
thicker and
more rigid

Blood pressure
increases to
compensate for
increased peripheral
resistance

Heart pigmented
with lipofuscin
granules

Less efficient
O₂ utilization

Less elasticity
of vessels

Figure 18-1. Cardiovascular changes with aging.

PULMONARY FUNCTION

There are certain changes that alter pulmonary function in the elderly patient. There is often a deformation and loss of elasticity in the thoracic cage. Many women have osteoporosis, with a decrease of 5 or 6 inches in height, and in some cases the rib cage rests on the iliac crest. This gives rise to serious problems with ventilation. Other changes in pulmonary function with age include diminution of vital capacity, breathing capacity, functional residual capacity, and pulmonary resistance. Superimposed disease, as well as the effects of heavy smoking, compound the problem. There is increased ventilation of dead space, diminished alveolar ventilation, decreased oxygen uptake, decreased arterial oxygen pressure, and reduced ventilatory reserve. Since the patient's pulmonary function is compromised, it is important that controlled respiration be performed in any surgical procedure that takes more than 1 hour. Assisted ventilation during anesthesia, and a generous oxygen supply postoperatively for a prolonged period, are prerequisites for the maintenance of undisturbed aerobic metabolism. In general, though, the usual age-related changes in arterial oxygen pressure and other tests of lung function without coincident cardiac or pulmonary disease do not appear to be severe enough to increase the risk of pulmonary complications significantly in elderly patients. It is known that pulmonary compliance, vital capacity, alveolar surface area, and resistance to infection diminish with age. Cigarette smoking and environ-

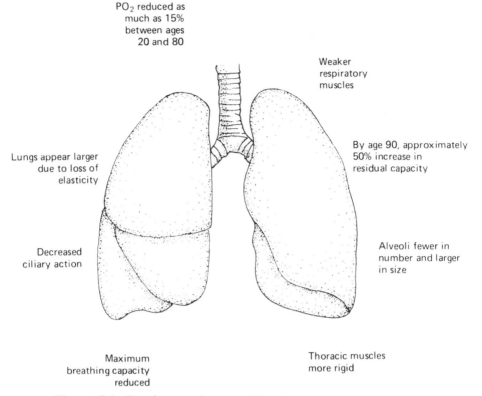

PO$_2$ reduced as much as 15% between ages 20 and 80

Weaker respiratory muscles

Lungs appear larger due to loss of elasticity

By age 90, approximately 50% increase in residual capacity

Decreased ciliary action

Alveoli fewer in number and larger in size

Maximum breathing capacity reduced

Thoracic muscles more rigid

Figure 18-2. Respiratory changes with aging.

mental pollutants significantly complicate the process, often precipitating superimposed emphysema or chronic bronchitis (Fig. 18-2).

RENAL FUNCTION

Renal function is altered after the age of 60. The glomerular filtration rate drops and changes in tubular function occur. Typical signs include gradual reduction of the glomerular filtration rate, renal plasma flow, and urine osmolality. With increasing age, the distal renal tubules become less responsive to antidiuretic hormone. The rate of creatinine clearance decreases with reduced renal function. However, serum creatinine concentrations may remain stable because of a concomitant decline in muscle mass. These changes in the glomerular filtration rate and the distal renal tubules result in a reduction in the renal clearance of medication and toxic substances. This is very important in the evaluation of the preoperative geriatric patient. Urinary tract infections are quite common in these patients. They should be evaluated and corrected before any elective surgery. During emergency surgery, the patient should be covered with the appropriate antibiotic. The consequence of the age-related decline in renal function is lack of reserve. It is easy for the geriatric patient to develop metabolic acidosis when there is a drop in the circulating volume of air or in the presence of shock. Since renal capacity after age 70 is decreased

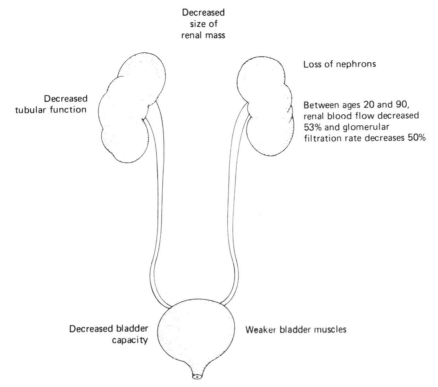

Figure 18-3. Urinary tract changes with aging.

considerably, it is important to regulate the doses of drugs and metabolites that are given to the patient. Although these patients have decreased sensitivity to antidiuretic hormone, there is concern that they may develop water retention. The elderly patient often suffers moderate dehydration due essentially to reduced water intake. Measuring the output and specific gravity, as well as the pH of the urine, is a most important postoperative consideration (Fig. 18-3).

PREOPERATIVE CARE

Advances in surgery during the past 25 years have been partially due to the development of new surgical techniques. However, improvements in preoperative and postoperative care have been equally important. Even the most superb technical skill does not obviate the necessity for excellent preoperative and postoperative management.

General Considerations

The patient and/or her family may ask about the particular risk involved. In the past, the surgeon assumed responsibility for explaining the risk, but in a society oriented to malpractice suits, the operative risk must be discussed clearly and completely in terms that the patient understands. It is important that the consent form for surgery include the state, nature, and extent of the operation. In addition, the complications that may arise from the operation should be included. If there is an alternative to the type of treatment selected, it should be explained to the patient, and the reasons for having selected a particular type of therapy should be clarified.

The operative risk is influenced by age, associated medical disorders (cardiovascular, respiratory, and metabolic), the familiarity of the surgeon with the natural history of the disease and the planned procedures, the experience of the anesthetist, the equipment and physical facilities necessary for the surgical procedure, the duration of the anesthesia for the operation, the staff of the recovery room, and the team for managing the patient's postoperative care.

The operative surgeon must assume the responsibility of caring for the patient and managing the postoperative care. Only one surgeon should write the postoperative orders.

It is important to evaluate the operative risk. The surgeon and anesthetist must institute proper and appropriate corrective measures in the preoperative period to establish optimal conditions before the surgical procedure. Training the patient preoperatively in the use of intermittent positive-pressure breathing (IPPB) is important, particularly for patients who smoke or who have a chronic lung problem. It is important that they be familiar with the technique prior to surgery so that it can be instituted when needed without delay and so that patients do not become frightened when they are told that it must be used.

In patients with suspected malignancy, the diagnostic workup and preoperative care can be carried out simultaneously. The workup is best accomplished at least 2 days prior to surgery. This must be individualized. Some patients will need hyperalimentation prior to surgery. It is therefore important for the surgeon to evaluate the status of the patient carefully at the time of the first visit so that plans can be made to expedite any preoperative treatment deemed necessary. It is the responsibility of the surgeon (shared with the surgical team) to evaluate the patient properly and to institute measures to prepare the patient for surgery. These measures must include a general evaluation of her physical status, as well as a detailed medical history.

The preoperative regimen should start before admission to the hospital. There should be a complete explanation of the workup and the anticipated surgery. It is important to reassure the patient and to prepare her psychologically. The patient who smokes should be advised to stop before admission to the hospital. A well-balanced diet is advised and iron supplements and vitamins should be prescribed. The patient should be encouraged to take long walks and to get as much exercise as possible.

Lower abdominal surgery is followed by clinically detectable abnormal pulmonary function in up to 30 percent of patients; this condition contributes significantly to postoperative morbidity. Unlike the internist, who is interested only in diagnosis and treatment, the anesthetist is primarily concerned with the pulmonary reserve of the patient and whether this reserve, if low, can be improved prior to anesthesia. Screening tests are mandatory in all patients suspected of having pulmonary abnormalities because effective preoperative treatment of airway diseases reduces the frequency of postoperative complications. It has been shown that 70 percent of patients with chronic obstructive pulmonary disease develop postoperative pulmonary complications, in contrast to 3 percent of patients who are negative symptomatically and had normal pulmonary function tests. Evaluating the pulmonary status of a patient prior to surgery does not require a battery of expensive, time-consuming tests.

HISTORY

The history is important. Knowledge of the patient's past illnesses and exposure to contagious diseases, type of work, tolerance of physical activity, and smoking habits is essential in helping to determine the patient's ventilatory reserve. It is important to question the patient about cough characteristics. Because exercise leads to increased oxygen consumption, CO_2 production, and lactic acid output, ventilatory reserve can be roughly estimated by having the patient walk briskly or climb one or two flights of stairs. If this can be accomplished without dyspnea, the respiratory reserve is obviously not seriously compromised and the following simple tests of pulmonary function will suffice.

Pulmonary Function Test

The match test establishes the ability to blow out a match held 3 inches from the patient's widely opened mouth (without pursing the lips) and correlates well with the maximum breathing capacity of more than 40 L/minute and a midexpiratory flow rate of more than 0.6 L/second. It is important that the patient not purse the lips, since an increased linear velocity due to flow through a narrow orifice may alter the results. It has been noted that 85 percent of the patients having a forced expiratory volume over the first second (FEV^1) of less than 1.6 L cannot extinguish the match. Thus, the match test, while requiring no sophisticated equipment, can select those patients in whom further evaluation is indicated.

Another test is to see how long the patient can hold her breath. The patient who is unable to do this for more than 10 seconds is considered to have a markedly reduced respiratory reserve. Additional information concerning ventilatory function as it is affected by muscular strength and/or bronchial caliber can be gained by measuring the maximum voluntary ventilation. This determines the greatest volume of air that a patient can move by the most rapid, deep breaths for a given period of time (12 seconds), expressed in liters per minute. When an obstructive element is present (as in asthma), a marked delay in expiration is seen. If a patient can exhale completely within 4 seconds, there is little obstruction present. To do this maneuver, place the stethoscope on the patient's chest and have her take a deep breath and then blow it out as hard and as fast as possible. If the patient requires more than 4 seconds to exhale, further studies should be performed prior to elective surgery. If the patient does have abnormal orifices or reduced bedside pulmonary function, some of the valuable tests that may be ordered from a pulmonary function laboratory include barometry and the measurement of flow rates. A conclusive determination of ventilatory insufficiency can be established only by arterial blood gas measurements. These will be discussed later.

General Workup

The patient admitted to the hospital for the treatment of cancer is subject to a general evaluation of physical status. A complete history is taken, and specific answers to the following questions are included: duration of present symptoms, a history of weight change, previous neoplastic disease, whether she is an identical twin, menstrual history, abortions, history of pregnancies, treatment with hormones, and previous operations. The history should be carefully reviewed for sensitivity to medications and anesthetic agents. It should be determined whether the patient is taking any long-term medication that might be a factor in anesthesia or result in an operative or postoperative complication. Antihypertensive drugs, diuretics, and tranquilizers are among the agents that may have such an influence.

Physical Examination

In the routine physical examination, pelvic and rectal examinations should be carried out and recorded. A Pap smear should be obtained and, if feasible, smears or biopsies of the endometrium should be secured. In addition to the hemoglobin, white blood cell count and differential, and red blood cell count, routine urinalysis should include the following blood chemistry factors: bleeding time, clotting time, tourniquet test, prothrombin time, prothrombin consumption time, clot retraction time, partial thromboplastin time, and a platelet count. An electrocardiogram and a chest x-ray, as well as an intravenous pyelogram, should be taken.

A patient who has cancer generally suspects the nature of her illness, for often she has been told the diagnosis or knows that such a diagnosis may be present. When entering the hospital she is apprehensive, regardless of her appearance. A well-organized admission routine can be most reassuring. The house officer and the nurse should refrain from a general discussion of neoplastic disease, methods of treatment, specific diagnosis of her case, and prognosis. The terms *tumor* or *growth* should be used in relation to her condition, not the word *cancer*. On admission, medication should be prescribed to allay apprehension, to ensure sleep, and to control pain.

Special Preoperative Orders

Prior to pelvic surgery, the general principles of preparation for laparotomy and major surgery are followed, with the addition of the procedures to be mentioned. Upon the return of the laboratory reports, any abnormal values are rectified by appropriate measures—that is, blood transfusions for anemia and hypoproteinemia and parenteral fluids for chloride, potassium, or sodium deficiencies. Because patients with advanced pelvic cancer are frequently debilitated and emaciated, hyperalimentation is being used more often in these patients and will be discussed later. In debilitated patients, preoperative blood volume studies may be carried out and blood replacement ordered as needed. Ordinarily such studies are not indicated.

Thorough preoperative bowel preparation is very important in preparing the patient suspected of having any malignancy that will necessitate bowel surgery or require removal of a tumor from the bowel. Although the mechanical bowel preparation is the most important part of the procedure, the addition of a sulfa preparation or an antibiotic may prove helpful. The bowel can be cleaned out and flattened by the administration of 50 mL of 50 percent magnesium sulfate for 2 days, followed by 45 mL of castor oil on the afternoon before surgery. Castor oil has the advantage not only of cleaning the large bowel but also of flattening the small bowel, making surgery easier.

The question of preoperative antibiotics has not been resolved but is included in some protocols. If time permits, one of the sulfa preparations in doses of up to 10 g/day for 5 to 7 days is given or a short course of neomycin and erythromycin is instituted at a rate of 1 g/hour, for a total of six to eight doses on the day before surgery. The vagina is prepared with an antibiotic suppository or one of the sulfa vaginal creams for 2 to 3 days prior to surgery. The night before surgery, the patient takes a shower, using Phisohex.

The evening before surgery, an infusion of glucose in water, or Ringer's lactate with 1000 units of heparin in each 1000 mL of infusion is started. This is allowed to run through the night, during surgery, and throughout the first few postoperative days.

Preoperative medication is given 30 to 45 minutes before the patient is taken to the operating room. Although the medication and dose are individualized for each patient, depending on her size, state of debilitation, and age, the average is usually 100 mg seconal and 0.4 mg atropine by hypodermic or 50 mg vistaril and 0.4 mg atropine or 50 mg of demerol and 0.4 mg atropine by hypodermic.

Aggressive surgery, chemotherapy, and/or radiation therapy for the treatment of pelvic malignancy has given rise to many complications. Among these are bowel fistulae with debilitation of the patient. This condition carries a high mortality. Parenteral hyperalimentation was originally used therapeutically, but more recently it has been used prophylactically to prepare patients for the anticipated treatment or in patients who have had a weight loss of 10 percent or more. Hyperalimentation is a unique form of intravenous therapy that parenterally provides all of the daily nutritional requirements. Parenteral hyperalimentation or total parenteral nutrition (TPN) is the technique of administrating enough calories, amino acids, and other nutrients to provide growth, weight gain, and normal healing. This technique has had a tremendous impact on the critically ill patient who faces slow starvation because of the inability to provide sufficient oral alimentation. If adequate nutrition is not available, the body will turn to itself for the energy necessary to remain alive. The rapid deterioration of lean tissue, muscle, and fat ensues. In the fasting state, the body breaks down approximately 75 g of protein per day (12 g of nitrogen). Liver glycogen stores are depleted within 24 hours. The catabolism of protein to glucogenic amino acids and finally to glucose is responsible for the maintenance of serum glucose in starvation. The body turns to stores of lean tissue and muscle for a source of glucose, rather than to fat stores. Therefore, a protein deficiency rapidly develops. As a result, secondary deficiencies develop in tissue synthesis, blood proteins, leukocytes, enzymes, hormones, and antibodies, with a consequent delay in healing and susceptibility to infection.

The significance of supplying adequate nutrition to the seriously ill patient is quite evident. A severe injury, sepsis secondary to surgery, or other trauma may cause an increased breakdown of body protein and/or nitrogen of up to 50 percent. Thus, when hyperalimentation is considered, the daily metabolic requirements should also be calculated as 50 percent greater than normal. Hyperalimentation should be used with extreme caution in patients with (1) impaired renal function, (2) hepatic insufficiency, and (3) diabetes. There are typical formulas for parenteral hyperalimentation, such as the protein hydrolysate solutions and free amino acid mixtures. Electrolytes, vitamins, and minerals should be added as needed. Heparin should be added to each infusion and insulin should be given as needed. It is extremely important that the regimen for each patient be individualized. It is good judgment to adjust the amount of fluid each day after the weight has been taken and the chemistries evaluated. The clinical response and appearance of the patient are also most important.

The basic guidelines for safe intravenous feeding include daily measurements of body weight and water balance. Serum electrolytes, blood sugar, and blood urea nitrogen should be measured daily until they are stabilized, and then every 2 to 3 days. The urine sugar concentration should be measured every 6 hours. Liver and kidney function should be evaluated every 2, 3, or 4 days, depending upon the stability of the patient. Periodic measurements should be made of the arterial and central venous pressures, blood acidity, and dissolved gases, which may be indicated in the management of patients with heart, kidney, liver or, metabolic disorders.

It is a cardinal rule that whenever an infection caused by a catheter is suspected, the catheter should be removed immediately and cultured. Blood cultures should be taken at the same time. It is important to avoid inducing hyperosmolar, hyperglycemic, and nonketotic diabetic coma. Adequate food intake must always be maintained and the urine carefully monitored for sugar and acetone. Insulin must be given as needed. A rapidly developing hyperglycemic syndrome may follow a too rapid infusion of glucose. The patient complains of frontal headaches, followed shortly by convulsions. Insufficient insulin and hyperglycemia complications can be avoided by preventing hyperglycemia; this is done by not allowing the blood sugar level to rise over 200 mg%. In those patients who seem to lose weight on hyperalimentation, it may be important to increase the amount of water given to the patient.

CARE OF THE PATIENT DURING SURGERY

Removal of Ascitic Fluid

During the surgical procedure, certain problems may be encountered. Two of these problems will be discussed. First, the removal of a great volume of ascitic fluid and the start of bleeding and/or oozing during the operation should receive special attention. The removal of 2 or more liters of ascitic fluid may lead to an unstable vasomotor system, which may result in shock. It is important to remove the peritoneal effusion slowly in order to prevent vasomotor instability. Therefore, enough plasma, fluids, and electrolytes should be given to correct the imbalance. In those patients in whom it is anticipated that a great amount of ascitic fluid may be removed, Ringer's lactate should be started and plasma given as needed.

Control of Intraoperative Bleeding

The second point concerns the diagnosis and therapy of hemorrhagic disorders that occur during surgery. Acute, unexpected bleeding during or shortly after an operation in the absence of an accountable surgical source is a vexing problem that may catch the surgeon unprepared, leaving him with no definite plan for management. In such an emergency, there is usually little time to run a battery of time-consuming hematologic tests. The discussion that follows is based on the assumption that the bleeding is not from a vessel but is related to a hemorrhagic disorder.

The plan of action suggested for the management of these patients is based upon three features: (1) clinical judgment, (2) rapid blood tests, and (3) selective therapy. Clinical judgment is based on a careful workup before the operation. Preexisting disorders, either congenital or acquired, would presumably be revealed by a thorough history, careful physical examination, and necessary preoperative tests. When preexisting hematologic defects have been ruled out, the causes of unexpected bleeding may be narrowed down to (1) bleeding from the surgical source, (2) fibrinolysis, (3) defibrination, (4) thrombocytopenia from massive blood transfusions, (5) anticoagulants and their antagonists, and (6) mixed clotting problems. Hemostasis involves an interdependence of the blood platelets, the coagulation mechanism, and the blood vessels. The least understood and the least studied factor in hemostasis is that involving the blood vessels. The platelet count may be normal, but there may be platelet dysfunction. This should be evaluated. In summary, clotting consists of platelet aggregation, the formation of the fibrin clot, clot retraction, and, in pathologic states, fibrinolysin. It can be assumed that blood loss sufficient to require almost constant transfusion to maintain the blood pressure is attributable to a surgical cause until proved otherwise. The circumstances before and at the time of bleeding may help to determine the cause. The onset of abnormal bleeding after massive blood transfusion is probably due to thrombocytopenia, which is associated with 5 or more units of bank blood. A precise or estimated platelet count may confirm that this is the cause of bleeding. Bleeding that follows one transfusion may be due to a mismatch of blood, and favors hemolysis and intravascular coagulation.

Rapid blood tests should be available within 10 to 15 minutes. Test tubes containing a 3.8 percent sodium citrate solution should be ready in the operating room at all times. There are five tests that can be done in all hospitals: (1) The partial thromboplastin time is a sensitive test used for identifying undiagnosed hemophilia, a variety of coagulation defects, and circulating anticoagulants. (2) Rapid estimation of platelets has helped in identifying the etiology of bleeding. (3) The bleeding time helps identify the reasons for the bleeding. In patients in whom the bleeding is prolonged beyond 4 minutes, attention must be directed to a platelet abnormality or vascular hemophilia (von Willebrand's disease). The bleeding time is normal in hemophilia. (4) A prothrombin time that is abnormal may indicate intravascular coagulation, fibrinolysis, or liver dysfunction. (5) A thrombin time that is prolonged indicates overheparinization, defibrination, or fibrinolysin.

Selective treatment depends upon the identification of all factors that contribute to the bleeding state. Because the emergency therapy available is rather limited, it is perhaps best to approach the diagnosis by selective treatment. In using this approach, one assumes that hemophilia or other severe, lifelong bleeding disorders would probably have been diagnosed preoperatively. There are indeed very few therapeutic modalities available clinically at this time: (1) Fresh frozen plasma will replace any plasma coagulation factor deficiency, as will antihemophilic plasma. (2) Platelet concentrates (or a poor second choice, fresh whole blood) will replace platelets deficient in number or function. (3) Epsilon aminocaproic acid, used to arrest fibrinolysins, probably acts by a competitive inhibition of plasminogen activators.

Disseminated Intravascular Coagulation

The triad of thrombocytopenia, hypofibrinogenemia, and lysis of blood clots within 2 hours points to the possibility of disseminated intravascular coagulation (DIC). Heparin may rapidly restore the platelet count and fibrinogen level, and thus attenuate the bleeding. After heparin has been given, the consumed clotting factors such as platelets and fibrinogen may have to be replaced in the form of plasma, platelet concentrates, or fresh blood. While the DIC is being treated, therapy for the precipitating cause (hypovolemic shock) should be carried out. In fact, DIC of short duration can be treated without heparin therapy by removing the precipitating cause. Only in profound and longstanding shock and DIC is heparin therapy necessary. Heparin therapy should be considered an adjunct to treatment but not a panacea for the patient in hypovolemic shock who needs a massive blood transfusion. In this situation, blood should be given in the quantity and at the rate that it is being lost.

INDICATIONS FOR GYNECOLOGIC SURGERY

A great majority of preoperative diagnoses in the elderly are breast cancer, genital prolapse with or without urinary incontinence, and genital cancer. Genital prolapse and pelvic and perineal relaxation are the main indications for surgery in the geriatric patient. Genital carcinoma makes up about one-third of the surgical cases, and benign gynecologic tumors contribute another 15 percent. Breast cancer is the most common cancer of the reproductive system but is not the most common cause of death from cancer among women, since cancer of the lung has surpassed it in the past year. However, since the breast is the major component of the upper genital tract, it should be considered in the operations performed on postmenopausal and geriatric patients.

By way of introduction, it may be stated that disorders of the female genital organs are not among the major causes of death. Yet they give rise to important illnesses, producing discomfort and disability, and therefore warrant treatment. Most of the gynecologic complaints of the elderly woman are related to genital prolapse. These conditions cause daily discomfort and anxiety. Contrary to the practice in younger patients, most of the operations in the elderly are carried out by the vaginal route. Vaginal hysterectomy is the preferred procedure in most cases of uterine prolapse.

Medical advances in diagnosis and treatment and a better understanding of the physiologic and pathophysiologic processes in the elderly now justify the performance of major operations in this group. Reports from numerous authors have shown that age alone is not a contraindication to surgical intervention if due regard is paid to the patient's general condition. Better anesthesia and antibiotic therapy result in greater security in the postoperative management of the geriatric patient. It is important for the physician to bear in mind that sexual activity in some women continues into very old age. Therefore, vaginal surgery should be performed with the recognition that the patient is or can be sexually active.

The operation should be kept as brief as possible, because a prolonged lithotomy position invites more complications than prolonged anesthesia. Mini-heparinization should be carried out in these patients. It should be started the evening before surgery and continued during surgery and for the first few days postoperatively.

As the geriatric population increases, women no longer accept age alone as a barrier to an active life; more elective surgery will be demanded by patients and performed by gynecologic surgeons. Contraindications to surgical intervention should not include chronologic age alone. Rather, the overall condition of the patient should be considered.

Cystourethrocele and Uterine Descensus

In general, a cystocele is a herniation of the retroureteric pouch that lies immediately behind Mercier's bar but occasionally may involve the bladder in front of it. In that case, the trigone muscle will be implicated, and since the sphincters are likely to be involved, the condition may not be cured merely by rebuilding the bladder supports. For clarification purposes, it must be stated that between the ureteric orifices there is a band of plain muscle fibers continuous with the longitudinal muscle codes of the ureters called the *interureteric ridge of Mercier's bar.* Similar fibers, known as *Bell's muscle,* commence at each ureteric orifice and, forming the lateral boundaries of the trigone, are continued in the wall of the urethral orifice. They end halfway down the urethra by merging with the longitudinal fibers on its posterior wall. There may be a prolapse of the anterior vaginal wall, resulting in prolapse of the urethra (urethrocele) or prolapse of the bladder (cystocele) or both. These conditions are not usually accompanied by stress incontinence. However, the patient may not be able to empty her bladder adequately and may have overflow incontinence. Prolapse of the anterior vaginal wall is much more common than prolapse of the posterior vaginal wall. This is because the posterior vaginal wall is well supported by muscles, while the anterior vaginal wall is not.

It is generally agreed that support of pelvic structures depends on the endopelvic fascia, uterosacral and cardinal ligaments, and levator ani muscles. This intact fascial system, with its attachment to the vaginal fornices and upper two-thirds of the lateral vaginal wall, provides a well-supported vaginal tube, which in turn is the most important structure for the uterus and the vaginal vault. Traumatic (obstetric) stretching, wear and tear of living, occupational and unusual athletic endeavors, heredity, and postmenopausal attenuation all contribute in varying degrees to the development of pelvic relaxation. Additional contributing factors that promote uterine descensus are obesity, asthma, and other chronic lung diseases.

Urethrocele is commonly associated with cystocele. A urethrocele is not a cause of urinary incontinence. It is interesting that women with large cystoceles usually never have stress incontinence. However, these patients often have repeated bouts of cystitis. A patient with a large cytocele that pulls on the trigone may give the patient a constant urge to urinate. Nothing short of surgery will correct this condition.

The essentials of diagnosis include (1) a sensation of vaginal fullness, pressure or falling out below, (2) a feeling of incomplete emptying of the bladder, with the sensation that soon after urinating, it is necessary to do so again; urinary frequency and perhaps a need to push the bladder up in order to empty the bladder completely, (3) the presence of a soft, reducible mass bulging into the anterior vagina and distending the vaginal introitus, and (4) with straining or coughing, increased bulging and descent of the anterior vaginal wall as well as the urethra.

The cystocele requires surgical repair if there are repeated bouts of cystitis or trigonitis, or if the cystocele becomes so large that the patient cannot empty her bladder adequately or the cystocele protrudes into the vaginal introitus and causes an ulceration of the vaginal wall. The presence of a large cystocele is often accompanied by repeated bouts of lower urinary tract infection. The various types of pessaries usually do not help manage cystoceles and often aggravate the situation by creating stress incontinence. Many older women tolerate large cystourethroceles and some degree of descensus without complaint, but massive procidentia (complete prolapse) is always disabling and occasionally is associated with trophic ulceration of the exposed vaginal mucosa, with kidney dysfunction caused by kinking of the displacement or pressure on both ureters. These conditions are probably best treated surgically, and even the very elderly patient can tolerate the surgery quite well. However, there are some women in whom surgery is not considered advisable. In these cases, a vaginal pessary of the Gellhorn, disc type or the Smith-Hodge type may support the uterus and bladder. Although the patient will require scheduled visits for removal and cleansing of the pessary, the need for an operation is decreased. The pessary is usually considered a measure of last resort. However, when indicated, it can be a great comfort to a very sick old woman with severe heart disease or emphysema when a procidentia is present.

Rectocele

There may be a prolapse of the posterior wall, resulting in herniation of the rectum into the vagina (rectocele)—a condition often associated with the type of constipation in which the patient experiences difficulty in emptying the herniated portion of the bowel. There may be a prolapse of the vaginal vault resulting in the falling of the uterus through the inverted vagina.

Bulging in the posterior vaginal wall and the underlying rectum through the rectovaginal septum results in a rectocele. A mild degree of rectocele (rarely causing symptoms) is usually present in all multiparous patients. A large rectocele may cause a sensation of pelvic pressure, rectal fullness, or incomplete evacuation of the stool. Occasionally a patient may find it necessary to reduce the posterior vaginal wall manually in a backward direction to evacuate the stool in the lower rectum. Distinguishing a high rectocele (including the entire rectovaginal septum) from an enterocele may sometimes be difficult. Generally with the patient straining, a rectovaginal examination will confirm the presence of abdominal contents sliding into the enterocele sac. Since pessaries are not helpful for this condition, symptomatic enteroceles should be surgically repaired.

Enterocele

An enterocele results when the small bowel pushes the peritoneum between the rectum and the vagina. The hernia of the rectovaginal peritoneal pouch through the posterior vaginal fornix is known as a *enterocele.* Elongation of the rectovaginal pouch inevitably accompanies uterine prolapse, and small intestine may be found behind the uterus in cases of procidentia. Enterocele may also occur without uterine prolapse, causing bulging of the upper part of the posterior vaginal wall that must be distinguished from a rectocele. Enterocele may occasionally occur after the uterus has been removed by either abdominal or vaginal hysterectomy, and is usually combined with some degree of prolapse of the vaginal vault.

Large enteroceles occasionally cause upper abdominal distress because of the pull on the mesentery of the bowel. The diagnosis of enterocele is made by having the patient stand and by inserting the index finger into the rectum and the thumb into the vagina and then asking the patient to strain or cough. An impulse of the small bowel is almost certain to be an enterocele. If the enterocele is large and bulges through the introitus, or if there is a great deal of abdominal discomfort, the enterocele should be repaired surgically. Since the enterocele is a true hernia, it is important to have a high ligation of the peritoneal sac, closure of the transversalis fascia, and approximation of the urosacral ligaments.

Uterine Prolapse

Prolapse of the uterus is accompanied by descent and inversion of the vaginal vault. In cases of procidentia, not only is there a prolapse of the uterus, but the bladder, the terminal part of the ureters, the tubes, ovaries, rectum, sigmoid colon, and part of the small bowel may also be included in the hernia. If the prolapse of the bladder is at all extensive, the ureters are bound to be involved. The involvement of the ureters by compression may lead to a hydroureter and hydronephrosis. It is, therefore, necessary to obtain a pyelogram in any patient with a marked prolapse.

Prolapse in at least 99 percent of the cases is the result of childbearing. In less than 1 percent, congenital weakness usually is associated with spina bifida occulta as the primary cause. Other factors, such as asthenia, malnutrition, and metabolic disturbances, may play an important part but are never the primary cause.

Three degrees of uterine prolapse are described: (1) the uterus becomes retroverted and descends in the axis of the vagina, or the cervix does not reach the introitus (first degree); (2) the cervix appears at or protrudes from the vaginal orifice (second degree); or (3) the vaginal walls are inverted to such a degree that the uterus lies outside the vulva; this complete form of uterine prolapse is known as *procidentia* (third degree). Cystocele or rectocele or both may occur without uterine descensus, but uterine prolapse is accompanied by descent of the bladder because of the close attachment of the bladder to the anterior aspect of the supravaginal cervix. The center of the rectum does not necessarily accompany uterine prolapse because the prolapsing vaginal wall easily becomes separated from the rectum.

The symptoms of prolapse can be explained by an analysis of the anatomic changes. Symptoms include a dragging sensation of the vulva and pain in the back due to the weight of the protrusion, frequency of urination, and stress incontinence. Some patients cannot empty the bladder until their fingers are placed in the vagina and the bladder is pushed forward; a type of constipation follows herniation of the rectum for the same reason. Finally, ulceration of the vaginal wall and chafed thighs develop because the organ is exposed.

Since most of these prolapses cannot be held in place with a pessary, surgery is required to correct the anatomic and functional disorders. Various techniques can be employed to correct the problem. These procedures include vaginal hysterectomy with anterior and posterior vaginal repair, the Manchester operation, and, in the very old and debilitated patient, the Le Fort operation. In selecting the best operative procedure for the individual patient, several factors must be taken into consideration. The most important of these factors are (1) the age and general physical condition of the patient, (2) the degree of descensus, (3) the condition of the cervix and the uterus, (4) the presence and degree of cystocele, and (5) the presence and degree of rectocele or enterocele. It is important for the gynecologist to be familiar with several types of procedures that will correct the problem and try to tailor the procedure to fit the needs of the patient and the extent of the prolapse.

Stress Incontinence

Urinary incontinence and lower tract disorders occur more frequently after the menopause. The lower urinary tract and the lower genital tract are of the same embryologic origin and influence each other in physiologic and pathophysiologic conditions. It is best to evaluate the patient as having a genitourinary problem.

Stress incontinence, an involuntary loss of urine due to a sudden increase in intraabdominal pressure, such as occurs with laughing, coughing or sneezing, is a common disorder. It must be distinguished from overflow incontinence, enuresis, and urge incontinence. Stress incontinence is most commonly seen in parous women, in whom it is usually the result of damage to the pelvic floor during delivery. In a few cases it may occur in nullipara, or it may appear for the first time or worsen after the menopause. About half of the patients who have a mild cystocele have stress incontinence, but this condition can also occur without evident prolapse.

The essential lesion is loss of muscular support at the vesicourethral junction combined with descent of the base of the bladder. It is possible that there is more than one defense against urinary leak. Even if the attachment of the pubococcygeous muscle to the urethra, which accounts for the posterior vesicourethral angle, is damaged, the patient may still have control if other mechanisms remain effective.

The causes of genuine stress incontinence are urethral (sphincter incompetence) or anatomic (scarred urethra—iatrogenic or traumatic—or urethral denervation). During the stress of coughing, the proximal portion of the urethra drops below the pelvic floor. The increase in intraabdominal pressure induced by coughing is transmitted to the bladder, not to the urethra. Since the urethral resistance is overcome by the increase in bladder pressure, leakage of urine results. On urodynamic evaluation there is a decreased functional length of the urethra, decreased urethral closure pressure and an abnormal response of the sphincteric mechanism in reaction to stress, assumption of the upright position, and bladder filling. Stress incontinence occurs when the urethra sags away from its attachment to the symphysis. With the descent of the bladder neck the upper urethra becomes extraabdominal, so that the normal external compression of the urethra does not occur. The urethra is also shorter and wider, so that urinary escape is easier.

Stress incontinence may appear before the menopause, but for many women it becomes increasingly distressing after the age of 60. Loosening of the pelvic supporting tissue, as well as damage caused early by vaginal delivery and aggravated by years of standing, becomes more marked after estrogen secretion decreases following menopause.

Half of the women with stress incontinence can avoid surgery if they have good pubococcygeal tone and faithfully practice pubococcygeal exercises (puckering the vagina and urethral supporting tissues in a manner comparable to that of stopping a stream of urine). The patient is advised to carry out these exercises for 2 minutes four times a day. It takes approximately 2 months before any positive results are seen in a great number of cases. The use of estrogen vaginal cream is often helpful, as are the Kegel exercises. Incontinence will recur if the exercises are not continued.

Three-fourths of the women with stress incontinence are asymptomatic after surgery to repair a cystourethrocele, with restoration of the urethra to its normal position above and behind the symphysis. This procedure is not effective if loss of urine is due to another cause. Therefore, it is most important to have a firm diagnosis before treatment is undertaken.

It is important to do a urinalysis as part of the workup, as well as an intravenous pyelogram. The best method of assessing these cases is by simultaneous radiographic cystourethrography and measurement of the intravesical pressure and urine flow—a video cystogram. A rectal catheter is used to record the intraperitoneal pressure. Another catheter in the bladder records the total bladder pressure, and subtraction of the intraperitoneal pressure gives the intrinsic bladder pressure. Since the procedure requires experience and the recording material is expensive, the patient should be referred to a urodynamic center for a workup. Treatment may be carried out either vaginally or by the suprapubic approach. In cases of cystocele, the first step in treatment is to do an anterior colporrhaphy, combined, if necessary, with other procedures for uterine prolapse. For those who are not relieved by this simple operation, a relatively simple procedure is a retropubic supporting operation such as the Marshall-Marchetti-Krantz procedure or one of its modifications.

Vulvar Carcinoma

The vulvar and vaginal tissues of every woman who is several years postmenopausal and who does not take estrogens are more or less atrophic. Shrinkage, loss of elasticity, and dryness of the vaginal mucosa are due to estrogen withdrawal. In situ lesions of the vulva can be treated with excision. If they are multicentric and not too widely scattered, the laser offers an excellent method of treatment. Vulvar cancer, unfortunately, is detected in an advanced state in many elderly women. However, if surgery is possible, it is the treatment of choice. Although the standard operation for years has been a radical vulvectomy, with superficial and deep node dissections, more recently there has been a trend toward scaling the procedure to the findings of the vulvar cancer. External x-ray therapy is being used with increasing frequency to treat the deep lymph nodes.

Vaginal Carcinoma

Primary vaginal carcinoma is uncommon, accounting for less than 1 percent of cancers of the female reproductive tract, compared to a 2, 3, or 4 percent incidence of vulvar cancer. Metastatic disease to the vagina is more common than primary carcinoma. Primary lesions are usually epidermoid, presenting as an ulcer high in the posterior vaginal fornix. Any persistent lesion in the vagina must be biopsied and the decision made regarding management. In the geriatric age group, radiation therapy is usually the treatment of choice. This may be combined external as well as intravaginal therapy.

Cervical Carcinoma

Carcinoma of the cervix is encountered less often in the postmenopausal patient than in the younger patient. The difference in incidence in these age groups is due in no small part to the widespread use of Papanicolaou smears. Even so, elderly patients should be examined for cervical carcinoma just as they are premenopausally.

After the age of 65, carcinoma of the cervix is usually treated by external therapy, as well as with a uterine applicator and vaginal colpostats. It is interesting that among white patients the observed median survival time by age is 6.8 years for all ages; for those 55 to 64 it is 5.5 years; and for those 65 and over, it is only 2.6 years. Black patients do not have as good a survival rate: for all ages, the observed median survival time is 3.5 years; for those 55 to 64 it is 2.8 years; and for those 65 and over, it is 1.8 years.

Endometrial Carcinoma

Carcinoma of the endometrium is the fifth most common cause of death from cancer in women 75 years of age or older. Diabetes mellitus, obesity, certain ovarian tumors, and hypertension are among the risk factors in cancer of the endometrium. In the elderly patient, it is very important to establish a firm diagnosis and to distinguish bleeding from the urethra, the vagina, and the anal canal. Therefore, it may be necessary to perform cystoscopy and sigmoidoscopy, in addition to investigating the reproductive tract, in order to determine the source of bleeding.

The management of endometrial carcinoma has evolved from using preoperative radiation followed by hysterectomy to doing surgery as an initial procedure and then making a decision about the type and extent of external therapy. Patients with carcinoma of the endometrium are given a radiation implant into the vagina. This has reduced the number of vaginal vault recurrences. Patients with a normal-sized uterus and well-differentiated adenocarcinoma confined to stage Ia, G1 can be treated with surgery alone, without any additional radiation therapy. In the geriatric age group, it is important to observe the patient carefully during radiation therapy. Many of these patients have diverticuli that are converted into diverticulitis during the treatment. At the first sign of symptoms, the treatment should be interrupted until the patient can be stabilized.

Ovarian Carcinoma

Ovarian cancer is the leading cause of death from gynecologic cancer. This is the most frustrating problem the physician faces in gynecology. It is not possible to make an early diagnosis, as evidenced by the fact that 60 or 70 percent of these patients are already in stages III and IV when they present for initial treatment and the 5-year survival for the truly invasive common epithelial cancer is seldom better than 25 percent.

Any woman who is more than 2 years postmenopausal and presents with a palpable ovary that is normal in size for the premenopausal years should have a careful workup. If on repeat examination this finding is confirmed, surgical exploration should be carried out without delay. This finding has been designated as the *postmenopausal palpable ovary syndrome (PMPO)*.

Treatment for carcinoma of the ovary consists of careful exploration with removal of the tubes, ovary, omentum, and appendix, with pelvic and abdominal washings before the removal of these organs begins. The surgery should be aggressive without creating inordinate morbidity and mortality. In the treatment of the common epithelial ovarian cancer, external radiation therapy is reserved for special findings. It should be used to treat supraclavicular or inguinal nodes, and if an area is found against the pelvic wall, it can be outlined by a metal clip and radiation directed to this location. However, radiation therapy has value in the management of germ cell tumors and gonadal stromal tumors. It is to be reemphasized that the geriatric patient does not tolerate radiation therapy as well as the premenopausal patient. This may be due in part to the arteriosclerotic changes in the blood vessels. These alterations produce anoxia early in the treatment phase, rendering the radiation therapy less successful in controlling the tumor. There is an increase in complications.

For the common epithelial ovarian cancer, the adjuvant therapy of choice is triple chemotherapy. The drugs most often employed are cyclophosphamide, cis-platinum, and adriamycin. In elderly patients, it is important to make sure that the ejection factor and the electrocardiogram are within normal limits before administering adriamycin and that renal function is normal before giving cis-platinum.

Carcinoma of the Fallopian Tubes

Primary cancer of the fallopian tubes is rare, constituting only 0.3 percent of all gynecologic malignancies. The mean age of occurrence is 55 years, with a range from 18 to 88 years. The disease is seldom diagnosed before laparotomy. Twenty-four percent of these tumors are bilateral. If confined to the tube, the clinical diagnosis of hydrosalpinx or pyosalpinx may be made. In this age group, however, these two conditions arc extremely rare. Only half of these patients show the classic triad of bleeding, abdominal pain, and pelvic or abdominal mass. The most common presenting symptom is abnormal bleeding or discharge. Dissemination is similar to that found with the common epithelial ovarian cancer, and the same treatment is employed for carcinoma of the tube as is used for carcinoma of the ovary. The results are about the same as those of ovarian cancer, and the follow-up is similar.

Breast Carcinoma

Carcinoma of the breast is the most common tumor that occurs in women and the second leading cause of death from cancer among women. Approximately 123,000 new cases are diagnosed each year, and for 1988, 39,900 deaths are anticipated.

Because cancer of the breast is increasing by 1 percent a year, it is important to reduce the mortality from this disease. The principles that should be followed are as follows: (1) breast examinations are an integral part of the routine gynecologic examination for all patients; (2) patients should receive instruction in lifelong periodic breast self-examination (BSE); (3) proper ambulatory surgical facilities suitable for performing breast biopsy should be developed; (4) the final diagnosis of pathology should rest on careful histologic examination of a biopsy specimen, (biopsy is necessary for all solid, three-dimensional masses); and (5) research, both basic and clinical, as well as on the etiology, diagnosis and treatment of breast cancer, is to be encouraged. Innovative screening programs for high-risk patients might be included in this effort. Residency training programs in obstetrics and gynecology should include specific instruction in early detection techniques of breast cancer. The American Cancer Society has published monographs on the technique breast examination by the physician, as well as monographs for the patient who wishes to learn BSE.

Indications for mammography have been fairly well established for the patient over age 50. The patient should have mammography every year, and definitely at intervals no longer than a year and a half. The patient should be told that it is important to do BSE, because approximately 10 percent of the cancers that show up are so-called interval cancers, appearing within a year of a negative mammography and breast examination by a physician. The patient should be advised to return in 6 months for a professional breast examination.

It is important to remove all lumps in the postmenopausal and geriatric patient. If the lumpectomy is positive on frozen section, the patient should have sampling or removal of the axillary nodes. Radiation therapy should be given to the breast; if the breast is estrogen positive and the nodes are positive, tamoxifen should be given. However, if the breast cancer has negative estrogen and progesterone receptors and the nodes are positive, chemotherapy probably should be given even though the patient is post-menopausal. There is some controversy about this, but chemotherapy is probably in the patient's best interest. However, if the patient is in a debilitated condition, chemotherapy is probably not wise. The other option for the patient, in consultation with her physician, is to have a modified radical mastectomy in which the pectoralis muscle is left intact. The indications for this are (1) lesions that are larger than 3 cm or (2) evidence of nests of tumor cells in the normal tissue surrounding the tumor on removal. The most common type of breast cancer by far is infiltrating duct cancer, and approximately 60 percent of these patients will have node involvement. Fortunately the geriatric patient usually is able to tolerate surgery on the breast with very little difficulty.

The crude 5-year survival is about 54 percent with this type of tumor.

The observed median survival time by ages for white patients is 6.6 years for all ages; for those 65 to 74 it is 5.9 years; and for those 75 and over, it is 3.3 years. The observed median survival rates by age for black patients are much more dismal. The use of chemotherapy and antiestrogen therapy is outlined in the chapter on breast tumors in the aging (Chap 11).

NONGYNECOLOGIC SURGERY

Persons who reach age 65 or more are subject to a wide range of disorders, many of which are best treated by surgery. A few decades ago, there was a tendency not to perform surgery because of the anticipated risk. However, the great progress that has been made in technology and in the training of physicians has changed the view about operating on the elderly.

The surgical principles to be applied to the aged individual, while not unlike those applied to patients in all other age groups, have many ramifications that require recognition, consideration, and meticulous management. While these may primarily involve diseases accompanying the aging process, which are often well defined, the patient's background, environment and his circumstances after surgery must be carefully analyzed.

Different problems are imposed by emergency and elective operations. Decision making by the attending physician, the family physician, the internist, and the surgeon is usually quite easy under emergency conditions. Emergencies often arise from trauma, and any procedure necessary to maintain life at that time must be carried out. This is generally accepted even if the patient's condition is precarious. The same attitude prevails in regard to such diseases as intestinal obstruction, hemorrhage from the gastrointestinal tract, or obstructive jaundice.

Elective surgery for chronic and recurrent conditions is an entirely different matter from the viewpoint of both the physician and the patient. If the physician and the patient knows what can be accomplished, there is little reluctance to accept surgery. However, when the experience of the attending physician is limited, or when the patient recalls disastrous results of surgery among members of her family and her friends, she too may be reluctant to accept surgery.

An increasing amount of surgery is being performed on the elderly. This surgery is largely elective. The two conditions that most commonly call for elective surgery are cancer in general and cancers of the gastrointestinal tract in particular. Another condition that has been controversial for some time is biliary colic. Biliary calculi are best treated conservatively, that is, nonsurgically, unless they produce symptoms or complications that are unbearable or incompatible with life. Ultrasound therapy is off in the future.

Many other general conditions also fall into this general category. Chronic peptic ulcer may weaken the patient because of malnutrition or blood loss. Hernias limit the individual's activity and pose the potential threat of obstruction. Disease of the large vessels insidiously restricts activity.

In addition to the various conditions requiring surgery, a whole new field has developed. The utilization of prosthetic devices to increase the blood supply to the lower extremities, as well as in the removal of aneurysms, is one of the most remarkable accomplishments of the past decade. Coronary bypass surgery is included in this group. Currently, many elderly patients are having replacements of hip and knee joints.

In acute abdomen in the elderly, the most frequent associated conditions are cholecystitis, appendicitis, diverticulitis, intestinal obstruction, mesenteric thrombosis, and massive gastrointestinal hemorrhage. These conditions all require immediate attention. If there is any hesitancy on the part of the patient or the family, they must be asked to weigh the accepted surgical morbidity and mortality of surgery against the almost certain mortality that would result from doing nothing. In evaluating the patient, the chronologic age is not nearly as important as the physiologic age.

SUMMARY

Gynecologic surgical treatment in the geriatric patient is possible. There are two important aspects of this problem: the management of the acute surgical problem and the decision to perform elective surgery. There is no question that in the patient with an acute surgical problem the treatment must be carried out and all of the risks accepted. The procedure should be to correct the immediate life-threatening problem without performing any additional surgery at that time. With the patients selected for elective surgery, there is an opportunity to evaluate their status, to correct any imbalances, and to regulate the medication, and to have an internist with special expertise in the care of the geriatric patient in attendance.

Often the geriatric patient is incapacitated by a large prolapse. Fortunately, the patient is usually well able to tolerate the vaginal surgery needed to correct it. Once the prolapse has been repaired, the patient has more mobility and gets greater enjoyment out of life. Dealing with cancer often requires a greater degree of judgment. However, the approach should be as radical as needed without introducing a great deal of morbidity and mortality. The physician must be conscious at all times that the risk of dying from cancer is not as great as that of dying from a stroke or a heart attack. This is particularly so if there is blood loss, a drop in blood pressure, or an increase in infection.

In general, the geriatric patient is able to tolerate operations that in the past would have been impossible. The support teams, the intensive care units, the hyperalimentation teams, the metabolic teams, better anesthesia, and improved technology have added a new dimension to the lives of geriatric patients who need surgery.

REFERENCES

Adkins, R. B., J. M. Whiteneck, and E. Woltering. 1984. Carcinoma of the breast in the extremes of age. *South. Med. J.* 77:554.

Atack, D. B., J. A. Nisker, H. H. Allen, et al. 1986. CA 125 surveillance and second look laparotomy in ovarian carcinoma. *Am. J. Obstet. Gynecol.* 154:287.

Barber, H. R. K. 1982. *Ovarian Carcinoma: Etiology, Diagnosis and Treatment,* 2nd ed. Masson Publishing USA, New York.

————. Geriatric gynecology, in: *Clinical Geriatrics,* 3rd ed. (J. Rossman, ed.). J. B. Lippincott Co., Philadelphia, p. 364.

Barber, H. R. K., and E. A. Graber. 1971. The PMPO syndrome (postmenopausal palpable ovary syndrome). *Obstet. Gynecol.* 38:921.

Bille-Brahe, N. E., and J. H. Eickhoff. 1980. Measurement of central haemodynamic parameters during preoperative exercise testing in patients suspected of arteriosclerotic heart disease: Value in predicting postoperative cardiac complications. *Acta Chir. Scand.* 502:38.

Birnbaum, S. J. 1973. Rational therapy for the prolapsed vagina. *Am. J. Obstet. Gynecol.* 115:411.

Blake, R., and J. Lynn. 1976. Emergency abdominal surgery in the aged. *Br. J. Surg.* 63:956.

Boley, S. J., A. DiBiase, I. J. Brandt, et al. 1979. Lower intestinal bleeding in the elderly. *Am. J. Surg.* 137:57.

Boyd, J. B., B. Bradford, Jr., and A. L. Watne. 1980. Operative risk factors of colon resection in the elderly. *Ann. Surg.* 192:743.

Brandt, L. J. 1984. *Gastrointestinal Disorders in the Elderly.* Raven Press, New York.

Cartwright, P. S., D. E. Pittaway, H. W. Jones III, et al. 1984. The use of prophylactic antibiotics in obstetrics and gynecology. A review. *Obstet. Gynecol. Surv.* 39:137.

Cortese, A. F., and G. N. Cornell. 1975. Radical mastectomy in the aged female. *J. Am. Geriatric Soc.* 23:337.

DelGuercio, L. R. M., and J. Cohn. 1980. Monitoring operative risk in the elderly. *JAMA* 243:1350.

Elkin, M., et al. 1974. Ureteral obstruction in patients with uterine prolapse. *Radiology* 110:289.

Fergal, D. W., and F. W. Blarsdell. 1979. The estimation of surgical risk. *Med. Clin. North Am.* 63:1131.

Glenn, F. 1973. Pre- and postoperative management of elderly surgical patients. *J. Am. Geriatric Soc.* 21:385.

————. 1983. Surgical principle for the aged patient, in: *Clinical Aspects of Aging,* (W. Reichel, ed.). Williams & Wilkins Co., Baltimore. 1976.

Gray, L. A. 1983. *Vaginal Hysterectomy,* 3rd ed. Charles C. Thomas Co., Springfield, Ill.

Hall, W. L., A. I. Sobel, C. P. Jones, et al. 1976. Anaerobic postoperative pelvic infections. *Obstet. Gynecol. 30:1.*

Herbsman, H. J., Feldman, J. Seldera, et al. 1981. Survival following breast cancer surgery in the elderly. *Cancer* 47:2358.

Hoffman, J. W. 1982. Gynecologic disorders in the geriatric patient: Geriatric gynecology. *Postgrad. Med.* 71:38.

———. 1983. The diagnosis and treatment of gynecologic disorders in elderly patients. *Compr. Ther.* 9:54.

Hofmeister, F. J. 1973. Prolapsed vagina (editorial). *Obstet. Gynecol.* 42:773.

Johnson, J. C. 1983. The medical evaluation and management of the elderly surgical patient. *J. Am. Geriatric Soc.* 31:621.

Josif, C. S., and Z. Bekassy. 1984. Prevalence of genitourinary symptoms in late menopause. *Acta Obstet. Gynecol. Scand.* 63:257.

Kessler, H. J., and J. Z. Seton. 1978. The treatment of operable breast cancer in the elderly female. *Am. J. Surg.* 135:664.

Linn, B. S., and J. Jensen. 1983. Age and immune response to a surgical stress. *Arch. Surg.* 118:405.

Linn, B. S., M. W. Linn, and N. Wallen. 1982. Evaluation of results of surgical procedures in the elderly. *Ann. Surg.* 195:90.

Macer, G. A. 1978. Transabdominal repair of cytocele, a 20 year experience, compared with the traditional vaginal approach. *Am. J. Obstet. Gynecol.* 131:203.

McKeithen, W. S. 1975. Major gynecologic surgery in the elderly female. *Am. J. Obstet. Gynecol.* 59:63.

Mohr, D. M. 1983. Estimation of surgical risk in the elderly: A correlative review. *J. Am. Geriatric Soc.* 31:99.

Nichols, D. H. 1978. Effects of pelvic relaxation on gynecologic urologic problems. *Clin. Obstet. Gynecol.* 21:759.

Panayiotis, G. A., Ellenbogen, and S. Grunstein. 1978. Major gynecologic surgery in the aged. *J. Am. Geriatric Soc.* 26(10):459.

Porges, R. F. 1980. Changing indication for vaginal hysterectomy. *Am. J. Obstet. Gynecol.* 136:153.

Schlueter, D. P. 1985. Pulmonary evaluation, in: *Operative Gynecology,* 6th ed. (R. F. Mattingly and J. D. Thompson, eds.). J. B. Lippincott Co., Philadelphia, p. 68.

Talbot, G. H., and N. J. Ehrenkranz. 1984. Nosocomial pneumonia in the surgical patient. *Infections Surg.* 3:557.

Warshaw, G. A. 1983. Hospital care for elderly patients, in: *Advances in Research,* vol. 7 (G. I. Maddox, ed.). Duke University Center for the Study of Aging and Human Development, Durham, N.C., p. 3.

Wiedermann, H. P., M. P. Matthay, and R. H. Matthay. 1984. Cardiovascular-pulmonary monitoring in the intensive care unit: Parts 1 and 2. *Chest* 5:537.

Wingate, M. B. 1982. Geriatric gynecology. *Primary Care* 9:53.

Yancik, R., L. G. Ries, and J. W. Yates. 1986. Ovarian cancer in the elderly: An analysis of surveillance, epidemiology and end results program data. *Am. J. Obstet. Gynecol.* 154:639.

Yarnell, G. W., and G. J. Voyle. 1981. The prevalence and severity of urinary incontinence in women. *J. Epidemiol. Commun. Health* 35:71.

Yates, M. J. 1975. An abdominal approach to the repair of posthysterectomy vaginal inversion. *Br. J. Obstet. Gynaecol.* 82:817.

19 Psychologic Problems and Mental Disorders

INTRODUCTION

The long life expectancy of humans is a decidedly modern achievement. The world population has reached 5 billion people. While the total population of the United States increased 3 times from 1900 to 1980, the number of persons aged 65 and over increased 7 times. This trend is expected to continue. Persons 65 and over now constitute about 10 percent of the U.S. population (about 22 million). Over the next 50 years, the proportion is expected to be between 12 and 16 percent. If zero population growth is reached within the next 50 or 60 years, there will be one person over 65 for every 1.5 persons under 20; the ratio is now 1:4. About one-third of the older population is very old, 75 years or more. This proportion will stay about the same for the foreseeable future if mortality rates remain constant. If they do, there will be about 12 million very old persons by the year 2000. If mortality rates decline, however, the number of very old persons may be as high as 16 or 18 million.

A 65-year-old man can now expect, on the average, to live to 78; a 65-year-old woman, to 82. By the year 2000, the life expectancy for 65-year-olds may increase by another 2 to 5 years. It is therefore important to assess the psychologic problems and mental disorders that occur among the elderly and try to separate minor problems caused by stress, environment, and the use of drugs from more serious conditions.

In today's youth-oriented society, most older adults are considered senile or psychotic. Actually, however, researchers estimate that only about 5 percent are psychotic or have severe intellectual impairment. About 20 percent have measurable memory impairment and approximately 20 percent have a psychologic disorder ranging from mild neurosis to psychosis.

It is vitally important to make an accurate diagnosis of the problem. The far-reaching changes accompanying aging probably have some psychologic effect. The elderly patient faces retirement, with an attendant loss of status and independence, and often the loss of a spouse, complicated by sensory loss and probably disease, pain, surgery, and, in certain instances, institutionalization. The strength of the person's coping mechanisms determines whether a serious psychologic problem will be precipitated. There is little doubt that the cumulative effect of many simultaneous problems may overwhelm even an emotionally strong, healthy person.

FUNCTIONAL DISORDERS

Researchers estimate that 15 to 20 percent of people over age 65 have some psychologic problem. The most common psychologic disorders affecting the elderly are functional disorders. The problems that are assumed to have an emotional basis, such as depression, neurosis, paranoia, and schizophrenia, are included in this group. Older adults probably experience depression more frequently than any other mental disorder. The major signs and symptoms include profound sadness, insomnia with early morning waking, anorexia and weight loss, helplessness, slow thinking, low self-esteem, self-reproach, decreased activity level, and hypochondria. These emotional disorders may give rise to psychosomatic physical symptoms. Most often, however, rather than causing a specific mental problem, old age may only intensify an inherent personality weakness or deficit.

It is often difficult to identify psychologic and mental problems in the elderly. The physician may attribute some of these changes to aging when in reality they are indications of physical illness, personality factors, and social-culture effects. In elderly persons, personality characteristics in a social milieu may prove to be as significant as laboratory results. It is important not to stereotype the elderly. It is obvious that maintaining good physical and mental health depends on many factors and forces, and the relative importance of any one of these varies from individual to individual. It is not sound judgment to predict an inevitable decline and a poor prognosis simply because a person is chronologically old.

In the postmenopausal patient, there are many nonspecific symptoms that have been rightfully or wrongfully identified with the menopausal age. These include fatigue, irritability, depression, headache, dizziness, palpitations, bloating, apprehension, insomnia, altered ego, apathy, difficulty concentrating, anxiety, tension, dyspnea, emotional lability, and feelings of inadequacy. Menopause is often identified with depression. It has been observed that treating patients in the immediate postmenopausal period with estrogen replacement therapy stops the flushes, flashes, insomnia, and night sweats. With a good night's rest, the patient often loses her depression, fatigue, irritability, and headaches. These symptoms may also occur in the geriatric patient, but they are extremely rare.

Medical History

If a problem has been reported, it is very important to get a good history. In taking a history from an older patient, it is extremely important to show special sensitivity. The patient should be made as comfortable as possible and an attempt made to establish a good relationship. In taking a history, one should begin by making a general observation about the overall behavior and physical appearance of the patient. The patient must also be addressed in respectful terms, and it is important to ask whether the patient wants to be addressed as "Mrs.," "Miss," or by the first name. If the patient is hard of hearing, it is important to sit in front of her so that she can read your lips as well as listening to what you are saying. The patient may take extra time to respond, and this should be permitted. Rather than force the history and fatigue the patient, it is better to determine how much can be obtained at one time and perhaps take the history in two or more sessions.

Patients often have a decrease in short-term memory with age, but they are able to verbalize fairly well. Questions may have to be reasked or restated in order to obtain a clear understanding of the mental and psychologic orientation of the patient. Some patients are poor historians. If this problem is detected, the history should be obtained from a relative or a close friend.

Elderly patients who seem to be confused or disoriented, or who have memory loss, slowed reaction time, or anxiety, may be suffering from the use of alcohol or drugs prescribed for physiologic or health purposes.

It is important to get a very good family history, including the age at which various members of the patient's first-degree blood relatives died and of what cause. In evaluating the problem, one must also know what medications have been and are being taken. The older patient metabolizes medication differently from the younger one, and there may be slowed metabolism due to decreased liver and kidney function, which makes the older patient more susceptible to toxicity from these drugs. The elderly tolerate sedatives, tranquilizers, and sleeping pills very poorly, leading to a variety of mental problems. Elderly patients often take laxatives, mineral oil and enemas, which can create electrolyte imbalances, and perhaps even malnutrition, by interfering with the absorption of food and vitamins. Alcohol use is also important to determine.

Elderly patients are very prone to eat a poor diet, particularly if they live alone. The poor diet often results in anemia, the cause of which cannot be determined on careful workup. Therefore, it is important to know the number of meals the patient eats, the type of food, and whether there is any difficulty in chewing and swallowing.

Elderly patients often have many gastrointestinal problems, ranging from constipation to diarrhea. It is important to determine the bowel habits of the patient and whether there has been any change in the last few months.

Urinary problems are fairly common in the elderly. Patients with a marked prolapse often have ureteral dilatation, with changes in their chemistry and elevated blood urea nitrogen. It is therefore important to determine whether the patient has frequency or burning or is unable to empty her bladder adequately.

By taking a careful history, it is possible to identify a physical problem that is being confused with a psychologic or mental problem. Older adults make up 16 to 25 percent of the suicides in this country. They have a suicide rate 40 to 60 percent higher than that of the total population. It is very important to keep this in mind when evaluating the patient.

Loneliness and depression are common emotional disturbances among the elderly. This may lead to suicide. The diagnostic criteria for a major depressive episode include several characteristics. Among these are a sad or depressed mood in which the elderly person complains of being very tired or down in the dumps. The patient may have a poor appetite, insomnia, loss of energy, psychomotor agitation, loss of interest or pleasure in usual activities, a feeling of self-reproach or inappropriate guilt, diminished ability to think or concentrate, and suicidal thoughts.

Diagnosis in the elderly is not easy. Many of the symptoms of depression are somatic. However, it should be remembered that depressive symptoms often accompany medical illnesses and, in fact, are a direct result of these illnesses. Therefore, it is important to make an accurate diagnosis.

Treatment

Once the diagnosis has been made, the major disorders in late life are predictably treatable. The tricyclic antidepressants can reverse the symptomatology in over 70 percent of affected patients. It is important to start with a small dose and work up to the level needed. It is imperative to bear in mind that the elderly do not tolerate medication as well as younger patients. The use of electric shock therapy is generally to be condemned because of the age of the patient, as well as any health problem that may be present. However, occasionally it is necessary to accept the risk in order to overcome the antidepressant-resistive severe depression that may exist.

Many of these elderly patients can be helped by a clinical psychologist, while others need psychiatric treatment. Often the greatest need of the elderly is to have a sympathetic listener. Besides depression, other types of neurosis can be observed in elderly persons, which often represent a reaction to the stresses peculiar to this period of life. Depression and physical disease often occur simultaneously. The clinician must always bear in mind the possibility of multiple etiologies when evaluating behavioral changes in old people. The patient with physical or mental impairment may communicate the need for attention and guidance with hypochondriacal complaints. Somatic distress may also be an expression of social and economic problems. Dissociative reactions may symbolize a denial of serious disability. Depression has often been called *pseudodementia* and must be differentiated from dementia. In depression there is often a rapid onset that can usually be accurately dated; cognitive function fluctuates markedly, the mood is consistently depressed, disabilities are exaggerated, and the patient doesn't know answers that are typical on the mental status examination. On the other hand, dementia is slow and indeterminate, while mental impairment is relatively stable. The mood is typically shallow and fluctuating.

CLINICAL ANXIETY

The elderly often present with clinical anxiety, anxiety with associated depressive symptoms, anxiety with associated cardiovascular symptoms, and anxiety with associated depression. After a careful workup to rule out more serious disorders, treatment can be instituted. Alprazolam (Xanax) is effective for the treatment of clinical anxiety and anxiety with associated depressive symptoms. It is well tolerated. Mild, transient drowsiness is the most commonly reported side effect. It does not cause cardiotoxicity and does not interact with propranolol, a commonly prescribed medication in the elderly. Most patients are controlled with 0.25 to 0.5 mg t.i.d.

PARANOID REACTIONS

Paranoid reactions may occur in the geriatric patient. These patients usually have a lifelong pattern of suspiciousness and aloofness or denial of intellectual or physical impairment. The geriatric patient with a failing memory may deny this fact but claim that things have been stolen. This often gives rise to other problems. The elderly suffering from loss of hearing often demonstrate a paranoid reaction. These patients often state that people whisper behind their back or that there is a plot to do away with them or place them in a mental hospital. A loss of hearing has two components—an inability to perceive and an inability to comprehend or integrate sounds, or both. Unless the patient is aware of this condition, psychiatric problems can arise and become irreversible. It is often difficult for a physician to differentiate hearing problems from confusion and disorientation, particularly if the patient is uncommunicative. This situation also makes it difficult to examine a patient for aphasia if there is a hearing defect. One way to identify a hearing defect is to observe the patient and note whether she functions adequately but appears disoriented. Patients with strong personalities and those who are very stubborn may have these traits aggravated by a hearing defect. It is a difficult situation, particularly if the elderly person is living with her family, with children and grandchildren present.

HYPOCHONDRIASIS

This is not an uncommon disorder in the elderly. It probably arises from a sense of decreased effectiveness and increased deterioration, as well as a decrease in the ability to communicate and interact with others. These people use hypochondriasis to transfer anxiety from other areas of concern to the body, and occasionally use this method to relate to members of the family who have physical ailments. Since most elderly people have at least one chronic illness, it is sometimes difficult to determine whether this is a hypochondriacal preoccupation or whether it represents a true disease state. The elderly suffering from hypochondriasis do not seem to be suffering, despite their frequent report of physical symptoms. They direct their anger towards others, and often in the physician's office get into an argument with the person who has brought them. They are difficult to treat because they complain of the side effects of medication. In reviewing their past medical history, it is not uncommon to find that in the midlife crisis there was a physical problem. These patients have some interference with social participation, but they not totally dysfunctional. Those with hypochondriasis can usually be separated from those with depression by their difference in response. Unlike the patient with hypochondriasis, who directs her anger toward other people, the patient with depression usually directs the anger toward herself.

ORGANIC BRAIN SYNDROME AND DEMENTIA

It is difficult to make a sharp differentiation between normal aging and very mild senility. Physicians sometimes consider these conditions as existing on a continuum that leads to organic mental disorder. The basic symptoms of organic brain disorders are impairment of orientation, memory, and judgment. Cognitive impairments including poor comprehension, calculation, and learning, as well as emotional lability and shallow affect, are also included in this group. These may occur in any age group.

Dementia is usually defined as a more or less sustained decline from a previously attained level of intellectual function. When this occurs in elderly persons, the diagnosis of *senile dementia* is made, and this term is sometimes used synonymously with the term *organic brain syndrome.* Of the various forms of dementia, one of the most feared is Alzheimer's disease. Multi-infarct dementia results in widespread death of brain tissue and is irreversible.

Alzheimer's Disease

Alzheimer's disease was first described in November 1906 at a meeting of the Southwest German Society of Alienists, at which Alois Alzheimer recounted the story of a 51-year-old patient. The woman first suffered loss of memory and disorientation, later was subject to depression and hallucinations, and progressed to severe dementia. At necropsy the patient's brain showed severe atrophy, and the cerebral cortex was marked by clumping and distortion of fibrous proteins and nerve fibers. Alzheimer called these jumbles of filaments *neurofibrillar tangles,* and they have since become the hallmark of Alzheimer's disease. Because it was a middle-aged woman whom Alzheimer described, and because other reports of similar findings in middle-aged patients soon followed, Alzheimer's disease is considered a presenile form of dementia. It can be confused with other dementias such as multiinfarct dementia, depression, Parkinson's disease, and a variety of infectious problems and drug-induced states. Because some of these diseases are reversible with treatment, it is extremely important to make an accurate diagnosis.

The CT scan has gained widespread acceptance as a valuable diagnostic tool in identifying structural defects, and a new technique, positron emission tomography (PET), is fast becoming known for its unique ability to monitor the biochemical activity of the human brain. Nuclear magnetic resonance also promises to make a significant contribution to the diagnosis of Alzheimer's-type senile dementia.

Many interesting studies of Alzheimer's disease are underway. Investigators are focusing on six conceptual models of the disease. The genetic model is based on the fact that there are families in which the incidence of Alzheimer's disease is unusually high, indicating the possibility of a hereditary factor. The incidence of Down's syndrome and lymphomas is also increased in families with a history of Alzheimer's disease. The association with the former disorder is especially relevant, as neuropathic changes identical to those in Alzheimer's disease develop in Down's syndrome patients who reach middle age.

Three pathologic signs of Alzheimer's disease have prompted researchers to base their work on the abnormal protein model. These signs are neurofibrillar tangles within neurons, the amyloid that surrounds and invades cerebral blood vessels, and the amyloid-rich plaques that replace degenerating nerve terminals. Each reflects an accumulation of proteins not normally found in the brain. In 1907, Alzheimer noted that the tangles take up silver stains that render them visible under the light microscope.

Alzheimer's disease patients often do not look sick. They never show signs of brain infection, such as fever or white blood cells and protein in the cerebrospinal fluid. But two other brain diseases, serapie and Creutzfeldt-Jakob disease, suggest that an infectious agent may be involved. Serapie is a slowly progressive, invariably fatal brain disease that is widespread in sheep and goats. Creutzfeldt-Jakob disease is a disease that usually affects people aged 55 to 70; it causes progressive dementia and, about a year after onset, disturbances in posture, vision, and control of movement. One of the theories behind these diseases—and suspected in Alzheimer's disease—is that a hidden or slow virus is responsible for the damage to the brain, producing symptoms only after a long period.

The toxin model is based—and some investigators believe—that salts of aluminum may contribute to the development of Alzheimer's disease. Such salts are present in drinking water or may be added to foods and drugs, including some processed cheeses, antiacids, and buffered aspirin. They may also be released from aluminum cans and utensils. This is a weak hypothesis because many people have been exposed to massive amounts of aluminum in the environment without developing Alzheimer's disease, and Alzheimer's victims have not been found to have experienced extraordinary exposure.

The blood flow model has been proposed by investigators who are studying the flow of blood in the brain. In persons with senile dementia, there is a definite overall decrease in the amount of blood reaching the brain. The obvious question is whether this decrease accounts for the disease or is secondary to it.

The acetylcholine model is receiving attention because it appears that in Alzheimer's disease neurons that secrete acetylcholine are selectively destroyed. Acetylcholine is one of a mere handful of chemical messengers in the brain. If cholinergic and, to a lesser extent, other neurotransmitter systems are selectively destroyed by Alzheimer's disease, the question is whether anything can be done about it.

One additional area that merits investigation for a possible relationship to Alzheimer's disease is the immune system. A great number of autoimmune disorders are now being identified. A variety of antigens and other substances constantly challenge the body's defenses and sometimes cause it to overrespond with an autoimmune disorder. Since autoimmunity plays such an important role in many degenerative disorders, such as rheumatoid arthritis and other collagen diseases, it must be given serious consideration as a contributing cause in Alzheimer's disease. No treatment of the basic disease process has yet proven effective for any primary dementia. However, some drugs may prove to be helpful. These include deanol, physostigmine, the ergoloid mesylates, and the neuropeptides.

Parkinsonism

Parkinsonism is a common condition in old people. It affects the central nervous system's ability to control body movement. It is most common in males and occurs frequently in the fifth decade of life. Although the exact cause is unknown, the disease is thought to be associated with a history of metalic poisoning, encephalitis, and cerebral vascular disease—especially arteriosclerosis—in older people.

Differential Diagnosis. Classic parkinsonism is the condition of paralysis agitans that commonly occurs in middle life, but which may have its onset in old age. The fully developed picture is one of akinesia, tremor, rigidity, and sialorrhea, with paucity of expression.

Postencephalitic parkinsonism. This is now becoming increasingly rare, but is still found in a small number of elderly people who have had it most of their lives. Postencephalitic parkinsonism was a complication of encephalitis or sleeping sickness, of which there were several epidemics in the years following 1919. Classic signs are present, as well as a number of special features—oculogyric crisis, sweating crisis, and marked skeletal deformity, such as scoliosis, wrist, and hand deformities.

Drug-induced parkinsonism. This is common in the elderly, particularly due to phenothiazines and tricyclic antidepressants. Secondary parkinsonism occurs in a few syndromes, such as the Shy-Drager syndrome.

Arteriosclerotic parkinsonism. This has been referred to as a clinical rather than a pathologic entity. The common clinical features are rigidity, akinesia, and loss of expression, whereas tremor, sialorrhea, and other autonomic effects associated with paralysis agitans are not usually found.

A faint tremor that progresses over a long period of time may be the first clue. The tremor is reduced when the patient attempts a purposeful movement. Muscle rigidity and weakness develop, witnessed by drooling, difficulty in swallowing, slow speech, and a monotone. The face of the patient has a mask-like appearance, and the skin is moist. Appetite frequently increases, and emotional instability may be demonstrated. A characteristic sign is a shuffling gait, with the trunk leaning forward. The rate of the patient's gait increases as he or she walks, and the patient may not be able to stop voluntarily. As the disease progresses, the patient may be unable to ambulate.

Parkinsonism is treated with L-dopa and its associated preparations. Effective treatment by L-dopa is limited mainly by nausea and vomiting. For these reasons, preparations with L-dopa and dopa-decarboxylase inhibitors are now widely used in geriatric practice. The dopa-decarboxylase inhibitor diminishes the peripheral breakdown of L-dopa to dopamine outside the central nervous system, thereby allowing a higher concentration of L-dopa (and so dopamine) within the central nervous system. Lower doses of L-dopa, which will lead to fewer side effects, may thus be used. The main side effects of L-dopa are those arising within the central nervous system, particularly dyskinesia (that is, bizarre movements).

L-dopa and similar drugs can precipitate severe confusion, sometimes with hallucinations, and they should be used cautiously in any old person already mildly confused. Hiccups and hematuria are two other unwanted side effects.

L-dopa should not be used in conjunction with any psychotrophic drugs that affect cerebral amine metabolism.

Anticholinergic, antiparkinsonian drugs (Benzhexol, Orphenadrine, etc.) have long been used in treating parkinsonism, but are not striking in their effect. The elderly are very sensitive to Benzhexol, which sometimes causes an acute confusional disturbance. An important alternative is to use Amantadine either alone or in combination with one of the preceding drugs.

As stated earlier, arteriosclerotic parkinsonism is a clinical rather than a pathologic entity. Its effects are not susceptible to treatment with any of the preceding antiparkinsonian drugs.

Since tension and frustration will aggravate the symptoms, it is important to offer psychologic support and minimize emotional upsets. Teaching is beneficial in helping patients and their families gain realistic insight into the disease. Patients and their families should be educated to the fact that the disease progresses slowly and that therapy can minimize disability. Although intellectual functioning is not impaired by this disease, speech problems and helpless appearance of patients may cause others to underestimate their mental abilities. This can be extremely frustrating and degrading to the patient who may react by becoming depressed or irritable. Communication and mental stimulation should be encouraged on a level that the patient always enjoyed.

USE OF MEDICINES BY OLDER PEOPLE

It is important to instruct the patient in the proper use of drugs. Family members should be involved in the conversation when drugs are prescribed for the elderly. Drugs sometimes produce effects that resemble personality changes or developing senility. Drugs can be wonderful tools for the care of patients of all ages. In fact, the growth of the over-65 population can be attributed, at least in part, to the availability of effective medicines and vaccines. But in older adults, drug use may involve a greater risk, especially when several drugs are taken at once.

People over 65 make up 11 percent of the U.S. population, yet they take 20 percent of all prescription drugs sold in this country. As a group, older people tend to have more long-term illnesses—arthritis, diabetes, high blood pressure, heart disease—than younger people. Because they often have a number of diseases or disabilities at the same time, it is very common for them to be taking many different drugs simultaneously.

Drugs taken by geriatric patients act differently from the way they do in young or middle-aged people. This is probably the result of the normal changes in body makeup that occur with age. As the body grows older, the percentage of water and lean tissue (mainly muscle) decreases, while the percentage of fat tissue increases. These changes can affect the length of time a drug stays in the body and the amount absorbed by body tissues.

The kidneys and liver are two important organs responsible for breaking down and removing most drugs from the body. With age, these organs begin to function less efficiently, and thus drugs leave the body more slowly. This may account for the fact that older people tend to have more undesirable reactions to drugs than do younger people. It is important to check on the intake of drugs by the elderly. These include not only prescription medicine but over-the-counter medicines as well. Drugs prescribed by a physician are usually more powerful and have more side effects than those sold over the counter. Yet many over-the-counter drugs contain strong agents, and when large amounts are taken, they can equal the dose of that normally available by prescription. Some substances, including vitamins, laxatives, cold remedies, antacids, and alcohol, can lead to serious problems if used too often or in combination with certain other drugs.

The elderly are at risk of reduced clearance and resulting accumulation of the parent drug and active metabolites of the benzodiazepines, flurazepan, and diazepan. The pharmakokinetics of oxazepan are not altered by age or liver disease, apparently making its use in the elderly relatively safe. However, the elimination half-life of oxazepan is increased from 10 to 25 hours in patients with renal insufficiency. Before passing judgment on the mental status of the patient, it is most important to evaluate the drugs that the patient is taking.

SUMMARY

In evaluating the elderly patient with a psychologic problem, it is important to realize that the person's sociologic, economic, psychologic, and physiologic factors are all interrelated. It takes a clinician with great diagnostic acumen to analyze the situation and to identify the psychologic problem precisely.

Senility is not a normal sign of growing old; in fact, it is not even a disease. *Senility* is the term commonly used to describe a large number of conditions with an equally large number of causes, many of which respond to prompt treatment. The symptoms of senility include serious forgetfulness, confusion, and certain other changes in personality and behavior. While physicians and patients alike once routinely dismissed these symptoms as the incurable effects of old age, this is not necessarily true. There are small memory lapses at all ages. Slight confusion or occasional forgetfulness throughout life may only signify an overload of facts in the brain's storehouse of information.

Mental decline in old age may be called *dementia, organic brain disorder, chronic brain syndrome, arteriosclerosis, cerebral atrophy,* or *pseudodementia.* It is important to recognize that some of the problems generally referred to under the medical description of senile dementia can be treated and cured, while others can only be treated, without hope of restoring lost brain function. Thus a complete, careful investigation of the source of the symptoms is necessary.

Diagnosis is very important in determining whether the elderly have irreversible changes or not. The most common incurable forms of mental impairment in old age are multiinfarct dementia and Alzheimer's disease. Multiinfarct dementia is caused by a series of minor strokes that result in widespread death of brain tissue. This condition accounts for about 20 percent of the irreversible cases of mental impairment. In Alzheimer's disease, changes in the nerve cells of the outer layer of the brain result in the death of many cells. Some 50 to 60 percent of all elderly patients with mental impairment have Alzheimer's disease.

Since many reversible conditions may mimic these disorders, a firm diagnosis is very important. A minor head injury, high fever, poor nutrition, or adverse drug reactions can temporarily upset the normal activity of extremely sensitive brain cells. If left untreated, such medical emergencies can result in permanent damage to the brain and possibly even death.

It is important to differentiate organic from emotional problems. Emotional problems can be mistakenly confused with irreversible brain disease. Depression, loss of self-esteem, loneliness, anxiety, and boredom can become more common as elderly persons face retirement, the death of relatives and friends, and other such crises. Unfortunately, these crises may occur at the same time.

A thorough workup is most important in persons suspected of having Alzheimer's disease and multiinfarct dementia. It is important to do a thorough physical, neurologic, and psychiatric evaluation. This includes a complete medical examination, as well as tests of the patient's mental state and highly specific tests such as a brain scan. The brain scan is useful in that it can rule out a curable disorder. The brain scan can also reveal signs of normal age-related changes in the brain, such as shrinkage, which are not necessarily a sign of disease.

Parkinsonism is a common condition in old people. The differential diagnosis includes *classic parkinsonism, postencephalitic parkinson's disease, drug-induced parkinsonism, secondary parkinsonism,* and *arteriosclerotic parkinsonism.* A characteristic sign is a shuffling gait, with the trunk leaning forward. The rate of the patient's gait increases as he or she walks, but the patient may not be able to stop voluntarily. As the disease progresses, the patient may be unable to ambulate.

The patient plays an important role in the diagnosis by giving information on her past medical history, use of drugs, diet, and general health. In performing the medical examination and taking the history, it is important to check the information with a close relative or friend.

It is very important to differentiate between delirium (or acute confusional state) and dementia. Delirium may arise from a variety of problems ranging from myocardial infarction to electrolyte imbalance, urinary tract infection, drug intoxication, alcohol intoxication, and other hidden medical problems. The treatment, of course, is proper recognition and management of the underlying medical disorder or drug problem. Dementia is often a more difficult problem to identify. However, with the new biochemical studies, the CT scan, positron emission tomography, and nuclear magnetic resonance, the diagnosis can be made with a fair amount of certainty.

The best treatment comes only after a complete medical examination by a physician who does not dismiss claims as just old age. If there is a diagnosis of a curable disease, the physician will know how to treat it or will have ready access to the best resources or specialists.

The diagnosis of an irreversible disorder is not a hopeless situation. Much can be done to treat the patient and to help the family cope with the problem. Careful use of drugs can lessen agitation, anxiety, and depression and can improve sleeping habits if this is needed. Proper nutrition is particularly important, although special diets or supplements are usually not necessary. The person should be encouraged to maintain her daily routines, physical activities, and social contacts, and should not be discouraged from trying new things. It is important to stimulate the patient by keeping her aware of important events that may be going on in her immediate environment. By challenging and stimulating the patient, it may be possible to keep brain activity from failing at a more rapid pace. It is important to provide memory aids to help patients in day-to-day living. Such aids may include a visible calendar, a list of daily activities, written notes about simple safety measures, and directions to and labeling of commonly used items.

A patient with an irreversible disorder must be under the care of a physician. The responsible physician may be a neurologist, psychiatrist, or family physician or internist who is willing to devote the time and interest required to monitor the treatment carefully, to treat the physical and emotional problems that may complicate the course of disease, and to answer the many questions of the patient and family. Since this is such a specialized field, the National Institute on Aging has established courses and training programs so that physicians can cope with this new group of patients with their unique problems and specific needs for therapy.

REFERENCES

Achong, M. R., D. Bayne, Jr., L. W. Gerson, and S. Golshani. 1978. Prescribing of psychoactive drugs for chronically ill elderly patients. *Can. Med. Assoc. J.* 118:1503.

Ancoli-Israel, S., D. F. Kripke, and W. J. Mason. 1984. Obstructive sleep apnea in a senior population. *Sleep Res.* 13:130.

Barnes, R. F., and M. A. Raskind, M. Scott, and C. Murphy. 1981. Problems of families caring for Alzheimer patients; use of a support group. *J. Am. Geriatric Soc.* 29:80.

Barton, R., and L. Hurst. 1966. Unnecessary use of tranquilizers in elderly patients. *Br. J. Psychiatry* 112:989.

Berger, K. S., and S. H. Arit. 1978. Late-life paranoid states. Assessment and treatment. *Am. J. Orthopsychiatry* 48:523.

Birren, J. E., and K. W. Schaie (eds). 1977. *Handbook of the Psychology of Aging.* Van Nostrand Reinhold, New York.

Botwinick, J. 1984. *Aging and Behavior,* 3rd ed. Springer Publishing Co., New York.

Butler, R. N. 1981. The medicine of the future—geriatrics. Joseph T. Freeman Lecture, 1980; presented at the 33rd Annual Meeting of the Gerontological Society. Quoted by R. W. Besdine: Health and illness behavior in the elderly, in: *Health, Behavior and Aging.* Institute of Medicine, National Academy Press.

Cole, J. 1980. Drug therapy in senile organic brain syndrome. *J. Psychol. Univ. Ottawa* 5:41.

Cotzias, G. C., P. S. Papavasiliou, and R. Gellene. 1969. Modification of parkinsonism—chronic treatment with L-dopa. *N. Engl. J. Med.* 280:337.

Craik, F. L. M., and E. Simon. 1980. Age differences in memory: The roles of attention and depth of processing, in: *New Directions in Memory and Aging* (L. W. Poon, J. F. Fozard, L. S. Cermak, D. Arenberg, and L. Thompson, eds.).

Craper, D., S. S. Krishman, and A. J. Dalton. 1973. Brain aluminum distribution in Alzheimer's disease and experimental neurofibrillary degeneration. *Science* 180:511.

Crooks, J. 1983. Rational therapeutics in the elderly. *J. Chronic. Dis.* 36:59.

———. 1983. Aging and drug disposition—pharmacodynamics. *J. Chronic Dis.* 36:85.

D'Arcy, P. F. 1982. Drug reactions and interactions in the elderly patient. *Drug. Intell. Clin. Pham.* 16:925.

Davis, K. L., R. C. Mohs, and J. R. Tinklenberg. 1979. Enhancement of memory by physostigmine. *N. Engl. J. Med.* 301:946.

Denerstein, L., and G. D. Burrows. 1978. A review of studies of the psychological symptoms found at the menopause. *Maturitas* 1:55.

Dominian, J. 1977. The role of psychiatry in the menopause. *Clin. Obstet. Gynaecol.* 4:241.

Eisdorfer, C., and D. Cohen 1981. Management of the patient and family coping with dementing illness. *J. Fam. Pract.* 12:831.

Finlayson, R. E., and L. M. Martin. 1982. Recognition and management of depression in the elderly. *Mayo Clin. Proc.* 57:115.

Ford, C. V., and J. Winter. 1981. Computerized axial tomograms and dementia in elderly patients. *J. Gerontol.* 36:164.

Gaitz, C. M., R. V. Varner, and J. E. Overall. 1977. Pharmacotherapy for organic brain syndromes in late life. Evaluation of an ergot derivative vs. placebo. *Arch. Gen. Psychiatry* 34:839.

Gallagher, D. E., and L. W. Thompson. 1982. Treatment of major depressive disorders in older adult outpatients with brief psychotherapies. *Psychotherapy* 19:482.

Gerard, P., K. Collins, C. Dore, and A. Exton-Smith. 1978. Subject characteristics of sleep in the elderly. *Age Ageing* 7(suppl):55.

Goudsmit, J., D. M. Morrow, R. T. Asher. et al. 1980. Evidence for and against the transmitability of Alzenheimer's disease. *Neurology* 30:945.

Guilleminault, C. (ed.). 1982. *Sleep and Waking Disorders: Indications and Techniques.* Weseley Publishing Co., Menlo Park, Calif.

Guttman, D. 1979. A survey of drug-taking behavior of the elderly, in: *Services Research Report,* National Institute of Drug Abuse, 1977. Cited in *Institute of Medicine: Sleeping Pills, Insomnia and Medical Practice.* National Academy of Sciences, Washington, D.C.

Heston, L. L. 1979. Alzheimer's disease and senile dementia: Genetic relationship to Down's syndrome and hematologic cancer, in: *Congenital and Acquired Cognitive Disorders* (R. Katzman, ed.). Raven Press, New York, p. 167.

Heston, L. L., and A. R. Mastri. 1977. The genetics of Alzheimer's disease: Associations with hematologic malignancy and Down's syndrome. *Arch. Gen. Psychiatry* 34:976.

Kierman, P. J., and J. B. Isaacs. 1981. Use of drugs by the elderly. *J. R. Soc. Med.* 74:196.

Lassier, L. B., and M. Gautitia. 1978. Depression in old age. *J. Am. Geriatric Soc.* 26:471.

Mace, N. L., and P. V. Rabins. 1981. *The 36-Hour Day. A Family Guide to Caring for Persons with Alzheimer's Disease, Related Dementing Illnesses and Memory Loss in Later Life.* Johns Hopkins University Press, Baltimore.

Miles, L. E., and W. C. Dement. 1980. Sleep and aging. *Sleep* 3:119.

Mendelson, W. 1978. *The Use and Misuse of Sleeping Pills.* Plenum Press, New York.

Pollak, C. P., M. R. Pressman, D. Appel, A. J. Spielman, R. D. Chervin, and E. D. Weitzman. 1981. Sleep apnea in elderly insomniacs and effects of flurazepam. *Sleep Res.* 10:222.

Pomara, N., B. Stanley, R. Block, J. Guido, D. Russ, and M. Stanley. 1983. Caution in the use of drugs in the elderly (letter). *N. Engl. J. Med.* 308:1600.

Raskind, M., and C. Eisdorfer. 1977. When elderly patients can't sleep. *Drug Ther.* 7:44.

Reynolds, C. F., P. A. Coble, R. S. Black, B. Holzer, R. Carroll, and D. J. Kupfer. 1980. Sleep disturbances in a series of elderly patients: Polysomnographic findings. *J. Am. Geriatric Soc.* 28:164.

Roehrs, T., F. Zonick, and T. Roth. 1984. Sleep disorders in the elderly. *Geriatric Med. Today* 3(6):76.

Salem, S. A. M., P. Rajjayabun, A. M. M. Shepherd, and I. H. Stevenson. 1978. Reduced induction of drug metabolism in the elderly. *Age Ageing* 7:68.

Schader, R. I., and D. J. Greenblatt. 1979. Pharmacokinetics and clinical drug effects in the elderly. *Psychopharmacol. Bull.* 15:8.

Scogin, F. 1983. Memory skills training for the elderly: The efficacy of self-instructional treatment on memory performance, memory complaints, and depression. Unpublished Ph.D. dissertation, Washington University, St. Louis, Mo.

Segal, H. J., and N. S. Bornstein. 1984. Drug use by the elderly in long-term facilities. *Ont. Med. Rev.* 51:15.

Spicer, C. C., S. A. Hare, and E. Slater. 1973. Neurotic and psychotic forms of depressive illness. *Br. J. Psychiatry* 123:53.

Stern, G. M., and A. J. Lees. 1977. Choice of treatment in Parkinson's disease. *Practitioner* 219:537.

Storandt, M. 1983. *Counseling and Therapy with Older Adults.* Little, Brown & Co., Boston.

Terry, R. D., and P. Davies. 1980. Dementia of the Alzhemier type. *Ann. Rev. Neurosci.* 3:77.

Thompson, J., and J. Oswarld. 1977. Effect of estrogen on the sleep, mood and anxiety of menopausal women. *Br. Med. J.* 2:1317.

Thompson, T. L., II, M. G. Moran, and A. S. Nies. 1983. Psychotropic drug use in the elderly; I and II. *N. Engl. J. Med.* 308:134.

Wade, O. L. 1972. Drug therapy in the elderly. *Age Ageing* 1:65.

Weissman, M. M. 1979. The myth of involutional melancholia. *JAMA* 242:742.

Weitzman, E. D. 1983. Sleep and aging, in: *Neurology of Aging,* F. A. Davis Co., Philadelphia.

Whitehouse, P. J., D. L. Price, and A. W. Clark. 1982. Alzheimer's disease and senile dementia: Loss of neurons in the basal forebrain. *Science* 215:1237.

Winokar, G. 1973. Depression in the menopause. *Am. J. Psychiatry* 130:92.

World Health Organization. 1981. Use of medicaments by the elderly. *Drugs* 22:279.

Yoshikawa, M., et al. 1983. A dose–response study with dihydroergotoxine mesylate in cerebrovascular disturbances. *J. Am. Geriatric. Soc.* 31:1.

The Overall Health Maintenance and Care of the Female Geriatric Population

20

INTRODUCTION

The most rapidly growing segment of the U.S. population is the elderly. Overall, there is a greater increase in the female than in the male population. The population at the time of the 1980 census contained 105.5 females for every 100 males. Boys outnumbered girls under the age of 18; however, from ages 18 to 44, that ratio became 104.7 females for every 100 males. Between 45 and 64, there were 109.1 females per 100 males; and after age 65, there were 138.5 females per 100 males. The 1960–1970 decade saw a widening in the female/male ratio in the aged from 120.7/100 to 138.5/100. Since females are living longer than males, it can be anticipated that this gap will widen. Currently, the population 65 years and older contains 69 males for every 100 females, with an estimated 65 males for every 100 females in the near future. These statistics highlight the importance of geriatric gynecology now and particularly in the future.

Since the gynecologist has been designated as the principal physician, many of his or her patients fall into this age group. Therefore, the gynecologist will have to carry out the role of the primary care physician. It will be impossible to send geriatric patients from physician to physician.

This new responsibility will require the physician to have a background in the overall problems encountered by the elderly, as well as a knowledge of the various services that the geriatric patient will require. The need for more services for the aged is intensifying at the same time that veritable costs are becoming more evident. Many areas will require the attention of the physician, including cultural factors, health factors, nutrition, transportation, social services, communication, legal services, recreation, civic participation, employment, and methods for the elderly to receive economic support.

A particularly important problem is that the life expectancy of women is now considerably greater than that of men. Basic research is required in the behavioral and social, as well as in the biomedical, sciences to understand the differences in life expectancy, how they compare with male/female mortality rates in other countries, and how the life expectancy of men can be improved. Research is also needed on the factors that underlie differential mortality rates among various socioeconomic groups.

There is one basic unsolved question to which social scientists are giving increased attention: whether young and old should be mixed or whether age homogeneity favors the development of interpersonal ties and increases morale among geriatric patients.

The extent to which age determines social interaction (such as the creation of in-groups and out-groups and the social barriers to interaction among persons of widely different ages) needs more refined analysis. Studies are needed of age-homogeneous communities (retirement communities, suburbs composed of young families, communities of students) with regard to the formal, social, and political patterns that differentiate them, as well as the informal patterns of interaction.

In a complex society such as that of the United States, defining systems for delivery of services is a difficult task. There are different ways of defining a *system*. One definition is that of a collection of activities resulting from programs primarily supported by public funds. These service programs are less than adequate because policies for the aging are affected by broad economic, political, and social trends and by shifts in society's values. Most of the programs in the human services delivery system can be categorized as either (1) providing income and things for which income is usually regarded as a surrogate (food, shelter, transportation, health care, entertainment, education) or (2) developing social roles (personal identification, purposeful activity, employment, interpersonal relationships, independence, personal growth). These concepts are interrelated and correlated with biologic, psychologic, cultural, and spiritual needs.

This discussion of the overall health maintenance and care of the female geriatric patient must be abbreviated because of the vastness of the subject. However, certain points will be briefly covered.

CULTURAL FACTORS

Cultural factors are particularly important in programs for the aged because aged populations are extremely heterogeneous. This heterogeneity includes education, class, race, income, and health. In addition, aging itself is a cultural as well as a biologic process. Culture invests the aging process with particular meanings and defines the appropriate relationship of the aged to themselves, to others, to social institutions, and to their environment. Aging in ethnic communities has received some attention. Intraethnic variations have also drawn some interest. Studies illustrate that groups such as Asian-Americans are not monolithic cultural entities but consist of distinct cultural groups. Furthermore, these ethnic communities are not static or immune to change from outside, although one cannot always predict the direction that change will take.

RELIGION

Spiritual and moral belief systems offer important supports to the aged, contributing to their well-being in both subtle and obvious ways. This field has to be explored and structured so that it will add another dimension to the care of the elderly. It is interesting to note that the Hindu, Thai, and Samoan elderly view death and dying as a transitional phase of life: the latter stages of life are a time of preparation for a good death. Much of the recent work on death and dying reflects Western cultural assumptions and calls into question the cross-cultural applicability of the goals of death counseling, as well as the cross-cultural implications of artificially prolonging life through the use of advanced medical technology.

HEALTH

This has been a favorite campaign slogan for many politicians. Over the past 50 years, some progress has been made but much of it has been misdirected and health care is often used as a political football. Certain problems must be addressed. First, the aged require more health care, especially long-term care, than younger persons; second, they are less capable, economically, physically and socially, of obtaining such care without assistance; and third, health care professionals have been less motivated, less well trained, and less financially rewarded in providing health care for the elderly than for other age groups. About 10 percent of the population aged 65 and over accounts for 20 to 25 percent of all short-term hospitalizations, 80 percent of nursing home beds, and 27 percent of annual expenditures for personal health care. Only recently has mental health in the aged been considered different from mental health in other age groups. Epidemiologic data show that 5 percent of the aged have severe psychiatric disorders, both organic and functional.

Providing dental care for the aged presents problems in many areas. In addition to prevention, diagnosis, and treatment of disease, there are other equally important concerns—for example, a system for delivering services in accordance with the nutritional, social, psychologic, financial, and educational status of the patient. Data from studies of nursing home populations indicate that two-thirds of these patients need dental treatment.

The problems of health must be divided into several categories. There are particular needs for mental health care delivery to geriatric patients.

Available short-term pharmacotherapy and individual or group psychotherapy are completely inadequate to meet the needs of our rapidly expanding geriatric population. Epidemiologic data indicate that approximately 15 percent of the population aged 65 and older are in need of mental health treatment. The incidence of suicide in depressed geriatric patients is at least three times as high as that of younger patients. The elderly who are mentally ill may be responsive to appropriate treatment.

Many long-term care facilities are poorly integrated with other facilities or community-based health and social service organizations and programs. All too often the utilization of long-term care patterns depends upon reimbursement patterns. Intermediate care facilities have been created, but since there is a lower rate of reimbursement than for long-term facilities, they are generally not used.

NUTRITION

Finding ways to provide geriatric patients with adequate nutrition should be a part of each patient's care plan. However, helping a patient develop a diet and follow it is not always easy. Before beginning, it is important to consider the physical condition of the patient, as well as the cultural background, previous eating habits, environment, and finances.

It is important to recognize some of the signs and symptoms of overnourishment, as well as to determine why an obese patient may be malnourished. A knowledge of how vitamins and minerals affect the patient's body is important. Overnutrition in a geriatric patient may follow the consumption of foods that lack essential nutrients but contain large amounts of sugar, saturated fat, salt, cholesterol, phosphates and calories —for example, potato chips, french fries and butter. Scientists have reported that an overnourished patient is more likely to develop such conditions as obesity, heart disease, high blood pressure, hardening of the arteries, stroke, arthritis, osteoporosis, cancer, diverticulitis, colitis, and cirrhosis of the liver. Subclinical nutrition is hard to detect. Because the patient consumes somewhat less than the required amounts of essential nutrients, she usually has low resistance to infection and is in less than good health.

A geriatric patient suffering from undernutrition consumes far less than adequate amounts of foods containing nutrients. This essential nutrient deficiency may predispose the patient to anemia, weakness, brittle bones, infection, gum disease, loss of teeth, and depression.

Essential foods that contain vitamins and minerals include dark green leafy vegetables, citrus fruits, and bananas for vitamin K. The sources of vitamin A include carrots and sweet potatoes; dark green leafy vegetables such as endive and collards; fish, liver oil, and egg yolks; cantaloupe; and animal fats such as butter, cream, and lard. Iodine, which increases circulation and boosts energy, is found in iodized table salt, seafood, and dark green leafy vegetables. The Vitamin B complex, which functions in normal metabolism, cell growth, and blood formation, is found in whole grain cereal, seeds, yogurt, buttermilk, cottage cheese, lean meat, fresh liver, kidney, and dark green leafy vegetables. Zinc promotes the synthesis of DNA, RNA, and, ultimately, protein and is found in seafood, oatmeal, wheat bran, meat, eggs, oysters, veal, and crabs. Choices of foods may also influence the absorption of zinc; this mineral is less readily absorbed from vegetable sources than from animal sources. Zinc may compete with phytate, wheat fibers, iron, phosphate, and total nitrogen, thus inhibiting its absorption. Vitamin C holds body cells together and strengthens blood vessel walls, helps keep bones strong, plays a role in healing wounds and bone fractures, and helps build resistance to infection. Vitamin C is found in cantaloupe, citrus fruits, strawberries, broccoli, brussel sprouts, peppers, and tomatoes. Iron functions in erythropoiesis and prevents anemia. It is found in raw meats, green vegetables, eggs, whole wheat bread, and iron-fortified milk. Vitamin D promotes absorption and regulates the metabolism of calcium and phosphorus. Good dietary sources of naturally occurring vitamin D are limited to relatively few foods, including fatty fish, eggs, and chicken liver. In the United States, milk is fortified with vitamin D. Calcium is essential for blood vasculature, heart and muscle function, and the development of healthy bones and teeth. The sources of calcium are milk, cheese, sardines, turnip greens, broccoli, kale, and citrus fruits. Vitamin E functions in the development of smooth muscle, skeletal muscle, and vascular tissues, and protects erythrocytes from ammonolysis. Vitamin E is found in vegetable oils, margarine, whole grains, dark green leafy vegetables, and nuts. Magnesium regulates body temperature and activates enzymes necessary for carbohydrate metabolism. It is found in milk, cheese, poultry, whole grain breads and cereals, and vegetables.

Because of the increased prevalence of chronic alcoholism among the elderly, the folate deficiency associated with alcoholism may be increased. Drugs other than alcohol may also lead to folate deficiency. Studies of folate absorption do not indicate that aging has a significant adverse effect. Malabsorptive disorders can significantly decrease folate absorption and should be taken into consideration in the management of such patients.

TRANSPORTATION

Transportation is the element of the physical environment that links elderly persons to the services, facilities, resources, and opportunities necessary for their existence. Transportation is critical and also influences the effectiveness of other services for the elderly. Public transportation is becoming increasingly important for this age group. On the other hand, public transportation is least adequate for those who need it most —physically frail individuals with no friends or relatives to drive them, members of minority groups, and the poor. It is important to help geriatric patients obtain transportation so that they can avail themselves of the health care and other services that are available for them.

SOCIAL SERVICES

The social services directed toward the overall population do not serve the elderly well. A study of state agencies on aging notes the divergence between the needs listed by older persons and the goals identified by the state agencies. Studies show that one-third of the elderly consumers listed priority needs that had no relation to those of state agencies; the needs of another one-third had only a tenuous connection to agency goals; and the needs of one-third had a clear and direct connection to agency goals. This pattern has been repeatedly documented. There must be methods for organizing and delivering services to the elderly, and the way services are offered must be reevaluated.

EMPLOYMENT

The participation of older persons in the labor force has decreased in every industrialized country since the turn of the century. This pattern is a result of compulsory retirement and age discrimination. Reports indicate that an increasing percentage of persons of age 55 and older are leaving the work force. This means increased years of retirement since there is an increase in longevity. The United States does have an Age Discrimination and Employment Act, which was passed in 1967. However, there is no systematic, nationwide knowledge of patterns and levels of discrimination by industry and occupation. The Employment Standards Administration of the Department of Labor is responsible for enforcing the act.

ECONOMIC SUPPORT

Very little work has been done on the economics of aging. Statistics indicate that geriatric patients are essentially a low-income group with a disproportionate amount of poverty, as defined by federal standards.

Social Security remains the major source of retirement income and is estimated to be one-third the amount of preretirement earnings. Actuarial projections predict problems in the relation of Social Security income to outgo in the future. Federal government policies will have to take into account demographic changes, inflation, economic growth, benefit level increases, and national priorities and equity.

Medicare, which provides third-party payment of certain health costs, has obviously helped, but it is now playing a decreasing role and seems to be most inadequate in the most serious area—long-term care. Supplemental private health insurance plays a very minor role. There is still a significant number of special public programs dealing with limited aspects of health care and health care delivery. With the growing increase in the geriatric population, this is a most important problem for the federal government to address.

Geriatrics is at about the level that pediatrics was in the 1920s, 1930s, and 1940s. Since life is a continuum, it can be said that geriatrics starts with pediatrics. It is increasingly clear that the gynecologist, who is the elderly person's principal physician and who often functions as the primary care physician, must become educated in the multiple problems of the aged. It is a challenge presented for the next decade.

SUMMARY

The elderly, perhaps more than any other group in society, rely heavily on health and welfare resources. Increased longevity and the lengthening of the retirement period have brought problems of providing social and health services, maintaining income, and maximizing the ability of the elderly to function in society.

Although a great deal of political attention has focused on organizing programs that will attract the votes of the elderly, very little concrete help is being provided. Communities are often unable to help the aged, and if services are available, the geriatric patient may be unaware of them.

One of the most significant improvements in the status of the aged or aging was the passage under the Social Security Act of the Federal Old Age Insurance in 1935, which provided some financial security for older persons. The past few years have brought a profound awakening of interest in older people as their numbers in society have grown. The Civil Rights Movement has brought a more humanistic attitude toward all people, including the aging.

It is obvious that geriatric persons will make up a significant part of the population after the turn of the twenty-first century. It is, therefore, necessary to start now to structure plans that will be cost effective for the care of this group. It must be broad-based and provide affordable care with dignity.

REFERENCES

Austin, M. J. 1976. A network of help for England's elderly. *Social Work* 21:114.

Blazer, D. 1978. Techniques for communicating with your elderly patient. *Geriatrics* 33:79.

Brocklehurst, J. C. (ed.). 1975. *Geriatric Care in Advanced Societies.* University Park Press, Baltimore.

Havighurst, R. J. 1975. The future aged: The use of time and money. *Gerontologist* 15(1, Part 2):10.

Kent, D. P., R. Kastenbaum, and S. Sherwood (eds.). 1972. *Research Planning and Action for the Elderly; The Power and Potential of Social Science.* Behavioral Publications, New York.

Klippel, R., E. Sweenye, and T. Sweeney. 1974. The use of information sources in the aged consumer. *Gerontolgist* 14:163.

Reichel, W. 1978. Multiple problems in the elderly, in: *The Geriatric Patient* (W. Reichel, ed.). Hospital Practice Publishers, New York, pp. 17–22.

Sherwood, S. (ed.). 1975. *Long-Term Care: A Handbook for Researchers, Planners and Providers.* Spectrum Publications, New York.

Tobin, S. S. 1975. Social and health services for the future aged. *Gerontologist* 15(1, Part 2):32.

Glossary

Adrenal glands the senescent adrenal gland exhibits morphologic alterations such as increased pigment deposition in collagen content, as well as vascular dilatation and hemorrhage in the cortex and the medulla mitochondrial fragmentation. Although the aging adrenal gland evidently maintains a relatively normal response to ACTH stimulation, the rate of adrenal cortical secretion decreases by 30 percent throughout the adult life span.

Adrenopause the time, usually around age 65, when the production of certain adrenal hormones slows down. This marked decrease in adrenal androgen secretion has been named the *adrenopause.* The responsible mechanism is unknown but is independent of ovarian function. It is an age-related phenomenon.

Age at menopause has been constant for more than 20 centuries and does not vary from one population to another. This suggests that the menopause in human beings is essentially an invariant biologic trait.

Alkaline phosphatase a liver enzyme involved in calcium metabolism.

Alzheimer's disease first described in November 1906 at a meeting of the Southwest German Society of Alienists, at which Alois Alzheimer recounted the story of a 51-year-old woman. The woman first suffered loss of memory and disorientation, later became subject to depression and hallucinations, and progressed to severe dementia. At necropsy the patient's brain showed severe atrophy, and the cerebral cortex was marked by clumping and distortion of fibers in nerve cells. Alzheimer called these jumbles of filaments *neurofibrillary tangles,* and they have since become the hallmark of Alzheimer's disease.

Antipruritic agent for hypertrophic dystrophy Urax combined with valisone cream. It is made up as a mixture of 30 percent Urax and 70 percent valisone and is applied twice a day.

Arteriosclerosis a general term referring to the thickening and hardening of arterial walls.

Atherosclerosis a particular type of arteriosclerosis characterized by patchy deposition of fatty streaks and fiber plaques on the walls of the large arteries. Factors that may be implicated in the pathogenesis of atherosclerosis include endothelial injury, intimal smooth muscle proliferation, and alterations in lysosomal function.

Atrophy of the vulva with persistent burning Application three times a day of an ointment consisting of 2 percent testosterone proprionate in white petrolatum seems to have the best effect. It should be continued daily for 6 weeks and then reduced to two or three times weekly and maintained, or the condition will recur. There may be symptoms of enlargement of the clitoris and masculinization if too much of the preparation is used.

Biofeedback a form of behavior therapy in which one specific body function is treated. It has been used to control heart rate and to lower high blood pressure. However, most of the studies on the applications of biofeedback to medicine are still in the laboratory stage. Biofeedback has been used to treat a variety of neurologic disorders and urinary incontinence.

Bladder training (bladder drill) advocated as the first treatment for detrusor instability. It is a psychologic approach to a condition the cause of which is often in doubt, and though it involves about 10 days in the hospital and much supervision, it is well worth a trial in resistant cases. After a full explanation, the patient is instructed to pass urine only at hourly intervals, which are gradually increased to every 3 hours if possible. Fluid balance and times of micturition are recorded, and obviously the patient must be motivated to persist with the treatment. This drill is followed only during the day but is continued in modified form after returning home from the hospital.

Bone mass the total amount of bone in the body. Overall bone mass increases from birth and reaches a peak at about the age of 30. Thereafter, it declines as bone is lost with age.

Calcitonin a calcium-sparing hormone released primarily by the thyroid gland. It acts to slow the breakdown of bone.

Cardiovascular system clearly reflects the course of senescence, although the severity of cardiac and peripheral vascular dysfunction varies, not only with age but also with diet, lifestyle, and genetic predisposition. Cardiovascular senescent changes include decreased cardiac output, progressive arteriosclerosis, increased peripheral vascular resistance, and hypertension.

Cell hybridization an excellent means for investigating age-related pathology of cellular organelles. Two types of

hybrids have been derived from mammalian cells: heterokaryons and synkaryons. It may be possible to develop cybrids.

Cell membrane the decreasing physiologic and biochemical functions of the aging organism may result from the declining ability of cells to carry on normal functions or to respond to stress. Cell membranes have leading roles in regulating cellular functions; thus, recent studies have focused on possible changes in the structure and function of membranes that may contribute to the overall deterioration of an aging organism.

Changing demographics about one third of the older population is very old, 75 years or more. This proportion will remain about the same for the foreseeable future if mortality rates remain constant. If they do, there will be about 12 million of the very old by the year 2000. If mortality rates decline, however, the number of the very old may grow to as much as 16 or 18 million. A 65-year-old man can now expect, on the average, to live to age 78; a 65-year-old woman, to 82. By the year 2000, the life expectancy for 65-year-olds may increase by another 2 to 5 years.

Cholesterol and triglycerides the concentrations of these substances increases with age, and there is an increased risk of coronary disease associated with cholesterol concentrations greater than 220 to 250 ml/dl. An increase in cholesterol values is associated with increased concentration of low-density lipoprotein cholesterol (LDL-C), whereas a rise in triglyceride values is associated with an increased concentration of very-low-density lipoproteins (VLDL). High-density lipoproteins (HDL), which carry about 50 percent of cholesterol, seem to protect against the development of atherosclerosis. A low HDL concentration is a more potent risk factor than a high concentration of cholesterol or LDL. HDL concentrations are decreased with smoking and increased with regular exercise or alcohol intake.

Climacteric the phase in the life of a woman that marks the transition from the reproductive age to the age at which reproductive function is lost.

Clinical types of osteoporosis (1) trabecular, characterized by loss of height, spinal curvature, and vertebral fracture; (2) cortical, characterized by fractures of the waist or hip.

Cortical bone the hard bone of the arms and legs.

Cybrids cells with cytoplasm from one parent and a nucleus from the other.

Cystocele prolapse of the bladder and anterior vaginal wall. Descent of the urethra and bladder neck may occur separately or accompany a cystocele; when sagging of the urethra occurs alone, it is sometimes known as a *urethrocele.*

Cystourethrocele and uterine descensus it is generally agreed that support of pelvic structures depends on the endopelvic fascia, the uterosacral and cardinal ligaments, and the levator muscle. An intact fascial system, with it attachments to the vaginal fornices in the upper two-thirds of the lateral vagina, provides a well-supported vaginal tube, which in turn is the most supporting structure for the uterus and the vaginal vault. Trauma secondary to obstetric delivery, occupational or unusual athletic endeavors, heredity, lack of estrogen, and postmenopausal attenuation all contribute in varying degrees to the development of pelvic relaxation. Additional contributing factors that promote uterine descensus are obesity, asthma, and other chronic lung diseases.

Demographic findings reductions in mortality and fertility have markedly changed the age distribution of the United States. While the total population increased 2.5 times from 1900 to 1970, the number of persons aged 65 and over increased 7 times. Persons aged 65 and over now constitute about 10 percent of the total population, but over the next 50 years, they are expected to make up 12 to 16 percent. There are now about four persons under age 20 for every one person over age 65. It is anticipated that in the United States in the next 50 to 60 years, this ratio will become 1.5:1.

Densitometer an instrument that measures the density of bones by determining the amount of radiation they can absorb.

Detrusor instability a contraction exceeding 15 cm of water and pressure, occurring during filling of the bladder or standing erect or coughing or straining. This may also cause involuntary incontinence, but the mechanism is altogether different from that of genuine stress incontinence.

Diseases and disability somewhere between the ages of 55 and 65, the number of people who have one or more chronic conditions skyrockets. There is evidence of this for all kinds of disease throughout the medical literature. Since a large number of people die between 65 and 75, the majority of the population over 65 is under 75. Also, this group is not nearly as sick as those over 75, a group that is growing even faster than the population aged 65 to 75.

Diseases of the breast the breast may be the site of contusions and lacerations secondary to trauma. Elderly women often fall against objects. It is not uncommon to see contusions of the breast with or without a hematoma, and fat necrosis may resemble a neoplastic process in the elderly female. Inflammatory lesions occur in the geriatric patient; most are secondary to scratching or insect bites. Fibrocystic disease, especially in the form of nodules, is occasionally seen in the postmenopausal woman. Intraductal papilloma and duct ectasia may occur postmenopausally. A nipple discharge, especially if accompanied by discoloration or blood, must be suspected of being a neoplastic process. Carcinoma of the breast is the second leading cause of death from cancer among women.

Dowager's hump a protuberance of the upper back caused by painful collapsing of the vertebrae and outward curvature of the upper spine.

Dual-photon absorptiometry a sensitive method of measuring the amount of trabecular bone in the spine.

Dysuria pain associated with micturition, which indicates either an infection of the bladder and urethra or of the vulval and perineal epithelium, which is irritated by the dribbling of urine.

Endoplasmic reticulum a system of membranes continuous with the nuclear envelope in the cell membrane and enclosing cisternae. The wall of the endoplasmic reticulum may be smooth or rough. The latter bears the ribosomes and polysomes, which are responsible for most of the protein synthesis within a cell.

Enterocele a hernia of the rectovaginal peritoneal pouch through the posterior vaginal fornix. Elongation of the rectovaginal pouch invariably accompanies uterine prolapse, and small intestine may be found in the peritoneal sac behind the uterus in cases of procidentia. Enterocele may also occur without uterine prolapse, causing a bulge in the upper part of the posterior vaginal wall that must be distinguished from a rectocele. Enterocele may occasionally occur after the uterus has been removed by abdominal or vaginal hysterectomy and is usually combined with some degree of prolapse of the vaginal vault. It is a true hernia in which there is peritoneal sac tearing of the fascia, usually with small bowel in its sac.

Epidemiologic studies these include (1) a randomized, prospective clinical trial, (2) a longitudinal cohort study, (3) a case control study, and (4) alternative analytic methods for case control studies.

Estrogen replacement therapy in postmenopausal women who do not have a contraindication, estrogen therapy is acceptable therapy. A progestational agent should be added to reduce endometrial hyperplasia and the potential for developing an endometrial malignancy.

Fibroblasts found in connective tissue. Because of their sustained growth and short life span in vitro, they are especially suitable to growth in tissue culture. They can proliferate rapidly in vitro for a number of divisions, usually about 40. Fibroblasts then enter a period of declining cell proliferation (the senescent phase) and finally, after a certain number of division (usually 50), stop proliferating.

Frequency increased frequency of urination is defined as the passage of urine seven or more times during the day and twice or more during the night. It may arise from any source of irritation, including infection, detrusor instability, tumor, and incomplete emptying.

Gastrointestinal system digestive disorders are common among the elderly. Anatomic changes include atrophy of the intestinal mucosa, which results in impaired absorption, decreased intestinal motility, diminished enzyme production, and increased bile viscosity. Gallstones, gastrointestinal cancer, diverticulosis, and constipation are also more prevalent with advancing age.

Genetics of aging involves the inheritance of longevity (life span) and the inherited difference in patterns of aging. From studies on identical twins, it has been estimated that 60 to 80 percent of an individual's tendency toward longevity is inherited.

Genitourinary atrophy specific atrophic changes in the genitalia and the urinary system can be directly related to estrogen deficiency and may be ameliorated with estrogen replacement therapy. Since mullerian and mesonephric structures arise in close embryonic proximity, it is not surprising that both may be similarly affected by estrogen. In fact, the vulva, vagina, cervix, endometrium, fallopian tube, urethra, and trigone of the bladder all have a large number of estrogen receptors and are sensitive to a decrease in available estrogen.

Geriatrics a term coined by J. L. Nascher and published in 1914 in the "Diseases of Old Age and Their Treatment" (P. Blakiston and Sons, Philadelphia). Chancellor Otto von Bismark of Germany first designated 70 as the age of retirement and then reduced it to 65, which is now considered the beginning of the geriatric period.

Golgi bodies a group of smooth membranes enclosing cisternae, responsible for processing and transporting proteins produced by the endoplasmic reticulum.

Gonadotropin-releasing hormone (GnRH) peripheral circulating concentrations of GnRH in postmenopausal women are reportedly increased, presumably because estrogen concentrations (and therefore negative feedback) are diminished. The development of sensitive assay techniques and controlled experimental studies are required to elucidate further the role of GnRH in the climacteric.

Gonadotropins a striking endocrinologic change in menopause is an increase in follicle-stimulating hormone (FSH) concentrations, the result of loss of negative feedback inhibition of estradiol (E_2) and possibly of inhibin. FSH serum values of 40 mIU/ml or more are generally associated with the failure of ovarian function, and values greater than 100 mIU/ml indicate menopause with relative certainty. Luteinizing hormone (LH) is a less sensitive indicator than FSH of the gonadotropic changes of the menopause.

Hayflick phenomenon vividly demonstrates the mortality of human diploid cell lines. Using cultured cells from fetal lung, Hayflick demonstrated an average of 50 doublings (range, 35 to 63) before the cells failed to replicate further. Cells from progressively older subjects exhibited fewer doublings, and adult cells showed only 20 population doublings (range, 14 to 29) before death. Hayflick estimated that approximately 54 population doublings would be required to produce from a single cell all of the erythrocytes and leukocytes needed for 60 years of life. His estimate corresponds remarkably to his findings of cell longevity in vitro.

Heterokaryons one of two types of hybrids derived from mammalian cells. They have two or more nuclei in a common pool of cytoplasm.

Hot flush it has been shown that in humans, LH, not FSH, showed pulsatile activity closely associated with the occurrence of symptoms and skin temperature increases during hot flushes. This association suggests that factors concerned with pulsatile releases of LH may be involved in the pathophysiology of hot flushes.

Hypertension in the elderly approximately 15 to 20 percent of all adults, and an even higher percentage of those over 65, have elevations in blood pressure, a leading cause of both morbidity and mortality in the United States. High blood pressure affects 40 percent of patients over age 65.

Ileococcygeus a bilateral muscle arising from the part of the white line that lies behind the obturator canal. It blends with the lateral fibers of the pubococcygeus proper and is inserted into the lateral margin of the coccyx.

Innervation of the bladder and urethra there is a intercommunicating sympathetic, parasympathetic, and somatic supply. The parasympathetic nerve stimulates the detrusor contraction, and the sympathetic fibers (chiefly through the alpha receptors) stimulate contraction of the bladder neck and urethra. There is thus some degree of reciprocal activity, but the precise function of each type of nerve and the exact control of the mechanism of bladder neck opening are not yet known.

Ischiococcygeus a bilateral muscle arising from the pelvic aspect to the ischial spine. It is inserted into the lateral border of the coccyx and the last piece of the sacrum. This muscle is now known as the *coccygeus muscle.*

Lactase an intestinal enzyme that breaks down lactose, a sugar, into small, easily digested components.

Lactase deficiency results in uncomfortable gastrointestinal symptoms when foods containing lactose are eaten. It may also be called *lactose intolerance.* The incidence of this deficiency increases with age.

Lactose a sugar found in milk and other dairy products.

Lipofuscin pigment the intracellular accumulation of these materials is a predominant characteristic of nondividing cells, such as nerve cells, in all organisms. Convincing evidence now links the presence of this pigment to lysosomes.

Lysosomes a special group of cytoplasmic particles found in all living cells. They are characterized by the presence of distinct enzymes, which are separated from external substances by a membrane-like lipoprotein barrier.

Maximum recorded life span of species humans, 111 years; horse, 46 years; goat, 20 years; guinea pig, 7.6 years; rat, 4.7 years; and mouse, 3.3 years.

Menopausal symptoms flushes, flashes, insomnia, night sweats, and dry vagina are characteristically identified with the withdrawal of estrogen. A variety of nonspecific symptoms have been alleged to become more prevalent during the menopausal age. These include fatigue, irritability, depression, headache, dizziness, palpitations, bloating, apprehension, insomnia, altered libido, apathy, difficulty in concentrating, anxiety, tension, dyspnea, emotional lability, and feelings of inadequacy. These complaints are often vague and ill-defined, and many of the symptoms may conform to the diagnosis of reactive depression or anxiety neurosis, which are multifactorial and do not represent a specific clinical syndrome. Relieving the symptoms of insomnia and night sweats often relieves the fatigue, depression, and anxiety associated with the menopause.

Menopause the final menstrual period that signals the end of cyclic ovarian function.

Mitochondria represent the energy-yielding enzyme packets in cells. Age-dependent changes in the structure and activity of the mitochondria have been observed in a variety of species.

Musculoskeletal system the structure of muscles is altered with age. With diminished activity and decreased neural stimulation, muscle fibers degenerate and are replaced by fat or collagen. The increased prevalence of arthritis among the elderly is at least partly due to degenerative changes in the articular surfaces and perichondrial margins of the joints.

Nervous system with increasing age, there is progressive loss of neuronal cells in the central nervous system. For example, by the ninth decade of life, the number of cells in the parietal and temporal areas of the cerebral cortex will have decreased by 40 percent. The age-related numerical diminution in the components of the nervous system in general is accompanied by a significant slowing in the transmission of impulses between neurons, whereas intraneuronal depolarization remains almost normal. The result is a slowing of reflexes and a diminution in the senses of smell, taste, touch, hearing, and vision.

Neurologic cause of incontinence failure of detrusor inhibition is the most common symptom and is the cause of senile incontinence. It is also a symptom, although not usually the presenting one, of multiple sclerosis. Full sensation is present, but the incontinence is of the urgency type and cannot be resisted.

Nucleus consists of DNA proteins (histones and acidic proteins) in one or more nucleoli (largely made up of RNA) and a surrounding membrane similar in composition to the endoplasmic reticulum. Age-associated alterations in chromatin composition have been noted in tissues of varying ages.

Oral estrogen the oral estrogen first-pass hepatic metabolism has been reported to be associated with an increase in HDL cholesterol. The patch technique for administering estrogen is not accompanied by a first pass through the liver, but later, of course, it does pass through the liver.

Osteoblast bone-forming cells, which fill in the cavities in bone with new bone cells. Many osteoblasts are required to replace the bone removed by one osteoclast.

Osteoclast bone-resorbing (bone breakdown) cells, which dig microscopic cavities along the inner surfaces of the bone.

Osteomalacia a bone disease in adults caused by vitamin D deficiency and characterized by inadequate mineralization of new bone.

Osteopenia the reduction in overall bone mass to a level below normal but still above that associated with fractures.

Osteoporosis not a disease but the end result of severe or prolonged bone loss. *Bone loss* refers to the gradual thinning and increased porosity of bones (hence the name *osteoporosis)* that occurs naturally with aging but that can be dangerously accelerated or beneficially slowed down by a multitude of factors. Osteoporosis is a painful, disfiguring, and debilitating disease.

Pancreas beta cell degeneration is a normal consequence of senescence, and carbohydrate tolerance gradually decreases with aging. Although 50 percent of the patients aged 65 or more have abnormal chemical responses to the glucose tolerance test, frank diabetes mellitus is clinically evident in only 7 percent.

Parathyroid hormone (PTH) a substance released by the parathyroid glands in response to low levels of calcium in the blood. It stimulates the breakdown of bone in order to release calcium and restore normal calcium levels in the blood.

Perimenopause defined arbitrarily to include the last few years of the climacteric and the first year after the menopause. After the menopause, there is gradual atrophy of the genital organs. The uterus diminishes in size; the endometrium becomes thin and atrophic; the vaginal wall becomes thin and smooth, with a fall in the acidity of the secretion; and the fornices become shallow around a small cervix. The labia are flatter and the growth of pubic hair is diminished. The ligaments and fascia that support the uterus atrophy, and prolapse may become evident if there has been previous damage during childbirth. Atrophic endometritis, atrophic vaginitis, and atrophic changes in the vulva may occur.

pH of less than 4.9 effectively excludes *Neisseria gonorrhoea, Gardnerella* *vaginalis, Hemophilus influenzae,* and *Trichomonas vaginalis.*

Postmenopausal bleeding any postmenopausal bleeding should be diagnosed by a fractional curettage and a thorough pelvic examination.

Postmenopausal ovaries exhibit an increase of connective tissue and a decrease of germinal elements. Although follicles, when present, appear to be undergoing atresia and the cells lining these follicles are in regression, activity in some cells is present. Theca internal cells from atretic follicles differentiate into stromal or interstitial cells. An abundance of stromal cells is seen in postmenopausal ovaries, and in vitro experiments indicate that these cells are the source of androgens. Within 2 years of the menopause, the ovary measures $2 \times 1.5 \times 0.5$ cm.

Postmenopausal palpable ovary syndrome (PMPO) what is interpreted as a normal-sized ovary in the premenopausal woman represents an ovarian tumor in the postmenopausal woman. This does not mean that anything that is felt is abnormal. The ovary must be the size of a premenopausal ovary, which is $3.5 \times 2 \times 1.5$ cm.

Principal organisms associated with an acid pH *Candida albicans* and groups A and B hemolytic streptococci, which usually function with a member of the Enterobaceteriaceae.

Progestogen a synthetic preparation that resembles the natural hormone progesterone.

Progestogen challenge test devised to identify postmenopausal women at greatest risk for endometrial cancer. Employment of this test in untreated postmenopausal women has identified many of those at increased risk. It is concluded that the use of this test and the continued use of progestogens in climacteric women who respond with withdrawal bleeding will reduce the risk of endometrial cancer in both estrogen-treated postmenopausal women and those with increased endogenous estrogens.

Psychopathology it has been estimated that approximately 15 percent of older adults in the United States demonstrate at least moderate psychopathology. Many do not seek treatment for a variety of reasons: cultural sanctions against many emotional problems, lack of economic resources, unavailability of outpatient treatment facilities and trained personnel to deal with the geriatric psychiatric patient, and fear of institutionalization. Thus, it falls to the geriatrician to be cognizant of the common forms of psychopathology of later life.

Pubococcygeus muscle by far the most important component of the pelvic floor and, significantly, the part that is best developed. It should be considered a single, centrally situated muscle that arises from the pelvic aspect of the body of the pubis and from the part of the white line of the pelvic fascia that lies in front of the obturator canal.

Rectocele prolapse of the rectum and posterior vaginal wall. It is usually accompanied by some deficiency of the perineal body.

Research on Aging Act signed into law on May 31, 1974. This legislation authorized establishment of the National Institute on Aging (NIA) for the conduct and support of biomedical, social, and behavior research and training related to the aging process and to diseases and other special problems and needs of the aged.

Resorption the process of bone breakdown in the bone remodeling process.

Respiratory system pulmonary compliance, vital capacity, alveolar surface area, and resistance to infection diminish with age.

Ribosomes concerned with general protein synthesis. Practically every aspect of the translational apparatus has been shown to be defective in the aging organism.

Senility the term commonly used to describe a large number of conditions and an equally large number of causes, many of which respond to prompt treatment. The symptoms include serious forgetfulness, confusion, and certain other changes in personality and behavior. Mental decline in old age may be called *dementia, organic brain disorder, chronic brain syndrome, arteriosclerosis, cerebral atrophy,* or *pseudodementia.* The important thing is that some of the problems that are generally referred to as senile dementia can be treated and cured, while others can only be treated, without hope of restoring lost brain function. Thus a complete, careful investigation of the source of the symptoms is necessary.

Serum aldosterone concentrations decreased by 50 percent in the elderly, causing a blunted response to sodium restriction in 30 to 40 percent of adults. Moreover, about one-third of the women older than 70 have low plasma renin concentrations, which fail to rise with sodium deprivation.

Sexual response Masters and Johnson have shown that all four stages of the response cycle (excitement, plateau, orgasm, and resolution) are somewhat diminished with increased age. In the excitement phase, breasts are less engorged and the sexual flush may be absent. The clitoris enlarges normally, but there is no noticeable change in the labia majora. Vaginal lubrication is reduced. Vaginal ballooning occurs later in the plateau phase and is often less marked. Orgasms continue to occur but its duration is shorter, and muscular contractions may also be less intense. Uterine spasms may render some orgasms painful. The resolution phase is rapid in elderly women, and occasionally, because of urethral trauma, is accompanied by a desire to void.

Single-photon absorptiometry a sensitive method of measuring the density of bone in the long bones of the body, usually the arm.

Stress incontinence involuntary leakage occurring in the absence of a detrusor contraction. This leakage is attributed to some displacement of the bladder neck so that it cannot respond normally to a sudden increase in intraabdominal pressure such as that following coughing, sneezing, or laughing. The cause is likely to be a pelvic floor weakness as a result of parturition, prolapse, aging, or a combination of all three.

Symptom in the later years, multiple disorders are present as the body's protective mechanisms, such as immunity, are compromised. Symptoms present differently in the old, and the untrained clinician often misses the diagnoses. An older person with hyperthyroidism, for example, may appear apathetic and hyperactive; tuberculosis may proceed in silence; appendicitis may occur without the characteristic abdominal tenderness at McBurney's point, without fever, and without an elevated white blood cell count; an older person may even have a heart attack without chest pain and may instead appear confused, disoriented, and may seem like a victim of a stroke.

Synkaryon a hybrid cell derived from mammalian cells. In these cells there has been nuclear fusion as well as cytoplasmic fusion.

Theories of aging molecular chemical research on the intracellular changes caused by aging have led to several theories. The cellular theories recognize the series of events within the cell that prevent the ordinary process of growth and metabolism. No single theory of human aging seems to be able to explain all these biologic phenomena. These theories include genetic, programming, somatic mutation, autoimmune, cross-linkage, and combination theories.

Tissue composed of a group of cells of the same kind working together. In complex animals such as humans, there are several kinds of tissue—including connective, muscular, and epithelial (skin and lining).

Tissue culture a laboratory method in which a dish or bottle is filled with culture medium (food for the cells, such as essential vitamins and minerals) so that cells can be grown.

Trabecular bone the spongy bone of the vertebrae. It lines the bone marrow cavity and is surrounded by cortical bone.

Trichomonas vaginalis thrives on an alkaline milieu, whereas *Candida albicans* is inhibited.

Trigeminal neuralgia (tic douloureaux) mostly affects the elderly with paroxysms of sudden pain in one side of the face, brought on by talking, washing, eating, or any sensory stimulus to the affected side. The onset of an attack is evident by the sudden screwing up of the patient's face on one side, accompanied by obvious pain: the true tic douloureaux. The pain is often absent at night. When asked to show the position of the pain, the patient will point to the spot but never touch the face. No other disorder can be confused with this one, although many patients with any sort of facial pain are often wrongly given this diagnosis.

Types of menopause there are two types: physiologic and induced or artificial. Physiologic menopause occurs in women because oocytes responsive to gonadotropin disappear from the ovary and the few remaining oocytes do not respond. Isolated occytes can be found in postmenopausal ovaries on very careful histologic inspection. Induced or artificial menopause is the permanent cessation of ovarian function caused by surgical removal of the ovaries or destruction of the ovaries by radiation.

Urethral syndrome includes complaints of frequency, dysuria, urgency, and a sensation of incomplete emptying in a patient in whose urine no evidence of infection can be demonstrated. The cause is not known but is usually due to an irritation of the urethra.

Urgency a desire to void before the bladder contains 50 ml of urine. True urgency occurs in the absence of a detrusor muscle contraction and is often associated with infection. Severe urgency leads to urge incontinence.

Urgency incontinence the patient experiences an irresistable desire to micturate. Detrusor instability is the most common cause, but the condition may also be due to inflammatory diseases of the bladder without detrusor contraction.

Urinary tract the most troublesome urinary symptoms of menopausal women are usually related to atrophic urethritis secondary to estrogen deprivation.

Uterine prolapse prolapse of the uterus is accompanied by descent and inversion of the vaginal vault. Three degrees of uterine prolapse are described: (1) the uterus become retroverted and descends in the axis of the vagina, though the cervix does not reach the introitus; (2) the cervix appears at or protrudes from the vaginal orifice; (3) the vaginal walls are averted to such a degree that the uterus lies outside the vulva; this complete form of uterine prolapse is known as *procidentia.*

Uterovaginal prolapse herniation of the genital tract through the pelvic diaphragm. The uterus and vagina are held in the pelvis by the cardinal and uterosacral ligaments and by the pelvic floor musculature, mainly the levator ani. When these ligaments and muscles become ineffective, the uterus and vagina descend (prolapse) through the gap between the muscles.

Vertigo peripheral vertigo is due to either intralabyrinthine or extralabyrinthine causes. The prototype intralabyrinthine auditory-vestibular disorder produces Meniere's disease. A number of other lesions can mimic Meniere's disease. The most significant extralabyrinthine lesions causing cochleovestibular disorders are eighth nerve tumors and lesions of the cerebellopontine angle.

Vestibular disorders producing only vertigo and nystagmus consist also of intralabyrinthine lesions (uncommon) and extralabyrinthine lesions such as viral vestibular neuronitis.

Vitamin B₁ deficiency chronic alcoholism is the most common cause of thiamine deficiency in the Western world, producing neuropathy, myopathy, and encephalopathy. The neuropathy is of the sensorimotor type, with pain in the legs, paresthesia in the hand, and peripheral weakness and wasting. It may be accompanied by heart failure and cardiomyopathy (beriberi). The encephalopathy is of two types. The first type is manifested as *Korsakoff's psychosis,* with disorientation in regard to time, place, and person; amnesia for recent events; and confabulation. The second type is known as *Wernicke's encephalopathy* with nystagmus, pupillary abnormality, ocular nerve palsy, ataxia, tremor, and stupor passing, in severe cases, into coma. This clinical picture is often of sudden onset and may be mistaken for virus encephalitis, meningitis, or intracranial tumor. An associated neuropathy, a history of high alcohol intake, cerebrospinal fluid in which there is no abnormality except for a modest protein increase, and a response to intravenously administered thiamine should make the diagnosis in the elderly patient clear.

Vitamin D considered to be both a vitamin and a hormone. It is produced in the skin during sun exposure and is available from several different foods. In the body, vitamin D is one of the three hormones of the calcium thermostat. Normal levels are beneficial to bone, and promote calcium absorption and limit calcium excretion. High levels can cause bone loss.

Vulvar dystrophies a term applied to noninfective, nonneoplastic diseases of vulvar skin. They are usually managed by the dermatologist and gynecologist. The symptoms of itching, soreness, and dyspareunia usually take the patient to the gynecologist. Dystrophic lesions can be classified into three pathologic entities: the lichen sclerosus; the hyperplastic or hypertrophic type; and the mixed type. Each of these types has a characteristic histologic and gross appearance. The hyperplastic and mixed types can occur with or without cellular atypia.

Wallenberg or lateral superior medullary syndrome —Posterior inferior cerebellar occlusion will produce a lateral superior medullary infarct known as *Wallenberg* or *lateral superior medullary syndrome.* It is characterized by a rather abrupt onset. The patient may be thrown to the ground with nausea and vomiting that are exaggerated by movement; these attacks may last for hours, days, or weeks. The lateral medullary syndrome has associated neurologic symptoms including difficulty in walking, Horner's syndrome, facial analgesia, and palate weakness.

Weber-Christian disease (mesenteric panniculitis) caused by a mass in the small bowel mesentery composed of inflammatory adipose tissue. Patients usually present with low-grade fever, malaise, and recurrent episodes of moderately severe abdominal pain. The long-term prognosis is excellent.

Winter itch (asteatosis or dermatitis hiemalis) there is a tendency for aged skin to dehydrate and chap more easily than the skin of younger persons.

Zenker's diverticulum and cricopharyngeal dyschalasia symptoms develop insidiously and are those of oral pharyngeal dysphagia in general; more specific complaints are noisy swallowing and postcibal or nocturnal regurgitation of undigested food because the diverticulum may empty in a retrograde direction when the patient is recumbent. Such diverticula are seen on upper gastrointestinal series, projecting posteriorly through an area of potential weakness at the back of the pharynx. An associated incoordination or incomplete relaxation of the upper esophageal sphincter with pharyngeal contraction supports the controversial theory that cricopharyngeal dysfunction leads to high pharyngeal pressure, which in turn result in the formation of a pulsion (Zenker's diverticulum) proximally.

Zeroderma pigmentosum despite the convincing evidence of genetic determinants, the manifestation of this hereditary predisposition to skin cancer clearly depends on exposure to ultraviolet readiation.

Index

Renal/urinary function, surgery, 250–251; *see also* Urologic/urinary dysfunctions
Research on Aging Act (1974), 1, 32
Ribosomes, theories of aging, 39–40

Scarpa's fascia, pelvic muscles and ligaments, 111
Scrapie, 277
Secondary aging, 5
Secretin, 81
Senile angiomata, 116–117
Sex
  and bone loss, 191
  ratio, population 65 and over, 14
Sexuality, aging women, 12–13, 235–244
  anatomic changes, 238–239
    lubrication, 238, 240
  drug effects, 242–243
  history and physical examination, 20–21, 23, 29, 236–237, 244
  hormone therapy, 239–240
    androgen, 239
    estrogen, 215, 239
  illness/disability effects, 241–242
  Kinsey on, 236
  libido, 236, 242
  long-term care facilities, 243
  Masters and Johnson on, 239–240
  masturbation, 239
  mental illness, 242
  orgasm, 240
  social-cultural factors, 240–241
  vaginal changes, 13
Shy-Drager syndrome, 278
Skin, changes at menopause, 9
Smoking, pulmonary function and surgery, 249, 252
Social-cultural factors, sexuality, aging women, 240–241
Social Security, 292, 293
Social services, health care/maintenance, 291–292
Somatic mutations, theories of aging, 36–37
Somatomedins, 80
Somatostatin, 61
  vulvar dystrophies, 171
Sonography, postmenopausal palpable ovary (PMPO), 185, 186
Specialties, medical, 2–5
  geriatrics, 1, 3–5
  gynecology, perimenopausal and geriatric, 5
Spine, osteoporosis, 192, 196–197, 199
  kyphosis, 188, 192, 203
Staging, breast cancer, 157, 158, 160
Staphylococcus aureus, 94, 134

Steiglitz, E.J., 4
Steroid hormone action, changes in aging, 71; *see also specific hormones*
Stress incontinence, 220, 222, 226, 228–229, 232
  drugs for, 229
  surgery, gynecologic, 260, 262–264
Stromal tumors, gonadal, 141
Superficial perineal pouch, 101
Surgery, 15–17, 247–269
  cardiovascular function, 248–249
  heparin, 255, 258, 259
  indications for, 258–267
    breast carcinoma, 157, 159–161, 258, 266–267
    cervical carcinoma, 264
    cystourethrocele and uterine descensus, 259–260
    endometrial carcinoma, 264–265
    enterocele, 261
    fallopian tube carcinoma, 264
    intraoperative care, 256–258
    ovarian cancer, 264–265
    rectocele, 260–261
    stress incontinence, 260, 262–264
    urologic/urinary dysfunctions, 229–230
    uterine prolapse, 261–262, 268–269
    vaginal carcinoma, 264
    vulvar carcinoma, 264
  intraoperative care, 256–258
  nongynecologic, 267–268
  patient history, 22–23, 253
  physical examination, 254
  preoperative care, 251–252
  preoperative orders, 254–256
  pulmonary function, 249–250, 252–253
  renal/urinary function, 250–251
Syphilis, 118

Telangiectasia, 50
Testosterone, 65, 239
Thecoma, 141
Thyroid gland, changes in aging, 70, 71–73, 83–84
Thyroid-stimulating hormone (TSH), 62, 66, 70–72, 80, 81, 84
Thyroid-stimulating immunoglobulin (TSI), 72
Thyrotropic hormone releasing hormone (TRH), 61, 62, 64, 66, 72, 81
Thyroxin-binding globulin (TBG), 71, 73
TNM staging, 157
Tokophyra and aging, 41, 42
Torulopsis (Candida) glabrata, 88, 89, 90, 122
Trabecular cf. cortical bone, 189, 191